PROFOUND STATES OF DESPAIR

PROFOUND STATES OF DESPAIR

A DEVELOPMENTAL AND SYSTEMS APPROACH TO TREATING EMPTINESS

CHARLES R. WANG, M.D.

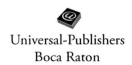

Universal-Publishers
Boca Raton

Profound States of Despair:
A Developmental and Systems Approach to Treating Emptiness

Universal-Publishers
Boca Raton, Florida • USA
2009

ISBN-10: 1-59942-943-8/ISBN-13: 978-1-59942-943-4 *(paperback)*
ISBN-10: 1-59942-942-X/ISBN-13: 978-1-59942-942-7 *(ebook)*

www.universal-publishers.com

The information in this book is accurate to the best of our knowledge.
The work presented here is intended as a general guide to the treatment of the pathology of
the self as described and not meant to replace sound medical and therapeutic advice from
mental health providers. Each case history is an amalgamation of a number of people and
do not represent any actual person, living or dead. Any resemblance to any actual person
is unintentional and purely coincidental. All recommendations herein are made without
guarantees on the part of the author or the publisher. The author and publisher disclaim all
liability, direct or consequential, in connection with the use of this work.

Library of Congress Cataloging-in-Publication Data

Wang, Charles R., 1960-
   Profound states of despair : a developmental and systems approach to treating emp-
tiness / Charles R. Wang.
      p. ; cm.
   Includes bibliographical references and index.
   ISBN-13: 978-1-59942-943-4 (pbk. : alk. paper)
   ISBN-10: 1-59942-943-8 (pbk. : alk. paper)
   1. Borderline personality disorder. 2. Despair. I. Title.
   [DNLM: 1. Borderline Personality Disorder--diagnosis. 2. Borderline Personality
Disorder--therapy. 3. Psychotherapy--methods. 4. Self Concept. WM 190 W246p
2008]
   RC569.5.B67W36 2009
   616.85'852--dc22

                              2008043535

TABLE OF CONTENTS

VII The Cup

VIII The Three Steps

PREFACE

In the stories of everyday life, there is a vicissitude of puzzling behaviors by each of us that at times confound others if not ourselves. Why, for some, the inconsequential frustrations and unhappiness about certain others turns into deep-rooted hatred or dislike; while, for others, the flirty crush can turn into an enduring infatuation? At times, such emotions seem painfully superficial to observers but intensely resolute to the holder of such sentiment. Although these feelings may seem highly incongruous to the situation at hand, the hosts of these emotions tend to be decidedly recalcitrant to advise otherwise. Frightfully, such scenarios of emotions are not restricted to certain strata of humanity; these operations of emotions are at play in every echelon of society where such emotions could well influence geopolitical decisions. Whether regarding individual happiness or world peace, there seems an urgent requirement for all of us to better understand this critical psychological pathology.

We face one of the greatest treatment challenges in the clinical work with individuals suffering from chronic pervasive sense of emotional emptiness. Such pathology would encompass individuals with difficulties in regulating emotions, experiencing constant interpersonal storms and acting out through highly self destructive behaviors. Furthermore, our society today lacks the collective insight to recognize the pathology of emptiness as insidiously ripping apart the fabric of humanity. Despite numerous therapeutic options today, clinicians continue the search for more effective and manageable approaches to treatment of conditions related to emptiness. Efficacious treatment requires a therapeutic language that can convey complex psychological dynamics and concepts in an easily comprehensible fashion for the patient and family.

In the clinical application of traditional transference based treatment work, a common frustration is the lack of balance between helping the patient reach a deep understanding of his conscious and unconscious mental functioning with that of general improvement in functioning and happiness and to achieve this in a timely fashion. On the other hand, many clinicians encounter insufficient consideration for the internal emotional life of the patient in the well respected work of dialectical behavior therapy. In addition, there is a lack of purposeful and productive methods of bringing about rapid stabilization of acutely suicidal patients and de-escalation of self destructive behaviors without further complicating treatment dynamics. A common clinical conundrum revolves around how best to help the acutely suicidal patient without the appearance of repeated emotional rescue that holds in paralysis any chance of therapeutic work.

Many eminent writers of our time have pointed out that even normative and innocent frustrations of early childhood can contribute to lifelong maladjustments. The fundamentals of these developmental processes in conjunction with possible misattunement and abuse may present as underpinning issues to many who seek mental health care today. Furthermore, these concerns may underlie the increasing social unrest that beset humanity. Of the vicissitude of individuals afflicted by this condition, patients with borderline personality disorder spearhead the call to the treatment community for an effective and readily applicable method of therapy. Fortunately, much of the needed knowledge for the treatment of emptiness have been widely available but never assembled into one cohesive manner of work that is accessible to providers and patients. The present work aspires to synthesize this information into an approachable model to the treatment of the self.

In assembling this work, I have had to constantly refocus my attention toward the central issue of how best to present the treatment of the self in a compact and digestible fashion without trivializing important axioms of psychotherapy and oversimplifying developmental principles. A pragmatic observation I made as a psychiatrist is the need for a unifying concept and approach to psychotherapy that can then be slightly modified to suit a variety of treatment scenarios for a broad range of the disorder of the self. The treatment described here places no blame for the pathology; therefore, it is a paradigm that is highly inviting for the patient and his family to engage in therapy.

This work incorporates an understanding of human development into a family systems approach to the treatment of individuals with underlying personality pathology. It uses classic developmental theories to help in the synthesis understanding of a patient in order to facilitate effective treatment planning. It is very specific about how all involved can best play a positive role in the patient's life. This approach is designed for acute stabilization phase (hospital care) of treatment for borderline patients as well as encourages the continuation and adjunct usage of many traditional modalities of psychotherapy and behavioral management work in outpatient therapy. Most importantly, despite conventional wisdom about hospitalization as un-therapeutic for borderline patients, DSA utilizes the most fundamental understanding of human development and weaves it into the fabric of the patient's daily life, whether in the hospital or in the community. As a consistent, effective and replicable model of treatment, this is work that can be applied to the daily life of every person.

In making observations about the patients I was working with at the time, it became quite obvious that the pathology of the self has to do with the individual's inability to hold steady the precious emotional contents, designated loosely as transference. Emptiness, an aversive inner tension, whether viewed psychoanalytically, existentially, or through religion and philosophy, echoes of the notion of impermanence. The preponderance of clinical evidence suggests a strong connection between the current state of emptiness and an individual's early history of anger and frustration. This treatment approach focuses on the central issue of emptiness while allowing interpersonal dynamics and transference issues to take its natural course in this arena.

In fashioning this work, I went back to examine the basic concepts in psychotherapy that I utilized in my daily work over many years. I started with what was comfortable for me and tried to understand why these particular concepts were of value. The essential factors contributing to healing are extrapolated from the idea that healthy development revolves around the concept of *person, place and time*. The emphasis of the *here and now* can be a powerful tool in therapy. Selfobject consistency is implicit in the therapeutic repair of developmental deficiency and damage. Conceptually, cognitive therapy and basic behavioral management are indispensable components in this work. The importance of the repetition of a task to inspire confidence and internalization seemed natural and critical to the task of therapy. These types of therapy tasks appear to improve interpersonal bond, trust and contribute to reworking of earlier developmental deficits.

In addressing the issue of emptiness, the fundamentals of several therapeutic modalities were combined in a specific order to form a highly effective treatment model. I have found in object relations school and self psychology, a theoretical foundation on which I could build a highly efficacious model of treatment for the disorders of the self. This is similar to the construction of a car from available and proven individual components. It is the engineering and planning of how components are selected and assembled that makes a tremendous difference in the final product.

Basic psychoanalytic and psychodynamic psychotherapy principles like therapeutic rapport, transference, countertransference, defense mechanisms and interpretation were all examined for inclusion in a refreshed approach to treatment. Although not in the sense of more traditional analysis, this work does utilize structured interactions to maximize transference based relationships. As is generally conceptualized, most modalities of therapy work are fundamentally a recapitulation and reworking of developmental issues played out in the context of psychotherapy. If so, why limit this work to just between the patient and the therapist? It would seem sensible to engage and involve the family system in a reparative process that involves a return to developmental basics.

Therapy is not easy; the preponderance of therapy work gets stalled or come to an impasse due to the patient's lack of true insight about his need to make changes. James Masterson noted that most, if not all, patients come into treatment to "feel good"; he goes on to explain that this expectation could actually derail treatment before it even starts. DSA places utmost emphasis in helping the patient to recognize the existence of his internal emotional world and how it affects his daily life. Once again, the focus of addressing the pervasive emptiness within takes center stage while the patient's acting out is handled in the context of the emptiness. Another common impasse in treatment comes in the form of therapist paralysis. We recognize this when, as the patient prepares to leave his session, the therapist ask the patient to recite the phone number he is to call in the case of any parasuicidal or suicidal ideas. Sometimes, the patient is given the therapist's private phone number. Patient safety is number one, but without a resolution to therapist paralysis, the work of treatment comes to a halt. DSA offers some important considerations for this obstacle to therapy.

Finally, as all therapists are well aware, learning techniques of therapy is a very personal endeavor. DSA is not meant to replace other treatment modalities, but is designed to integrate well with most of the accepted mainstream schools of therapy. It can be envisioned as a fundamental skeletal structure to which other modalities of therapy could hang. The DSA therapist seeks to help the patient to earnestly identify emptiness and become aware of the transitory nature of his sense of the self in order to have the patient achieve true motivation for change. While examining this work, the reader must pay particular attention to the implementation of the 3-steps, beyond which, this approach to treatment should be quite flexible. The goal of this treatment is to help the patient increasingly experience the self as integrated, without experiencing the self as separately good or bad. In theory, ego integration is achieved through the repair of leakage at the bottom of the metaphoric cup, and in practice, the selfobject experience helps to evoke the emergence and maintenance of the self.

·I·
INTRODUCTION

"From error to error one discovers the entire truth."

-Sigmund Freud

Clinical Challenges in the Treatment of the Self

When psychotherapy is at an impasse, the most fundamental concern is almost always the patient's lack of basic insight about the need for change. As fundamental as it may seem, few patients in treatment have sufficient insight about the need for personal change. Realizing this dilemma, the therapist should always be vigilant about the real reason that a patient has entered into treatment, such as the search for subjective gratification and temporary cohesion of the self. In effect, treatment has to first of all convince the patient that he has to make changes within and secondly, the patient has to be willing to accept the hard work of repetitive practice in achieving a corrective emotional experience. These two criteria are rarely accomplished in the course of psychotherapy.

Developmental and systems approach (DSA) is a highly compelling method of helping the acutely ill patient to rapidly reach an awareness of his psychological pain as well as come to an integrated understanding of his pathological ways of coping. Understanding the importance of individual history, the patient will come to recognize his earliest developmental frustrations and the resultant false self that vacillates with the true self around the core self, represented by the central cup. (Fig. 1.1) Following the path to the development of the false self, the patient then comes to appreciate the damage sustained by the central emotional structure of the "cup" and the precarious manner in which the transference input from others plus the acting out input of intense activities balance against the steady leakage. Through his insight about treatment, he will also understand the need to accept the pain of emptiness and all of its accompanying risks while allowing for treatment to take place. Finally, the patient will be given a simple and direct tool to negotiate improved object relations with important others in his surroundings.

Treatment must contribute to the effective introjection of the selfobjects. For many, the suffering of psychological pain comes primarily from the lack of adequate internalization of important others. Thus, the inability to hold steady this symbolic maternal image leads to tremendous instability in our creativity, relatedness, confidence and happiness. This deep-rooted disequilibrium can not be easily corrected through focused problem solving or in-depth inquiry into the psyche unless such exercises are coupled to a system of treatment that directs the patient toward the internalization of the selfobject. Selfobject introject can only take place in the context of an environment that offers secure sense of independence, conceptualized by the toddler exploring his surrounding while periodically looking back to check that his mother is still there.

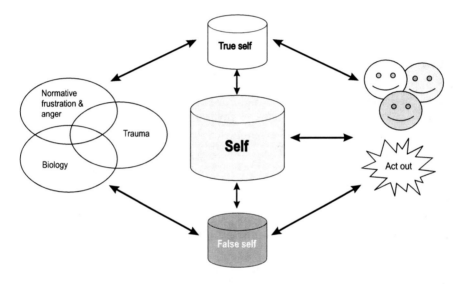

Fig. 1.1 *Emptiness is seen as the central feature for treatment. Bio-psycho-social factors can affect the health of the self. The core self consist of the vacillation between true self and false self. Each of us is prone to use of others and acting out behaviors to satisfy the needs of the self. DSA seeks to describe how all of these factors impact the self.*

The term borderline or borderline personality disorder (BPD) will be used throughout this text because this term is synonymous with the most common concept of the pathology of the self as described in DSM IV. In the following chapters, the reader will find the term, borderline, used in a very broad sense that encompasses a wide degree of the pathology related to the self.

In a sharp moment of discontent with his mentor, Goldmund felt, "He was still feeling deeply, desperately wounded, as though his friend had plunged a knife into breast." In a dejected state, he considered, "This was old pain, only considerably sharper, the same inner choking, the feeling that something frightful had to be looked in the eye, something unbearable." Thus, Goldmund began a long journey of self discovery in which he indulged in extreme adventurous wandering, drinking, fighting, womanizing and a life of impulse and unpredictability. Several times he attempted to settle down but found the wanderlust of his heart demand that he return to the adventurer's life. Hermann Hesse created in the character, Goldmund, a young man of physical beauty, intellect, artistic discrimination and sexual prowess, arising out of a background of a loveless and chaotic family. Despite ongoing acting out and the incessant search for meaning that transcends the mundane of life, at the conclusion of a period of fervent creativity, Goldmund felt only further questions and doubt, "He remained behind, empty." Finally, at the end of his life, old and ill, he dreamed of his mother reaching in and plucking his heart out, a mother he never got to know well since she too was lost and searched for extreme adventures by running away from home (Hesse 1968, p.44, 171).

Concerned about the safety and wellbeing of the distraught patient newly admitted to the hospital milieu, the staff set aside a few minutes to comfort and coaches this patient through the apparent distress. Few minutes turned quickly to an hour and the staff looked at his watch anxiously with his other responsibilities in mind; he is conflicted about what to do next. Since he has already spent an hour with this patient, he feels that he should be able to return to his usual duties but he is now even more concerned that this patient would surely act out impulsively and perhaps, cause self-harm. Not wanting to allow a sentinel event to occur during his watch, he reluctantly promised the patient that he will quickly find someone to cover his responsibilities and will return momentarily to carry on their "therapeutic" conversation.

Another common challenge is illustrated by the scenario in which an individual embraces his or her abuser as someone who is vital and indispensable to his wellbeing. A patient might even identify such a relationship as "love"; this leaves very little room for insight or treatment. Alternately, there are those who hold great contempt or enmity for others while unable to reasonably account for such emotions. It is as if this individual experiences specific others as having been highly contaminated somehow; that is, they are contaminated with his own incessant original anger (to be discussed in a later chapter). In clinical terms, these manners of relating points to acting out, dependence, enmeshment, splitting and projective identification. Regardless, treatment has to address such an issue rapidly, especially when this type of behavior can have detrimental consequences.

A psychotherapist's greatest challenge is the prospect of convincing the borderline patient that his "acting out" behavior is not just in response to irritations from his environment but that it is indicative of the need to resolve original anger and appease the evocation of pathologic defense mechanisms. Frequently, patients enter into and remain in psychotherapy without adequate insight about the need for change. Lacking such insight, it is like feeding a hunger without an understanding of the long term nutritional needs of the body. In therapy, this translates to ongoing frustration for both the patient and the therapist. Most likely, the borderline patient blames others for inducing the negative feelings that swarms within. It is all too easy to react to these internal feelings by connecting them to some external event. In so doing, this patient will have great difficulty recognizing his own roles in the myriad of endless conflicts in life. At other times, the individual may attribute the negative internal feelings to just another "bad day" and remains oblivious to why he is exhibiting another episode of lashing out at others.

Individuals spanning the continuum from the elite athlete hoping to achieve performance perfection to the psychotherapist pursuing clarity in therapeutic neutrality, we all look inwardly toward an aversive inner tension that can potentially confuse our ability to truly function. A March 2008 Seattle Times article was about the "metacongitive" ability of Ichiro, a Seattle Mariner baseball player. "It's the ability to observe yourself as if you're observing your own internal state from the outside." It is speculated that, in so doing, Ichiro is able to fine tune his batting through his analysis of every experience of inner feelings at the plate. To him, allowing such feelings to remain elusive is to function at a "deficient state." Most of us will never achieve such heightened sense of awareness of our inner feelings but such work should be practiced by all people.

Extremes of inability to regulate one's emotions can be due to a number of reasons. Of course, the differential diagnosis can cover a wide range of psychiatric diagnoses as well as medical etiology. In this writing, we will make the assumption that *any possible lead for medical issues has been exhausted by a thorough medical evaluation.* Interestingly, an individual is likely to go directly to his primary care physician if he felt that there was something physically ill within his body but how would one recognize one's behavior as arising out of the pathology of the self in order to seek appropriate help?

The emotional experiences of the borderline patient are often epitomized by the frantic search for some degree of stability, even fleetingly. The constant negotiation for emotional rescue and the inevitable turning toward intense and high risk behaviors have obvious ramification in the design for clinical care. Many eloquent and thoughtful theoretical constructs fall prey to highly defended and resistant patients operating out of such intense internal emotional pain that their single minded pursuit of relief precludes them from the benefits of most all traditional work today.

Psychotherapy is an exploration of some of the hidden recesses of the mind. It can be characterized by the analogy of an individual holding a lone candle walking up and down dark stairways and hallways; opening mysterious doors to discover what is behind. Few patients are really ready to find out what is behind those doors. In such a situation, the more in-depth psychotherapeutic exploration may have to be put off until the patient has completed some type of treatment work that has allowed him to be more emotionally stabilized. It is not difficult to see that some forms of psychotherapy may actually worsen matters for these patients. Matching the right type of therapy to the right patient is especially critical. I hold strong respect for psychotherapists who guide individuals in longer-term therapy work to foster better understanding and coping of issues ranging from trauma to the subtle nuances of life. But doing this work with an individual who can not tolerate even the smallest of life's daily challenges without becoming self-destructive can be highly risky and unproductive.

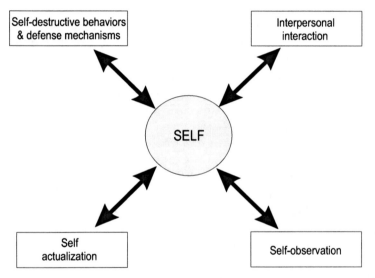

Fig. 1.2 *In the work described here, the self is seen as intersected by four critical areas that affect its functioning. Each of these areas represented by interpersonal interaction, self-observation, self actualization and self-destructive behaviors has to be consistently addressed for productive treatment.*

Although there have been some developments in the management of BPD over the past few decades, many treatment facilities designed to address this condition have come and gone without any methodology to treatment standing out as practical and replicable from patient to patient and from facility to facility. There are many disparate theories and ideas but no one cohesive method that can be easily introduced and elegantly applied. Unquestionably, the stalwarts of current mainstream treatment have merits in the hands of experts and conscientious application; while a complex method such as dialectical behavior therapy (DBT) is challenging to implement in the constraints of psychiatric residency setting without greater exposure for the trainees (Sharma 2007). Such is the frustrations that are likely to complicate most methods of work with the borderline patients.

Psychotherapy with borderline patients requires a great deal of experiences, skills and the will to persevere. Perhaps the complexities of issues related to the individual with BPD require a very different approach to traditional psychotherapy. (Fig. 1.2) Psychotherapy is an important armament in the tool chest for anyone working in mental health. Highly respected therapy modalities include such variety as psychoanalysis, psychodynamic psychotherapy, time-limited therapy, interpersonal therapy, family systems therapy and cognitive behavioral therapy to name just a few. The psychotherapeutic literature is full of seductive theories and techniques. Psychoanalytic formulation offers synthesis understanding of the pathology of the self whether related to anxiety, depression, phobias or sexual dysfunction. Quite often, elegant case formulations lack readily applicable treatment solutions. It is difficult to absorb and integrate a theoretical construct into a consistent way of working when an intellectual discussion could not be easily translated into daily clinical work.

At the present time, I am not aware of any treatment methods in existence that meets the exceedingly difficult challenges presented by the borderline patient in an acute crisis. Numerous modalities of therapy today have long term merits although therapy can often be easily derailed by the characteristics of borderline pathology. The intensity of borderline symptoms often paralyzes treatment from the start and this pattern of therapeutic relationship often defeats available methods of treatment today. Within this conundrum, transference based therapy can seem frustratingly time consuming while cognitive behavioral skills (i.e. dialectical behavior therapy) can appear intellectually unattainable and interpersonally distant to the acutely ill patient. The approach to treatment introduced here should serve as a fundamental skeletal structure to psychotherapy and is the platform in which many other modalities of work can be attached.

There are a number of prominent works on the subject of developmental psychology and the self that have inspired me and guided my own work with borderline patients. Some of these works focus on the theoretical description of the self. Some of these works focus on the treatment aspect of the deficiencies of the self. Cognitive behavioral therapy (CBT) and some of the variations around this theme have also come into prominence since the 1980s. CBT has been highly touted in the treatment of depression and anxiety disorders as well as in BPD in modified forms. Despite the important academic foundation that these works contribute to our understanding of the self and the condition of BPD, there is the lack of practical and easily applicable methods of addressing the treatment of BPD.

Any treatment modality or method would have to be taken out of the complex academic discussions and described in a cohesive and easily applicable system to be implemented at all levels of care. In the last few decades, there have been a number of experimental programs for the treatment of BPD as well as some highly respected work that is being implemented in a variety of treatment settings. In a landmark 1991 study by Linehan and colleagues, a reduction of parasuicide episodes and inpatient psychiatric days was shown with patients assigned to treatment with dialectical behavior therapy as compared to treatment as usual group over a one year period. Many institutions are currently looking at whether DBT can be effectively implemented across a variety of settings (Linehan 2006). Intensive three-week outpatient DBT for borderline patients in crisis was found to be an effective treatment that allows therapists to treat a large number of patients in a short time (McQuillan 2005).

On occasion, one hears about the patient, undergoing a particularly sophisticated form of cognitive behavioral therapy, comment with frustration that others expect him to reason himself out of his troubled emotional state. Commenting about this work, he says, "It's alright but I don't believe it." He may express feeling outraged and incredulous regarding the perceived message that, as an intelligent person, he should be able to take what he has learned and use reasoning and logic to work himself out of a moment of emotional dysregulation. The patient may draw the conclusion that his therapist has a simplified solution to his problems; the therapist must be oblivious to the severity of his psychological pain. Thus, feeling frustrated, he may decide that his therapist is irrelevant. Thus follows an exceptionally fervent period of work to no avail. He generally comes away from therapy feeling disheartened, discouraged and with the resolve to reenact behaviors to meet internal emotional pain as well as reentering into the status quo of his conflict with family.

Some modalities of treatment attempt to modify an individual's reaction and response to the current conditions in life have been shown to improve the current and future experiences in a similar or related context. However, this may be best applied to more isolated and specific traumatic events occurring later in life rather than trauma contributing to early developmental hurt. I also do not believe that treatment can be based solely on intellectual discussion or analysis. In-depth behavioral and psychological changes require an embraceable understanding of the root cause of one's emotional pain. This is not easily achievable through a play of words or an exercise in perspectives. Approaching the false self requires greater trepidation and care in order to help an individual take a risk in trusting others. It is hoped that a modality of therapy addresses current acuity of impulse as well as the eventual resolution of dysphoria and issues of dependence.

Not that any one method is likely to remain unchallenged, one recent study made a comparison of dialectical behavior therapy, transference-focused psychotherapy and a dynamic supportive treatment. For patients with borderline personality disorder, "A structured dynamic treatment, transference-focused psychotherapy was associated with change in multiple constructs across six domain; dialectical behavior therapy and supportive treatment were associated with fewer changes" (Clarkin et al. 2007). Furthermore, modalities of treatment that are more effective in addressing core areas of impulsivity and interpersonal difficulties often leave chronic dysphoria and dependency issues unresolved (Zanarini et al. 2007). Frequently, while reviewing available materials regarding the treatment of the disorders of the self, one gets the impression that it would take a tremendously experienced and masterful clinician with a large supportive team to achieve adequate success. In the meanwhile, most clinicians are faced with the daily challenges of therapy work without an immediate solution and long-term guideline to the treatment of these patients or an experienced treatment team regularly available for consultation.

Judging the effectiveness of any modality of treatment is always difficult. It is exceedingly difficult but perhaps not impossible to design studies that can reliably determine the effectiveness of a model of psychotherapy in treatment. A common criticism of many studies of personality disorder is the lack of parity between treatment modality under study when compared to control group receiving treatment as usual by expert therapists. Specifically, the challenge of empirical study is the difficulty in pinpointing the aspect of the work that brings about improvement and determining if this progress has longevity. Until a truly suitable methodology for empirical study in psychotherapy can be formulated, judging the effectiveness of a model of therapy will have to rely on clinical experiences based on work founded on solid theoretical foundation.

Treatment is obviously complex and delicate. I do feel that some treatment options may even be overly complex and time consuming; many clinicians are only able to implement components of such programs which can lead to questionable effectiveness. The acute needs of these individuals often exhaust the available mental health resources in a community. Because of the long and intensive work needed to achieve stability for these individuals using more traditional therapy, few patients could afford such complex treatment and few indeed receive adequate treatment; yet, effective treatment should not just be reserved for the privileged. Without effective treatment, these individuals remain in tenuous stability and often require more restrictive levels of care.

The High Cost of Inaction

Treatment of the individual with a disorder of the self is becoming an increasingly urgent issue in any clinical setting. For the informed reader, many news reports of homicides, suicides and terrorism around the globe reflect the crisis of the self. Many teens and pre-teens are engaged in self-mutilation as well as other self destructive behaviors. This is not a disorder limited to young adults; most "cutters" start cutting in their teens. At times, the cuts are so severe that the term self-mutilation no longer suffices and parasuicide seems to be the more appropriate description. Beyond cutting, many other types of acting out behaviors are taking a toll on individuals, communities, schools, jails and so on.

The Center for Disease Control and Prevention provided the data that more people died of suicide than homicide in 1999. Suicide was the eleventh leading cause of death (homicide was fourteenth), and the third leading cause of death between ages 15 and 24 years. In 1999, in America, 29,199 individuals died of suicide (Hoyert et al. 2001). It has been estimated that 90% or more of them can be shown to have a major psychiatric illness (Henriksson et al. 1993, Mann 2002).

Self-injurious behavior (SIB) is self-harm without suicidal intent. However, it has been suggested that self-injurious behavior may have elements in common with suicidality, despite differences in intent. SIB are common among young women and are associated with a wide spectrum of other types of direct and indirect self-harming behaviors such as alcohol and drug abuse, eating disorders and suicide attempts (Favaro 2007). In one study, patients with BPD tend to misjudge the lethality of their attempts and believed they would be saved and viewed death as less irrevocable, which increases the risk of accidental death (Stanley et al. 2001). One in ten patients with borderline personality disorder does complete suicide. A 15-year follow-up of 162 patients treated at a general hospital in Montreal found a rate of 9 percent (Paris J, 1987, 1989); after 27 years, the rate of suicide completion in this group increases to more than 10 percent (Paris J, 2001). Contrary to conventional wisdom that borderline patients are less likely to die of suicide after age 30, the mean age of those who completed suicide in the New York study was 30 years (Stone MH, 1990), and in the Montreal study it was 37 years (Paris J, 2001). Even if completed suicide is excluded from the ultimate outcome, the affective symptoms of BPD represent more enduring aspects of the disorder. Of the 24 symptoms of BPD followed for 10 years, symptoms reflecting core areas of impulsivity (self-mutilation and suicide efforts) and interpersonal difficulties seemed to resolve more quickly while chronic dysphoria such as anger, loneliness and emptiness as well as abandonment and dependency issues remain most stable (Zanarini et al. 2007).

In a 1987 study of treatment-resistant hospitalized patients, 71% of this population had an Axis II diagnosis, a cluster consisting of personality disorders, in addition to the readily apparent Axis I diagnosis such as anxiety, depression, bipolar disorder and schizophrenia (Marcus and Bradley). Individuals with suicidal behavior tend to experience affective lability, anger impulsivity, and disruption in interpersonal relationships. Hopelessness and impulsivity were found to independently contribute to suicide risk in individuals with BPD (Black 2004). Suicidal ideation and suicide attempts are part of the diagnostic criteria for BPD in the DSM IV. In a study comparing 32 patients with BPD, 77 with depression, and 49 with both diagnosis, 84% of the 81 patients with BPD had attempted suicide. Observer-rated depression scores were higher for depressed and comorbid patients but the patients with BPD had earlier onset and more suicide attempts (Soloff et al. 2000). There appears to be no significant difference between the suicidal behaviors of patients with BPD as compared to patients with major depression (Soloff 2000). In one study, it was found that the only clinical criteria for BPD that correlated with the number of previous attempts was impulsivity after controlling for major depression and substance abuse (Brodsky et al. 1997).

Many suffer from trauma ranging from verbal, emotional, physical and sexual. A small percentage of them may already be receiving help as a result of alarmed parents and school officials. These individuals tend to languish in treatment for many years without apparent improvement. They usually test the limits of the family, friends and community's resources for support and safety net. They are high utilizers of services in both the outpatient as well as inpatient setting. Because they often exhibit co-morbidity of depression, bipolar disorder, anxiety and many other psychiatric diagnoses, they are often tried on many medications over many years of treatment without success. Alcohol abuse is common amongst this population and "among a variety of variables, only presence of a personality disorder and chronicity of addiction were independently associated with a decrease of cumulative four-year abstinence probability." The authors felt that contemporary treatment for addiction can be successful in interrupting current alcohol use or alleviate symptoms of dependence, but it does not really address the underlying disorder (Krampe et al. 2006). As a category of patients, this is a group of individuals that challenges the most seasoned of mental health providers as well as the community's ability to meet their needs (Hayward et al. 2006). This is a condition often referred to as borderline personality disorder.

The Current Paralysis in Treatment

As I entered into practice in 1994, following fellowship training in child and adolescent psychiatry, I focused mainly in working with young people. In doing this work, I encountered a surprisingly large number of young people who present with classic symptoms and signs consistent with BPD. It is interesting to note that the symptoms of BPD are often quite prominent in teens and even occasionally in pre-teens. The prevalence of "attachment work" often prescribed for children with certain behavioral difficulties may reflect a preponderance of the pathology of the self.

I believe the developmental needs of the teen with borderline symptoms are nearly identical with the young adult with borderline pathology. Although emptiness is the common denominator to multiple disease states in mental health, the different developmental stage of the individual presents the therapist with some unique challenges. Without a practical and effective model of treatment, most clinicians are in fact rendered ineffective through their own paralysis as a result of the anxiety posed by working with such a challenging population of patients.

It should not come as a surprise that the teen who does not address his symptoms will grow up to be a young adult with much the same problems and issues. Regardless of the early onset of such highly disruptive symptoms, one can reasonably expect that these are young people who will continue to exhibit such symptoms into their young adult years. Nevertheless, the formal diagnostic label of BPD should be reserved for diagnostic use with adults. For this reason, I feel that the term Borderline Symptoms Cluster (BSC) or Borderline Personality Organization (BPO) as Otto Kernberg suggested, would be more appropriate to the work that I will describe here given the age range that I will mostly cover. However, for the sake of simplicity and familiarity, I will continue to use the term Borderline Personality Disorder (BPD) in this discussion.

These are the cases in which we go sleepless at night. These are the cases that make us jump when the phone rings. These are the cases that cause us to wonder if we fell asleep while in class when the most important lecture was delivered. Often, these are the cases that take away our courage to be a therapist and humble us as clinicians. Is this not the point where we feel that we are never going to take another vacation? Is this not the point when we gave our mobile phone number to a few of our special patients out of our own anxieties about their well-being? We do it because we want to help although such help does not necessarily promote independence and the growth of the self for our patients.

Within the confines of paralysis, the therapist is more likely to resort to what it takes to help get the patient to "feel good" as opposed to "get better". The therapist has to examine his or her contact with the patient with a critical eye toward defining what constitutes treatment. Therapist "burn-out" reflects the incongruence of attempting to maintain therapeutic stance while feeling pulled toward "filling the patient up", suggestive of a poor treatment model. Subsequently, without true improvement, the patient continues to experience one crisis after another. Deep down in the clinical recess of our mind, we all have many such experiences to tell.

Few of us got into this line of work knowing just how challenging it would be to work with such a special population. Proper precaution must be taken by the therapist in a period of impasse or paralysis in treatment to avoid destructive countertransference issues from further interfering with treatment. It is not uncommon for the therapist to seek consultation or supervision in order to work through clinical issues as well as possible personal issues. It is imperative that a therapist follow a model of treatment that can guide the treatment of the patient and prevent the development of therapist paralysis. Avoidance of paralysis is important because paralysis is born out of fear and fear makes us less human and less compassionate. Without compassion, there could be no treatment work.

A Treatment Relevant to Many

It is my belief that a myriad of patients presenting on the inpatient unit as well as outpatient office suffer from significant pathology of the self. My clinical experiences would suggest that many of the patients on the inpatient unit can best be categorized as quasi-borderline. These are individuals who presents with acting out behaviors, chronic mood disorders and unstable interpersonal relationships but do not fit the classic clinical picture of the depressive and parasuicidal behaviors of the mostly female borderline patients. Even so, on close inspection, many of these individuals hold the same emotional and psychological dynamic as the borderline patient.

Some teens and young men have perhaps been transferred from detention centers for psychiatric stabilization but have very poor insight about their behavior and its consequences; labeled as antisocial or borderline pathology, hope should involve some type of forthcoming treatment. For some of them, exercise of bravado and aggression is a matter of daily existence. Without regard for the feelings and needs of others, these individuals seemingly transgress without remorse. Often, these young men are labeled as antisocial and given diagnosis such as conduct or antisocial personality disorder and dismissed as beyond available treatment. These patients are frequently marginalized by society and likely become a part of the growing incarcerated population. There is a need for a treatment method that can help bring about insight development and acceptance of change in a very challenging patient population. If viewed through the scope of the psychological pain of emptiness, this population too may have hope of treatment.

I have not been able to find existing treatments for BPD that meets my personal requirements in clinical work. I needed a method that can be used in both the inpatient and outpatient setting. (Fig. 1.3) Most of my case discussions are limited to the types of cases of BPD that one is likely to encounter in the inpatient setting. The majority of this discussion will be focused on the acute intervention and stabilization in the inpatient arena. Acute inpatient intervention should ideally enhance long term stability, which is the perennial debate in the mental health community about the benefits of hospitalization for borderline patients. The intervention of choice should be elegantly applicable to both the inpatient and outpatient settings. Some discussion will be given to the treatment of BPD in the outpatient setting but this is mainly a discussion of how to extrapolate the acute intervention into some type of continuity for outpatient care.

Especially in the inpatient hospital setting, the treatment protocol has to bring about rapid stabilization of the patient while allowing for sustained benefits in treatment that can be further strengthened on an outpatient basis. Many individuals seeking treatment may already feel poorly about themselves while therapy that is overly complex and difficult to master will only contribute to the patient feeling even more incompetent, frustrated and alienated. It has to be a method that involves helping the patient and the families understand the condition of BPD and develop a realistic understanding of the acuity of such a disorder. The aggregate benefit of treatment should include the long term resolution of chronic dysphoria and dependence.

A program for inpatient treatment would have to take into consideration the severe constraints in terms of patient to staff ratio. There is of course the challenge of the managed care system that severely limits the length of stay for inpatient care but this is a necessary reality of healthcare today. An inpatient treatment protocol has to work within the constraints of this reality or it has little chance of becoming adopted for implementation.

The treatment has to emphasize patient safety as the number one goal and also help the patient and families understand the risk of death is very high for those suffering from BPD. It is my strong feeling that most family members of the patient are already aware of how deadly this patient can be. In entering into treatment, the family and relatives of this patient want to know that the therapist is realistically aware of this issue and is willing and able to handle this challenge.

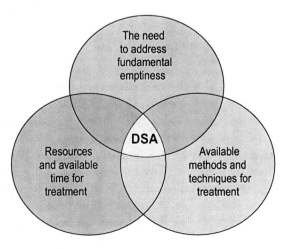

Fig. 1.3 *DSA exists at the confluence of three major considerations for successful and efficient mental health treatment of a multitude of clinical pathology.*

I believe that a treatment protocol that meets the criteria for acute inpatient intervention should also function well in the outpatient setting. It has to be treatment protocols that can be easily taught to the patient and actively involve the patient. It needs to be a method that promotes healthy boundaries between therapist and patient. Most of all, of course, it needs to be a method of treatment that can be easily repeated in a clinical setting so as to allow the maximum number of patients to benefit. Program of treatment would warrant replicable implementation by general practitioners of mental health care in the institutional setting as well as in the private practice setting. An ideal program would be one in which the application in the inpatient and outpatient settings are actually fairly similar.

In approaching the treatment of the self, I see it as divided into two phases. The first phase is often applied in the acute psychiatric hospital setting. The second phase is generally part of the ongoing psychotherapeutic work that extends far into the outpatient clinical setting. This is not to say that the work I will describe here is not applicable to the outpatient setting but simply to raise the awareness that much of the work of the initial phase of this treatment method involves individuals who are very ill and emotionally unstable. Stabilization may require a degree of psychiatric inpatient care or partial hospital program in order to initiate the patient into this therapy approach and treatment insight. Once the patient has been initiated into this model of work, it is hoped that the treatment can be generalized into the patient's psychotherapy and life in the community. Further resolution of the primitive defenses toward an improved integration of the self would be the eventual goal. To effect this change, the pre-3-steps work in conjunction with the 3-steps prime the self for developmental repair with appropriate and consistent mirroring and idealizing transference.

A Plan for Introductory Work

Inpatient hospital care has its own set of special challenges and requirements. Because of the higher level of acuity in the inpatient environment, this is arguably the most challenging and demanding setting for any type of treatment work with the borderline patient. From the standpoint of the inpatient setting, we are faced with the most acute of psychiatric emergencies. The work that I will introduce here is shaped by lessons learned in the front lines of treatment work with BPD. These patients are all highly unstable and at great risk of severe self harm or suicide. There is insufficient time to develop any reasonable degree of rapport or trust in the therapeutic relationship. In this setting, there is a need for quick stabilization before any further treatment considerations can begin. Therefore, any method of treatment would have to be approached in three phases.

Phase one is to partner with the patient in identifying the precise nature of his pathology as well as forming a goal for treatment. Most patients are able to identify their daily stress in life such as those related to finance, relationships, family, job and school. They can easily describe how all these events and people in life cause them distress and how this stress feels internally. Even though they could be exquisitely in touch with these types of feelings, they may be oblivious or ignore the deeper sets of fundamental pain of existence that fester at the core of the self. Lacking a basic sense of this core emotional pain prevents this individual from addressing the most fundamental axiom of his pathology in treatment.

Preparing the patient for treatment in a time limited setting without the precedent of therapeutic rapport is one of the most challenging issues in the initial portion of any therapeutic work. In the initial phase, there is little or no time to truly develop good rapport and trust in this treatment relationship; empathy may not yet have taken place but compassion shall be sufficient in carrying on the work of treatment. Patients do respond to empathy but they may be distrustful of the therapist's empathic intentions at such an early stage in treatment; naturally, the therapist could only rely on simple compassion in the early phase of work.

With the acuity at hand, some type of treatment must be implemented despite the lack of a solid treatment relationship. One may question the feasibility of doing any treatment work under such a condition. Such is the daily reality of attempting to stabilize an acute patient in the psychiatric inpatient program. One must also remember that the professional therapist and patient relationship is a very powerful entity to begin with and we also rely on this initial relationship to carry us in the beginnings of treatment. Traditionally, the healthcare provider is offered a status of respect in our society, this provider and patient relationship can be a good starting point in beginning treatment.

Phase two is the process of presenting the DSA model of treatment to the patient and his family. The patient learns to see himself in orbit around important people in his life and begins to practice his treatment work with select selfobjects. In this phase, the treatment work contributes to his becoming more engaged in treatment and trust is built upon some of the initial success.

Phase three is to help the patient transition back to the more conventional concept of psychotherapy while still embracing and retaining the initial benefits of stabilization with this approach. I would like to introduce you to this method of treatment that has been developed through my clinical work both in the outpatient and inpatient setting.

Program Requirements for Inpatient Implementation:
The following is a summary of the minimum requirements for a treatment protocol to be useful in an inpatient setting.

1. The protocol has to contribute to increasing patient safety in treatment.

2. This model of treatment has to enlighten all staff toward a more compassionate and non-judgmental way of working with the patient.

3. The protocol can not demand a dramatic increase in existing and available staff schedule.

4. The protocol has to complement and work with existing knowledge base of working staff. This means that one would not have to send a whole cadre of working staff back to school for special training. The protocol of treatment has to be compact and easily adoptable in most any psychiatric inpatient setting. In-services and practice work should be implemented in the clinical environment.

5. The method of treatment has to take effect rather rapidly. The very short stays of inpatient care today do not allow for lengthy introduction to any modality of treatment. This does not mean that treatment has to be completed in the short inpatient stay but that a degree of stability has to be attained for the brief inpatient treatment to be safe and productive.

6. The work introduced to the patient during the hospital stay has to compliment the existing work he or she is doing on an outpatient basis, engage the patient in sober understanding for the need of treatment, and perhaps instruct the patient in a more effective modality of treatment work. Furthermore, this work should maintain compatibility with any form of outpatient therapy work even if the outpatient provider is not completely familiar with the inpatient work introduced.

Developmental and Systems Approach (DSA)

I have devoted a good portion of the past decade in search of a viable method of working with individuals with BPD. It is through this focus on all things related to this topic that has shaped this rather eclectic method of treatment for BPD. I will call this method Developmental and Systems Approach (DSA). This is an approach to treatment that is based on many accepted and standard of practices that are utilized in the mental health community today. I would reason that the effectiveness of this approach is based on the execution of the whole as opposed to the piecemeal use of the parts. In addition, I would argue that it is the implementation of this approach in a specific sequence that makes it unique and effective in the treatment of borderline personality disorder.

Micro-corrective Reenactment

In part, DSA is a reflection of the most traditional of psychotherapy in that it works to systematically intensify the same dynamics evoked in long term treatment. Long term psychotherapy relies on the consistent, neutral, supportive, and validating presence of the therapist. Corrective reenactment can be a powerful therapeutic entity consistent with the general practice of psychotherapy. DSA borrows from this tradition and through *micro-corrective reenactment* magnifies the therapeutic effect for improved efficacy.

The well regarded study by Silbersweig et al. (2007) produced some compelling evidence that supports the need to address the impulse control issue in borderline personality disorder with contextual factors in therapy. In this study, it was shown that healthy subjects displayed good impulse control through increased activity in the orbitofrontal and subgenual cingulated cortices, brain regions associated with emotion regulation (Ochsner 2004) and inhibition of limbic regions, including the amygdale (Drevets 1999). Borderline patients displayed decreased change in subgenual cingulate activity and increased limbic activity under the stress of the same negative words in the study. It has been shown that stimulation of the subgenual cingulated region is effective for treatment-resistant depression (Mayberg 2005) and cognitive therapy is helpful in those with increased amygdala and decreased subgenual cingulated activity (Siegle 2006).

The aforementioned works offer hope for designing a type of treatment that can specifically target the various symptoms of borderline personality disorder, of which impulse control issue being a particular challenge (Siegle 2007). Given that the borderline patient's difficulty in impulse control is likely to be worse in the context of negative emotions, treatment has to address those negative moments repeatedly. In addition, thinking about such negative moments may not be quite comparable to experiencing of negative emotions in the context of daily life. As an example of therapy design, treatment of impulse control in BPD will have to be taken out of the therapy sessions and experienced as they occur in the emotionality of living.

Micro-corrective reenactment, the 3-steps, is the magnification of the benefits of learning through high repetition. Through this repetitive and reciprocal interpersonal interaction is achieved the integration of the internal emotional world. As is perceived in general psychotherapy, it is through insight development as well as corrective reenactment that bring about psychological repair. I am reminded of the benefits of practice by the way young musicians are asked by their teachers to practice for two hours daily and prepare for a recital six months to a year ahead; this means one piece of work is played an inconceivable number of times. This can be very lonely work at times, but it is only through such repetition can mastery be achieved.

Making Use of the Family System

Regardless of the methodology used in treatment, developing a synthesis understanding of the individual patient is critical before proceeding with treatment. An understanding of the early development as well as subsequent developmental phases of the individual can contribute to our overall integrated understanding of this individual. "Systems" is a term representing the involvement of the patient's world sphere. Many individuals suffering from the pathology of the self may need to work within the context of the family to address earlier patterns and styles of relating to one another. Initial therapy for this individual has to offer a fairly rapid way for him to experience some stability and security in the treatment environment. The involvement of the family and his world sphere serves to keep him grounded in the reality of life as well as serving as a constant reminder of the need to integrate "the good, the bad and the ugly" into a cohesive whole that is consistent with the reality of life.

This is the use of the resource of the therapist, family and others involved, to maximize the efforts of treatment. Treatment in this fashion is a team effort. DSA was developed out of the need to have an integrated system of treatment that takes family system, object relations and cognitive behavioral work and shapes it into an easily applicable work that all involved can embrace. DSA starts with the important notion of the role that the "object", the critical mother figure, plays in one's life and makes the natural assumption that family system is going to be inextricably linked to the successful treatment outcome of the patient. The object or more specifically, selfobject means the self has a certain degree of investment in another. One can not fully comprehend the treatment needs of a patient without an adequate understanding of the developmental and the systems impacts in this individual's life.

Calling Attention to Defense Mechanisms

Taking from traditional technique in psychodynamic psychotherapy, I do believe that a stable therapeutic relationship that weathers the storms of therapy can help the patient work through many selfobject issues. However, I believe the sole reliance on this relationship raises the risk of escalating the dynamics of splitting, projective identification and so on. Splitting, as discussed in the language of object relations, is an intense dynamic that, in the early stages of treatment, can be highly disruptive in therapy. The intense emotional demand that splitting sets up in the therapeutic environment can be extremely exhausting for the patient and the therapist; few can withstand it in the early stages of therapeutic engagement.

Rather than working through the issue of splitting in therapy, a patient may come into therapy to seek reward or play out aggression and afterwards, therapy comes to a halt. Similarly, projective identification has to be recognized early in therapy and addressed accordingly. "Projective identification is a primitive form of projection, mainly called upon to externalize aggressive self and object-images; 'empathy' is maintained with the real objects onto which the projection has occurred, and is linked with an effort to control the object now feared because of this projection" (Kernberg 1985).

This is one of the most difficult defensive operations to recognize in therapy. Often, the therapist may be annoyed by a persistent unsettling feeling that accompanies the frustrations of the patient's ongoing resistance in treatment; only to be caught off guard by the projected aggression of the patient. DSA offers the therapist a treatment model and structure that highlights the inevitable development of splitting and projective identification.

Repetition is a Key to Learning

One would expect that the therapist's devotion and attention to the patient would naturally bring about a temporary improvement in the patient. This is a basic tenet of psychotherapy. However, an experienced therapist understands that such an improvement is usually brief. Even though the all important therapeutic relationship should account for much of the positive results of psychotherapy, many important constructs in therapy makes use of the benefits of repeated learning a critical part of treatment. Therefore, therapeutic rapport and therapeutic insight may play an important role in treatment, but one must be mindful of the benefit of repetition in internalization of learning.

Repetitive experiencing, micro-corrective reenactment, is one of the emphasis in DSA. DSA offers some key tools to provide treatment structure and interpersonal boundary as well as addressing behaviors that may sabotage treatment. As in cognitive-behavioral therapy, DSA involves the patient in much self directed experiencing and learning. DSA can be used to initiate treatment and then maintained in treatment as sort of a backbone to treatment. For use in the inpatient psychiatric setting, this treatment protocol functions as short-term stabilization of the patient. Other therapeutic interventions can be seen as pieces that one would affix to the basic framework of DSA. In such a scenario, DSA continues to be an integral part of the longer-term treatment process.

Of the many psychotherapeutic methods available today, when used by skillful therapists, some of these methods can be highly effective in the long-term treatment of BPD. Most clinicians interpret the available theories and discussions into a personal style of working in their individual clinical settings. Often, because of the complexities of a treatment method or the lengthy time required in treatment, many therapists find themselves facing the limitations of the various treatment methods. As a result, providers of varying experiences and training apply many of these methods with various degrees of proficiency. Many frustrated patients and their families give up on psychotherapy and turn to medications as the sole solution. A search for medication help can often lead the patient and his family down a convoluted path of going from one provider to another and trying many powerful medications with high potential side effects. Most psychiatrists will agree that medication utilization with the patient with BPD can be helpful but it rarely addresses the short-term acuity and the long term healing that these individuals suffer. Through repetition in micro-corrective reenactment, a therapist can guide the patient and his family toward developmental growth.

The Five Primary Foci of DSA

Of the countless patients who have worked with me in this method of treatment, I believe a significant portion of these individuals became sufficiently stabilized to continue in treatment in a safer and more productive fashion. They were then able to continue in treatment with more traditional models of therapy. After leaving the inpatient setting, many patients who were stabilized using DSA in treatment are then able to generalize this work and integrate it with other work in the community with minimal prompting.

The development of this work is an exercise in understanding what aspects of treatment tends to be the weakest link in most modalities of treatment and to make a punctuated emphasis to correct this deficit in the treatment with DSA. I have identified several areas of focus that will be emphasized in the work using DSA.

- Firstly, the patient has to become aware of his emptiness within as a driving force in many of his behaviors in daily life.

- Secondly, he has to develop an accurate sense of his relationship with all the people around him.

- Thirdly, he has to recognize the true purpose of his acting out behavior.

- Fourthly, he has to find the motivation to accept his internal emotional pain in order to focus on treatment.

- Fifthly, he has to be empowered to pursue healing.

·II·
BORDERLINE PERSONALITY DISORDER

Diagnostic Criteria

As varied as the opinions may be on the validity and values of the diagnostic criteria for borderline personality disorder (BPD), I find it quite useful. Labels are not necessarily kind or reassuring. Labels tend also to produce preconceived ideas about an individual. However, most mental health professionals would agree that diagnostic criteria allows us to be able to describe a specific clinical picture and be able to focus our collective knowledge on it; therefore, negating the need to reinvent the wheel each time. It is also a short hand way of communication amongst professionals.

Borderline Personality Disorder
301.83

A pervasive pattern of instability of interpersonal relationships, self-image, and affects, and marked impulsivity beginning by early adulthood and present in a variety of contexts, as indicated by five (or more) of the following:

(1) frantic efforts to avoid real or imagined abandonment. **Note:** Do not include suicidal or self-mutilating behavior covered in Criterion 5.

(2) a pattern of unstable and intense interpersonal relationships characterized by alternating between extremes or idealization and devaluation.

(3) identity disturbance: markedly and persistently unstable self-image or sense of self.

(4) impulsivity in at least two areas that are potentially self-damaging (e.g., spending, sex, substance abuse, reckless driving, binge eating). **Note:** Do not include suicidal or self-mutilating behavior covered in Criterion 5.

(5) recurrent suicidal behavior, gestures, or threats, or self-mutilating behavior.

(6) affective instability due to a marked reactivity of mood (e.g. intense episodic dysphoria, irritability, or anxiety usually lasting a few hours and only rarely more than a few days.)

(7) chronic feelings of emptiness.

(8) inappropriate, intense anger or difficulty controlling anger. (e.g. frequent displays of temper, constant anger, recurrent physical fights.)

(9) transient, stress-related paranoid ideation or severe dissociative symptoms.

Fig. 2.1 *Diagnostic and Statistical Manual of Mental Disorders, Fourth Edition, Text Revision*

The Emergence of the Self

"More and more, psychoanalysts have become aware of the fact that the pathologies of many of their adult (and, of course, also child) patients derive from the earliest years of life. (Mahler 1974, p103)" The theoretical understanding of the self is paramount in our endeavor to comprehend the treatment needs of the borderline patient. Whether to design a treatment effort targeting a particular traumatic event in an individual's life or to devise a counter measure to modify physiological response of our biology would hinge on our theoretical view of the pathology. Primary to our treatment concern, how do we understand the developmental path toward the development of emptiness? How we view the potential for the development of emptiness has a bearing on how we would approach the treatment of this condition. DSA makes the hypothetical assumption that emotional emptiness is highly prevalent and therefore, this treatment approach is designed for rapid and broad implementation. Perhaps we do have to travel back in time to the very beginning of the patient's life to take a look at what environmental impact has made upon the design of nature, the bio-psycho-social view of psychopathology. Therefore, I have selected the object relations school as a helpful starting point in our understanding of the pathology of the self.

Whether through a nod of acknowledgement or a heart felt expression of interest in the events in a child's life, these are the kernels of building blocks for a healthy self. If instead, it is the chronic unconstructive criticism, frequent vote of no confidence or the contemptuous tolerance that relegates the child to a tertiary role by his primary selfobject, then the developmental trajectory of a child can be damagingly altered. When parents are emotionally unavailable, the frustrations of unreturned love can bring about a sense of inadequacy, shame and self hatred in the child. Conversely, the child who was made to feel that love is not forthcoming without achievement will go on in life to despise others and hold a grandiose sense of his own achievement (Miller 1997). For most, it is probably not difficult to imagine that the frustrations of early childhood can result in the vicissitude of perverse and self destructive behavior of adulthood but it may take a leap of faith to see that the infant is already a highly interactive being within his environment.

Is there evidence that the infant is sufficiently aware of his environment to suffer frustration in reaction to his surroundings? If the infant cries, does this signal a frustration so profound that it should have an impact on the rest of his life? Is this crying just a physiological response to hunger and discomfort or does it have deeper meaning and molding of his character? If he laughs at the triumph of achieving a goal, does he expect to be recognized and empathically understood? How does this impact him as a person in later life? Although I do not feel that we have all of the answers, infant researchers such as Daniel Stern give us a glimpse into the very non-autistic world of the infant.

Daniel Stern wrote, "The sense of being with an other with whom we are interacting can be one of the most forceful experiences of social life." This would mean that at some point, early on in the life of the infant, he develops a sense of a "separate mind." It has been suggested that the acquisition of the realization that inner subjective experience can be shareable occurs between the seventh and ninth month of age. "Only when infants can sense that others distinct from themselves can hold or entertain a mental state that is similar to one they sense themselves to be holding is the sharing of subjective experience or intersubjectivity possible." At this stage in development, the possibility of sharing subjective experience becomes meaningful due to the distinction of self and other. "The caretaker's empathy, that process crucial to the infant's development, now becomes a direct subject of the infant's experience." Once sharing can take place, "The sharing of affective states is the most pervasive and clinically germane feature of intersubjective relatedness." Stern uses "interaffectivity" to describe parental mirroring and empathic responsiveness. The infant makes a face and the mother then takes this expression and thematically modifies it before returning with an affectively attuned expression of her own. Stern gives the following example as illustration of affect attunement (Stern 1985, p. 124-140).

> A nine-month-old girl becomes very excited about a toy and reaches for it. As she grabs it, she lets our an exuberant "aaaah!" and looks at her mother. Her mother looks back, scrunches up her shoulders, and performs a terrific shimmy with her upper body, like a go-go dancer. The shimmy lasts only about as long as her daughter's "aaaah!" but is equally excited, joyful, and intense."

With this information, it is a very exciting time to note about the life of the infant. It seems the infant is actively engaging the caretaker and taking note of all the subtle movements, gestures, and sounds of his caretaker. Stern refutes the notion of "normal autism" in describing early infancy and states "the infant becomes more social, but that is not the same as becoming less autistic" (Stern 1985, p. 234). Having thus accepted the early infant as an active and engaging being through all of his senses, one could then appreciate the huge enthusiasm in which classical writers of analysis heaped on the infant.

Hence, with the certainty of knowing the infant is capable of sharing of affective states, one can then examine the frustrations in the life of the infant. Frustrations likely take shape in many forms for the infant. Even without outright abuse or neglect, it is possible to imagine that the infant can face a great number of frustrations in daily life. First of all, communication without the use of words means that, whatever the manner of communication, it would have to be done with intensity. Smiling does not get one's hunger resolved. Even crying would have to be dramatic and the butting of the nipple done with ferocity for the need to be obvious for the caretaker. Next, what goes in must come out; it may be easy going in, but it may not be easy coming out. As a resident rotating through the pediatric program, one gets the idea that dealing with infant diarrhea and constipation practically defines infant pediatrics. An innocent mismatch of the feeding formula can lead to endless bowl discomfort for the infant. Any parent could describe in detail the agony they observe as the infant strains at stool with his body completely contorted and his face crimson while holding his breath. Then there is colic, for which the cause can be many, and accompanied by inordinate frustrations.

Hypothetically, I believe that it is possible that everything from the feel of the nipple to the discomfort of colic and perhaps, the anger of uneasy bowl movements can all be a source of daily frustration for the infant. I do not suggest that such routine frustrations can have pathological impact on the developing psychic of the infant. However, under certain circumstances such as that of the particularly vulnerable individual, I would entertain the possibility that even this type of routine daily activity can pose as potential anger and frustration that complicates the healthy formation of the self. As the anal musculature becomes more mature, the infant's battle of autonomy rests with the conflicting impulses of retention and elimination. The balance of mutual regulation between the adult and child brings about the determination of a healthy identity and adjustments later in life (Erikson 1968 p. 109).

Brazelton et al looked at the neurophysiological fit of infant and mother through their engagement with each other. When exposed to an irrelevant noise, some mothers were able to quickly screen it out of their consciousness while others habituated more slowly. The mother and child pairing in which the mother showed more reaction to the noise tended to have babies who showed relatively little social orientation; they tended to have brief periods of gazing at each other, indicative of poor attunement (Als 1977). In addition to such frustrations, I would also propose that some types of predispositions such as anxious temperament, attention deficit, perhaps with hyperactivity, aggressive temperament and autistic characteristics are but a few of the possible etiologies leading to a pathological development of the self. In a 2006 study, Anckarsäter and colleagues suggested just such a possibility that ADHD and autism spectrum disorders are associated with increased risk of personality disorders.

Beyond the frustrations connected to daily routines of feeding, sleeping and defecating, we now have to take a look at the frustration of intersubjective relatedness. Once we are certain that the infant can experience the self as physically distinct from others, he is ready to sense the quality of psychic and physical intimacy. "The caregiver's empathy, that process crucial to the infant's development, now becomes a direct subject of the infant's experience. The desire to know and be known in this sense of mutually revealing subjective experience is great" (Stern 1985, p. 126).

Additionally, attunement between the mother and child can now take place. "Attunement permits the parents to convey to the infant what is shareable, that is, which subjective experiences are within and which are beyond the pale of mutual consideration and acceptance" (Stern 1985, p. 208). Through selective attunement by the caregiver, the infant can then determine which behaviors fall within the bounds acceptable to his caregiver. His learning can range from how much noise he should make to his preference for people. "Her response is analogous to naming the formless experience that inhabits the baby. She gives it a reality." If the mother does not provide a response, the child is left with a diminished sense of the reality and meaning of his existence, resulting in the disruption of the self (Meares 1993, p.143-144). With this, I recall an observation Dr. Young Soon Lukoff shared with me during one of my supervisions as a fellow. She said to me, as I paraphrase, "next time you go to a party in which the host is a woman holding her one year old infant, as she stands at the doorway receiving her guests, pay particular attention to the infant and you will realize who this woman favors and who she dislikes." Whether one considers this to be attunement or a specialized kind of bidirectional projective identification, there is clearly something special happening here to hint at the critical nature of the relationship between a caregiver and the infant. At the height of such a bidirectional interchange, it is like a mystical experience between the two. Granted that this is an interaction that is difficult to study, it is nevertheless an observation readily available to anyone who has paid attention to such a dyad. The quality of such a relationship can be vulnerable to misattunement, intentional tuning as well as abuse.

It is known that some parents are aware of their ability to manipulate their attunement to the infant as to elicit a particular reaction from the infant that somehow meets the desire and fantasies of the parents. This, for example, may be the mother who attempts to undermatch the affective behavior of her ten-month-old infant son feeling that he should focus more on his initiative rather than shift toward her. She did not want the infant to rely on her to experience a bout of excited emotion. As a result, she responds to his excitement with an understated "Yes, honey." In so doing, she hopes to make sure that he does not grow up to be passive like his father. The paradox may be that this under-attunement tends to create a lower-keyed child who was less inclined to share his spunk.

"Attunement and misattunement exist at the interface between attitude or fantasy and behavior..." An even more powerful act of misattunement is "emotional theft." In this instance, the mother behaves as if she is attuned to his experience at the moment and attempts to use this entry into his world to further her own agenda. Stern gives the example of the mother who attunes to her infant's behavior in chewing on his doll's shoe and as she gains entry into his moment of pleasure, she takes the doll from him and hugs it; in effect, she teaches the infant that dolls are to be hugged, not chewed. The infant is left feeling let down by this interchange. "She slips inside the infant's experience by way of attunement and then steals the affective experience away from the child." "This is likely to be the point of origin of the long developmental line that later results in older children's need for lying, secrets, and evasions, to keep their own subjective experience intact" (Stern 1985, p. 211-214).

One has to ponder the multitude of possible causes in the development of severe pathology of the self. It is easier to establish the cause when there is evidence of severe early neglect or trauma. However, the work of infant psychologists have furthered our understanding of the interpersonal world of the infant and raised some interesting considerations for the development of pathology of the self. It is a remarkable fact that infants are very keenly aware of their surroundings from the beginning. There is sharp attunement bilaterally between the infant and his mother which sets the stage for attunement to be both a blessing and a curse. Most attunements in this dyad are probably innocent and with good intentions; but when attunement is our tool to act out our attitude and fantasy, it can inadvertently become misused.

By most account, misattunements are probably unintentional. Parents can easily be distracted by the franticness of daily life or perhaps, acting through their own emotional pathology that interferes with their ability for empathy. This and a host of issues in life can spill over from the adults to affect the child. Hence, it is important to recognize that the psychological pain of emptiness is rather pervasive and the need to address this pathology in most every individual suffering unhappiness in life.

As the infant now becomes a teenager, his mother questions the therapist as to the reason her son continues to behave in such a self destructive and threatening fashion. "I did everything in my power to give him what he needed." Even while she was being given a synthesis understanding from the evaluation, she was unable to quiet her own anxiety and tune into the messages in this discussion. The pain of this misattunement can be visible through the eyes of every member of this family present. No overt abuse has happened to this teen but other than his mother, no one uttered a single word in this family conference.

The Resilient Child

It is fitting to mention at this juncture that the developmental theories discussed in the following section are to provide a reference point for our understanding of BPD and related disorders. I find, in particular, object relations theory to be of immense help in laying the foundation for developing a sensible way to work with disorders of the self. Object relations school teaches us the importance of the reciprocal interpersonal interaction in the self and object experience. In a related discipline, self psychology offers us a very optimistic view of the possibilities and the flexibilities of human development. Through self psychology, one is able to glimpse a world in which the self has many options to meeting selfobject requirements through a multitude of alternative objects.

It may indeed take a village to raise a child, especially in periods of human history in which disease and war can easily claim the lives of parents, leaving a child to survive with alternative selfobjects. This seems sensible in the natural world in which the survival of the species is of primary agenda. Hence, for the healthy survival of the species, having multiple object supplies would seem practical and enrich the chances of healthier survival of mankind. In this discussion, as in any text about object relations, there may be conveyed a heavy sense of responsibility on the mother as an object playing a near exclusive role in the developmental health of the infant. One must keep in mind that the mental health of the child is only as healthy as that of his surroundings. When a child suffers, it is the failure of the society and we all collectively suffer one day. Beyond the parents, the village needs to realize the logarithmic importance of raising a healthy child in order to avoid the cumulative catastrophe of the following generations.

Melanie Klein, a contemporary of Freud, found the mother and child relationship most intriguing in her studies. Klein's basic theoretical assumption was, in agreement with Freud's (1920) dual instinct life and death theory that proposed the inner struggle between the natural forces of life and death that was ultimately projected onto the external world. There is a kind of an "archetype" of the mother that exists in the child. "It is the primal maternal image of the mother that guides the child's interaction with a flesh and blood caretaker, i.e., the real mother, rather than the other way round" (Cashdan 1988, p. 6). In this view offered by Klein, the infant arrives at birth with a preconceived idea of the mother that is based on the instinctual concept of the death instinct. Here, the infant's grappling with the struggles of life and death splits his world view into good and bad. Through this frightening developmental view, the infant has to contend with an extremely polarized idea about life that sets the tone of his beginning interactions with the external object world.

Even without the threat of the death instinct, it is tragically true that many unfortunate individuals do start out life in less than ideal circumstances and thus, suffer the impairments of development with lasting emotional pain. In view of object relations theory as a basis for understanding the intricacies of the infant and mother interactions, one might surmise that many factors in development can interfere with a child's natural resiliency. One in five women and one in ten men suffer depression at some point in their lives (Blehar 1995). Depressed mothers may be less nurturing in their interactions (Sameroff 1982). Such statistics leave children at risk of developing depression and related maladaptive emotional functioning (Downey 1990). Diurnal pattern of cortisol production is disrupted in young children who are placed in foster care. Researchers have made the conjecture that certain types of atypical cortisol production are related to conduct disorder, substance abuse, depression and anxiety (Dozier 2007).

Once again, I would remind the reader that not all borderline patients started life angered and frustrated by misguided parents. It is of common expectation that not all parents are created equal and that most imperfections of parents are merely blemishes on otherwise normal developmental milestone for most children. There is also the concept of the mechanism of "fit" and "misfit" between the infant and parent dyad. In this instance, if the infant is at all frustrated by his caretaker, it is purely innocent on the part of the parent due simply to a lack of fit between the dyad. Clinically, it is quite clear that some individuals suffer the symptoms of BPD without evidence of significant traumatic or frustrated childhood. Studies have shown that certain neuropsychiatric disorders can interfere with proper development and this issue will be touched upon in a later chapter. Is it possible that certain temperament or personality traits predispose some individuals to the frustrations of poor attunement?

My own clinical explorations and studies of developmental issues have persuaded me toward the belief that human emotional health is at best resilient in its mastery of survival. Even as we acknowledge the resilience of the child, resilience may mean that the individual is capable of making every effort to face the day but our true ability to cope with the conflicts of daily life is highly modified by the frustrations of early life. Speaking about the problems of early development, Erikson states, "Familiarity with such radical regressions as well as with the deepest and most infantile propensities in our not-so-sick patients has taught us to regard basic trust as the cornerstone of a vital personality" (1968 p.97). Hence, it is critical to recognize the potential for pathological emptiness in all. Although many appear to function in daily living but as attested to by the endless parade of books on the search for happiness, few achieve such virtue.

People from all walks of life are apt to suffer developmental hurt manifested in the pain of emotional emptiness. Witness the number of individuals who holds unfathomable distain for another or a group. Life is full of stories of irreconcilable differences that reach beyond simple logic. The endless bickering and paranoia between small groups and large groups of people all harks back to individual mishaps in the building blocks of development. Although the variances in emptiness of most do not manifest in borderline character pathology but the resulting activation of pathological defense mechanisms in the average individual is sufficient in wrecking havoc in all institutions of mankind.

Can particular types of personality characteristics predispose some individuals to suffer greater developmental and life frustrations? This is the same question many researchers have asked about post traumatic stress disorder; survivors of the same trauma do not all suffer the symptoms of PTSD. Numerous studies have indicated that only a small subset of individuals exposed to a specific traumatic event goes on to develop disorders such as depression, anxiety or PTSD (Yehuda 1998). Certain pre-existing personality traits such as higher level of hostility and anger as well as low levels of self-efficacy, when presented together, are associated with the development of PTSD for those whose work put them in the line of traumatic stress (Heinrichs 2005). This would suggest a genetic predisposition toward experiencing life as greatly frustrating or not meeting one's needs. Authors from the aforementioned work discussed that theses characteristics reduce an individual's ability to preserve a social support network and tends to experience life as unpredictable and uncontrollable, thereby increasing the risk of long-term trauma-related psychopathology.

Under unfortunate circumstances of genetics as well as life, leading to the inability for some individuals to meet his selfobject needs, self psychology teaches that the individual is able to salvage his selfobject mishap through the use of alternative objects. "A workable definition of mental health may be the capacity to choose from a number of psychic mechanisms according to need" (Kohut in Elson, 1987, p.82). Self psychology subscribes to the idea that selfobject experiences emanate from objects, which can include people, symbols and other experiences. Just like the infant using a transitional object like the blanket to experience a sense of maternal security, as adults, we continue to rely on such a symbolic experience to maintain cohesion of the self. A writer may find that he is particularly creative and productive when using his favorite fountain pen. Having the option to utilize other symbolic means toward cohesion of the self has distinct advantages in allowing for greater chances of maintaining good function. Kohut has discovered what nature has intended; make each being as resilient as possible.

A Historical Timeline

Since the pioneering work by Sigmund Freud, his psychoanalytical techniques and case studies have crossed path with the more modern empirical schools, gave birth to the use of the term borderline personality disorder in the Diagnostic and Statistical Manual. Some people today believe that many of Freud's case histories may actually describe what is known as borderline personality disorder in the DSM. Many writers and researchers through the intervening years have variously described a schizophrenic-like disorder that straddles both neurotic features as well as psychotic features. In 1938, Adolph Stern, coined the term ***borderline*** to describe a group of patients who did not seem to fit nicely into the primary diagnostic classifications of "neuroses" and "psychoses."

The attempt by researchers to develop a succinct description and delineation lead to different emphasis of important clinical symptoms as seen by different researchers. In 1953, Robert Knight utilized the term "borderline states" in his recognition that even though patients presented markedly different symptoms and were categorized with different diagnosis, they were in fact expressing the same pathology. For a period of time, the diagnosis of borderline personality was considered a "waste-basket diagnosis" where many resistant patients or poorly understood patients were placed. Researchers today might suggest, perhaps, that many of the diagnostic categories described in the DSM-IV-TR are in fact expressions of some types of fundamental pathology with a common pathway. This was in fact what Otto Kernberg suggested in 1967 with the term Borderline Personality Organization (BPO).

Of Neurosis and Beyond

Kernberg pointed out that many individuals with neurotic symptoms and character pathology have peculiarities that suggest borderline personality organization. He urged that the term "borderline" should be reserved for those patients presenting a chronic characterological organization which is neither typically neurotic nor typically psychotic. It was felt that transient psychotic episodes may develop in patients with BPO when under stress or under the influence of drugs and alcohol. Borderline patients have "alterations in their relationship with reality and in their feelings of reality, their capacity to test reality is preserved, in contrast to patients with psychotic reactions."

Kernberg suggest the "presumptive" diagnostic elements of borderline personality organization includes an individual with chronic, diffuse, free-floating anxiety, who may also suffer from multiple phobias, obsessive-compulsive symptoms, bizarre conversion symptoms, dissociative reactions and hypochondriasis. Kernberg's diagnostic elements would also include individuals who manifest sexual deviation within which several perverse trends coexist. This could also be an individual with "classical" prepsychotic personality structure such as schizoid personality, hypomanic personality and cyclothymic personality organization. Furthermore, this group also includes impulsive acting out behavior, devaluation of others, as well as addictions.

Finally, the "lower level" character disorder includes the hysterical, infantile and narcissistic personality as part of the high to low level character disorder in this order. " What distinguishes many of the patients with narcissistic personalities from the usual borderline patient is their relatively good social functioning, their better impulse control, and what may be described as a "pseudosublimatory" potential, namely, the capacity for active consistent work in some area which permits them partially to fulfill their ambitions of greatness and of obtaining admiration from others." Nevertheless, the narcissistic individual utilizes some of the same defenses as that of the borderline personality organization. These are namely the mechanism of splitting, denial, projective identification, omnipotence, and primitive idealization (Kernberg 1985, p. 4-20).

In his not so subtle way, Kernberg appears to be suggesting the application of the dynamics in borderline personality organization to that of a number of other character pathology. In a sense, the DSM IV-TR is reflective of the broad expanse of disorders that Kernberg covered with his use of the term borderline personality organization. I see the potential to understand the pathology of disorders such as some types of anxiety, obsessive compulsive symptoms, eating disorders, substance use disorders, and aggressive acting out behavior in the same vein as the borderline personality organization.

In exploring the psychodynamics of BPD in the context of DSA, it became inevitable for me to examine the application of this model of treatment to numerous other psychiatric conditions. This is both exciting and encouraging in relating to the search for solutions to many of the disorders encountered in the clinical setting. If the myriad of disorders and character pathology can be comprehended through the scope of one theoretical underpinning, this would greatly improve our chances of arriving at a solid solution to treatment.

Developmental Pathways

In the style of work that we pursue here, the awareness of the various developmental understandings serves to help us comprehend the existence and significance of emptiness. Once again, I wish to stress that the pathology of emptiness is likely more pervasive than is conceptually accepted by the psychiatric establishment today. In many ways, numerous existing literatures about early development offer us an insightful look into the presence of a myriad of potential frustrations in early life. If so, it appears that adequate resolution of these developmental frustrations are requirement toward healthy adjustments in adulthood. However, developmental pathways can be a wild ride of sort and traumatic as well as inadvertent circumstances in life frequently leave us in psychological quandary.

If Kernberg points the way to the understanding that multiple types of character pathology can all be classified under one banner, how then do we hypothesize about the origin of such a disorder? Kernberg relates that the history of the patient with borderline personality organization often suggest extreme *frustration* and intense *aggression* during the first few years of life. Melanie Klein elaborated on the infant's destructive fantasies that are based on Sigmund Freud's hypothesis of the *death instinct*. For much of the first year of life, the infant struggles with his impulses of aggression toward his only source of sustenance which leads to a great deal of turmoil and apprehension. At times, I will refer to this as *original anger* in this work; it represents the remnants of poor resolution of early frustrations and aggression.

In beginning his introduction on identity, Erikson suggest that we "start out from Freud's far-reaching discovery that neurotic conflict is not very different in content from the "normative" conflicts which every child must live through in his childhood, and the residues of which every adult carries with him in the recesses of his personality" (1968 p.91). Furthermore, with a nod toward Freud's primeval instincts, Erikson points out, "I refer to the *rage* which is aroused whenever action vital to the individual's sense of mastery is prevented or inhibited. What becomes of such rage when it, in turn, must be suppressed and what its contributions are to man's irrational enmity and eagerness to destroy, is obviously one of the most fateful questions facing psychology" (1950 p.68).

Kernberg writes that the pregenital and oral aggression resulting from the denial of oral gratification by the dangerous, frustrating mother is projected and extended to both parents. In an effort to escape from oral rage and fears, premature development of genital strivings takes place. These oedipal strivings then leads to the presence of "several of the pathological compromise solutions which give rise to a typical persistence of polymorphous perverse sexual trends in patients presenting borderline personality organization" (Kernberg 1985, p.4-20).

In response to experiences of extreme frustration and intense aggression in infancy and early childhood, this child develops *oral aggression* which is a distortion of early parental image and views parents as dangerous. The effort to escape from oral rage leads to the development of premature genital strivings. For the boy, this brings on the pregenital fear of mother, seen as the dangerous castrating mother and oedipal fear of father; both of these positions contribute to the generation of fierce anxiety. For the girl, the premature genital striving leads to the anxiety of experiencing the dangerous castrating mother and the anxiety of longing for the father's penis. The development of premature genital striving worsens the child's predicament; he or she is now faced with tremendous anxiety, fear and guilt.

As would be expected, having long term fear of one's primary object is not conducive to survival. This is not fundamentally acceptable to personality organization. Klein suggests that the infant had to deal with such malignant images by mentally separating it into a representational world consisting of the good and bad components. By the second year of life, the child has undergone rapid psychological growth and some degree of the integration of the good object and bad object would have to take place for the child to recognize that the mother can be both good and bad (Klein 1952, p.63).

Aaron Beck (1976) proposed the cognitive model of psychopathology stating that disorders such as depression, anxiety disorder, personality disturbances and other psychiatric conditions are grounded in characteristic errors in information processing. He then introduced the concepts of automatic thoughts and the maladaptive schemas that often lie dormant until triggered by life events; schemas being the cognitive structures containing the rules for screening, filtering, and decoding information from the environment (Beck et al. 1979). These organizing constructs developed through early childhood experiences and subsequent formative influences can help in assimilation of data and appropriate decision making as well as contribute to self-defeating behaviors and perpetuate dysphoric mood. In cognitive theory, it is generally believed that schemas pertaining to the self may be more resistant to change than schemas in depression or anxiety disorders (Beck and Freeman 1990; Beck and Rush 1992).

Elaborating on Freud's theories, Erik Erikson (1950) did some pioneering work on identity and drew attention to the idea that human development can only be understood through taking into account the social forces that influence and interact with the developing person. He places the developmental stage of autonomy vs. shame and doubt at age one year to three years. It could be suggested that each of his stages of development from infancy to old age constitute a reworking of shame involving subsequent crisis. Shame is a prominent emotion in women with BPD and associated with poorer quality of life and self-esteem and greater anger-hostility (Rüsch 2007). Silvan Tomkins further elaborated on shame by presenting the model for an affect theory of motivation. Here he ascribes facial and bodily behavior as primary to our awareness of affect (1962). He viewed affect as a greater motivating factor "more urgent than drive deprivation and pleasure, and more urgent than physical pain" (1987 p.137). Tomkin accounts for the differential activation of affect by the various density of neural firing and conceives of "stress" as resulting from the suppression of the innate affects. "The failure to fully, openly validate, and understand another's need by directly communicating its validity can sever the interpersonal bridge and thereby activate shame" (Kaufman 1989, p.34).

Interestingly, there are now some recent considerations about the contribution of neuropsychiatric conditions such as ADHD and autism toward that of personality disorders and deficits in character maturation. "Hypothetically, neuropsychiatric diagnoses designate dysfunctional extremes of normally distributed abilities, such as attention and impulse control; adaptive decision-making strategies; adequate perception and control of voice, posture, mimicry, and interpersonal skills and mentalizing." Observations have suggested that deficits in neurocognitive development or certain childhood temperament profiles may impair healthy character development, producing personality disorder in adulthood (Anckarsäter 2006). The division of neuropsychiatric conditions from developmental psychology seems an unnecessary obstacle in the attempt to understand borderline pathology. Neuropsychiatric disorders likely contribute further insult upon what is already a precarious state of anger and frustration arising from a primitive need for gratification.

A Failure to Resolve Original Anger

Classic developmental psychology as delineated specifically by Klein, Kernberg, Kohut and others have inspired my interest in the fundamental formation of personality pathology although my own clinical work gave rise to my current view of object relations as implemented in DSA. In addition, each of these models of work impressed me with the sense of the pathology of the self as a fluid state rather than that of static psychopathology. This state would suggest that the inner workings of the self and ultimately, the pathology of the self resides in an emotional place occupied by an intangible quality of flux that governs our very being.

Whether due to developmental frustrations, pathologic schemas, neurocognitive deficits or original scenes related to shame, the various developmental pathways of the borderline individual appear to suggest that innate drives or schemas are further influenced by events and surroundings. The essence of the works by the early pioneers of psychoanalysis sets a tantalizing stage for the understanding of the importance of resolving original anger. The theory of the death instinct opens the door to the possibility for the existence of inborn or early anger and frustration. It appears that, even within normal parameters for developmental growth, the failure to address original anger can have serious pathological consequences. Bowen suggested the idea of an "emotional system" (Kerr, Bowen, 1988) that can be attributed to most organisms seems to lead us to the consideration of instinctual and universal emotions at a primitive and perhaps, infantile level. If so, the theory of the emotional system could be thought of as the precursor of death instinct. Whether or not these theories bear true, I am persuaded by clinical work that points to the existence of a certain instinct of anxiety in early life that seeks developmental resolution.

In my work, I have included a dimension of our internal psychic makeup that functions to drive us in the fervent pursuit to reduce emotional pain. Whether this early emotion is the result of the instincts related to death, a primitive emotional system, frustrations of infancy, or some other natural state, developmental resolution appears both critical as well as beneficial. When early frustration and anger are unresolved, some sort of psychic injury or developmental delay occurs which contributes to one's life long pursuit to counter this pain.

Borderline and narcissistic individuals do not function consistently across all spheres in life; in other words, they have no consistency in function over person, place or time. At times, these individuals appear and reports of feeling "never been better" while even shortly after, he may report feeling completely in distress. In yet other cases, an individual who appears to function well for much of his life time can suddenly exhibit all of the hallmarks of character pathology. What about the cases in which classical borderline pathology is accompanied by the appearance of a lack of any known trauma or abuse? The DSA model of treatment takes into consideration such etiology as original anger to contribute to our understanding of emotional fragmentation and emptiness pain. Depending on the child's success at the task of developmental integration, the most important of borderline defenses are formed; understanding the defensive operations of splitting and projective identification will help us better comprehend the self in the context of DSA.

Splitting

Splitting, as understood through object relations, is the extreme separation of the self and the object into "all good" and "all bad" in order to protect the good self and good object from the anger, hatred and aggression of the bad self and bad object. It is also a fear of *contamination* of the good object by the bad object. "Excessive aggression results in excessive splitting mechanisms in order to protect the good internal and external objects from contamination and badness" (Kernberg 1980, p. 27). The term selfobject can be quite confusing in the discussions of object relations and self psychology. Essentially, the self is considered a selfobject and the object is also considered as selfobject due to the intertwined nature of the self and the object, an important other. In this work, I will use object and selfobject interchangeably and any differences in the usage of the term will be left up to the different context in which it is used. Selfobject will generally connote a set of characteristics that are being shared by both the self and the object. Use of the term object will generally mean that I am attempting to denote a concern that is more specific about the external.

How we then actually perceive the object hinges on our own projective identification toward the object as well as the transference projection by the object in a delicate dance of sort. Splitting becomes a survival function when one's frustration and anger in early life leads one to the predominant belief that our very survival may be dependent on bad objects who are incapable of responding to our needs. At the core of our being, we all yearn for the all loving and all giving mother like object. "Splitting is also linked with idealization, an exaggeration of the good qualities of internal and external objects, together with a denial and splitting off of contradictory evidence regarding the object's real characteristics" (Kernberg 1980, p.28).

If in contrast to this idealized fantasy of infancy, the individual is highly frustrated by the vicissitude and perhaps the stress of misfortunes of life, the reality can be extremely frightening. Such hardship gives rise to the original anger that can cast a shadow over the infant's outlook about the security of his survival. In the mind's eye of the young child, the objects (In this case, the caregivers) can be viewed with much detest and fear. As a result, our inherent ideal and longing likely contributes to the polarization of objects into distinct good and bad.

Essentially, this is to protect one from the notion that all objects are bad or negative. By having such a polarity, one is assured of the partial existence of the object as good and not all bad. "Only at later stages of development, when splitting mechanisms decrease, is a synthesis of good and bad aspects of objects possible and the coming into existence of ambivalence toward whole objects" (Kernberg 1980, p.25). Thus, splitting can be viewed as a natural part of infant development; as a primitive defense, it serves to help the infant and young child cope with frustration derived anger and aggression. In normal development, the use of splitting is decreased as the individual ages and the simultaneous existence of good and bad is accepted in the self and objects.

Not only is the object separated into the good and the bad but the self is also compartmentalized into the good and the bad as well. In the case of the developmental passage through tremendous frustration and aggression, the individual then develops great intolerance for the self. He is fearful that his anger and aggression will ultimately destroy anything at all of value in his life. Given that this is not an acceptable position, he needs to escape from such a highly anxiety provoking sense of the self. Therefore, from early life, he began to see and experience himself as being distinctly good or bad in a mutually exclusive way. In this fashion, the borderline individual is being cautious of the destructive potential of his aggressive self. By separating his self into distinct portions of good and bad, he could spare himself the great anxiety of feeling as if his sole purpose in life is to be aggressive and destructive. This allows him to experience himself or at least the good selfobject, as someone who is worthy of being loved.

Interference in Learning

Having separated the self and the object into compartments of good and bad, another consequence of this diathesis presents as the borderline's inability to learn from past mistakes and experiences. To a keen observer of the dynamic of splitting, it is a defense of overwhelming proportion in the reality of the patient's daily life. When this patient experiences himself as "good", he is likely to see the self as totally "good" and in this compartment, it is simply the truth at that very moment. When he experiences himself as "bad", it is a very real and very dominant state and it too is the truth at that very moment. Quite often, when in a positive state about the self, the borderline patient presents as if he has never known himself in any other state.

He is living in the here and now and when feeling upbeat, seems unable to accurately recall recent states of feeling very negative about the self. When he switches to experiencing the self as negative and deserving of rejection from others, he seems completely unable to recall that he had enjoyed a very positive state with himself and others in the recent past. He may claim to not have remembered a recent event or that he recalls it as if it is a memory about someone else's life; in effect, he is just having great difficulty in re-experiencing and re-living that past moment. The reader must keep in mind that the states that we discuss here are emotional feeling states and this has to be differentiated from that of actual memory of an event. Whether or not the emotional state of the moment can cloud the memory of an event is of course open to much debate.

At times, the borderline patient may clearly recall an event from the day before but insist that consequences should not be applied to him because it is no longer relevant. He may truly feel that consequences are not applicable because he is unable to reconcile current feelings to that of the recalled memory. It is as if he experienced yesterday as a totally different person. This is the result of internal emotional splitting.

Given his propensity to view the selfobject in similarly compartmentalized boxes of "good" and "bad", it is not surprising that he should have difficulty in integrating his interaction with others on a continuum of time with past, present and future. In this lack of continuum with time, it is probably the inability to experience the self as continuous entity that causes him to have the most trouble in learning from experience. This unique defensive dynamic is clearly not conducive to helping the borderline patient in learning from experiences. This *state dependent learning* is often related to the defense dynamics of splitting.

Because of the dynamics of splitting, he is unable to experience the specifics of an event accurately; it is also difficult for him to properly process about it at a later time. This does pose a dilemma in treatment. It means that any processing that relies on the patient's own memory about the event may have to occur at the very moment that it occurred. Even then, his experiences may not be accurate. This has little to do with his memory since his cognition is just fine but his experiences of the event may be skewed. However, instant processing is simply not always feasible in daily life; it is also not possible on the inpatient unit. This is but one of the reasons that instant processing is not usually recommended in the daily work with a borderline patient. In the transitional state of life being polarized between the good and the bad objects, it is exceedingly difficult for him to experience an interpersonal interaction accurately and he is also going to be challenged in his ability to recall much of this event for posterity.

Rather than argue with him about the inaccuracies of his recall about a given event, it is perhaps more therapeutic for the borderline patient to develop a degree of insight about his own involvement through the metaphor used in DSA. In this work, the borderline patient is taught to understand the variability of his emotional state through the metaphor of the cup. He is made aware of the existence of the split states of good and bad that can easily cause him to experience life as based on one state or the other. As such, it makes it easier for him to understand his challenge in accurate recall as well as embrace responsibility.

In DSA, the patient is encouraged to journal in accordance to the treatment protocol as soon as possible and as accurately as possible after an episode of emotional difficulty or external conflict. When there is an opportunity to process, the patient is then asked to first relate about his internal emotional state and then explain how he has managed to cope before any attempt is made to help him recall the recent event. In so doing, this patient can truly benefit from each and every contact with his therapist (or object figure) even if he is unable to accurately recall and process a recent event.

In the next section, projective identification will be looked at in terms of its relevance to the model of work here. As will be emphasize throughout this work, the state of emptiness is accepted as variable and therefore, state dependent learning will also be applied to projective identification. As such, this defense mechanism occurs fluidly depending on the condition of emotional emptiness; it is activated greatly in times of severe emptiness. Hence, one might expect the borderline individual to suffer increased activation of splitting as well as projective identification in emotional crisis. Because of the state dependent nature of this pathology, it contributes to the patient's difficulties in being able to accurately account for his feelings and responses during an episode of particular distress.

As is frequently the case, people in the life of the borderline patient look on with incredulous concern regarding his repetition of past mistakes. People wonder why he is not getting "wiser and smarter" in his handling and coping with even mundane life issues. People are apt to comment, "He just can't learn from mistakes." "He never sees it as his problem." "He has his way of looking at things and he thinks he is always right." It is easy to come to the conclusion that, perhaps, he is simply not interested in learning from current problems and issues. Alternately, recognizing the powerful borderline defensive dynamics that can cloud his judgment and learning, one learns to be patient and compassionate in relating to him. Productive learning from experiences will be further elaborated in chapter 8 under event analysis.

Projective Identification

It is through the world of projective identification that our universe becomes populated by angels and demons. Having taken into account the possible existence of aggressive and destructive instincts, we can now turn our attention to another psychological dynamic that uses such internal drives. The aggressive and destructive instincts (original anger) can be viewed as the fuel that propels projective identification in the daily functioning in all people but more intensely in borderline individuals. Kernberg relates, "The main purpose of projection here is to externalize the all-bad, aggressive self and object images, and the main consequence of this need is the development of dangerous, retaliatory objects against which the patient has to defend himself" (Kernberg 1985, p. 30). In chapter 9, projective identification will be integrated into a DSA manner of understanding and visualizing this defensive dynamic in clinical cases.

Melanie Klein (1946) defined projective identification as a process by which unconscious information, largely unwanted parts of the self, is projected from the sender to the recipient, described by Klein as a massive invasion of someone else's personality (1955). "Therefore, they have to control the object in order to prevent it from attacking them under the influence of the (projected) aggressive impulses; they have to attack and control the object before (as they fear) they themselves are attacked and destroyed. In summary, projective identification is characterized by the lack of differentiation between self and object in that particular area, by continuing to experience the impulse as well as the fear of that impulse while the projection is active, and by the need to control the external object" (Kernberg 1985, p. 31).

More than the projection of unwanted parts of the self, projective identification has the propensity to create great confusion between the self and object. "A consequence or parallel development of the operation of the mechanism of projective identification is the blurring of the limits between the self and the object (a loss of ego boundaries), since part of the projected impulse is still recognized within the ego, and thus the self and object fuse in a rather chaotic way" (Kernberg 1985, p. 56). This dynamic illustrates an interesting case of a young man with a tremendous sense of emptiness and loneliness, which manifested in the inability to attend school while engaged in perpetual battles with his parents. On further examination, this example demonstrates two possible conceptions of projective identification. One, his original anger was projected not only toward individual objects but can also be projected in a general direction toward an entity such as school. This would suggest that a broader projection is possible and opens up a larger area of consideration for the use of the concept of projective identification. Two, whether it is a group of people or a specific individual, the recipient of the projection may take note of such an impulse and respond accordingly.

Quite often, an individual arises out of a life full of frustrations and anger that was never resolved to finally project this indignation externally on a world that could not see it coming. The external world then responds with outrage, which in turn, gives this individual the justification for his fury. It would seem plausible that, in more severe cases of projective identification, one can identify some of the more notorious and news worthy characters in human history. In abject poverty or oppression, narcissism is likely to be suppressed. Curiously, narcissism in a society may follow a hierarchy that determines its expression based on various factors of oppression. Thus, many in our society have suffered the injuries to predispose them to narcissism but the pathology is more likely to be expressed when this individual reaches a certain level of social status or power; at which point, the hidden anger resulting from projective identification is no longer contained and is unleashed with full fury. Once again, earlier authors of the object relations school suggests to us the wide possibilities of using the dynamics of projective identification to further understand a multitude of human ills as well as, perhaps, human evil in our world.

Not all projective identification should be viewed as negative. "Klein originally described projective identification as the projection of an unwanted part of the self onto an important other, together with identification of that part with the other." "Klein also spoke about the role of projective identification in the child's positive relationship with the mother, stating that this process also involves the projection of a much-valued part of the self into another" (Alhanati 2002, p.9). In both the developmental and therapeutic context, projective identification can be viewed as bi-directional process that involves mutual reciprocal influence characterized by the mother and infant communication. The securely attached child is able to induce in the other, the object, an affect-regulating and empathic mutual regulatory process that allows the self to project "valued" parts of the self into the mother which forms adaptive projective identification (Alhanati 2002, p. 11-12).

Mirroring and Idealizing Transference

The precarious conditions of the infant is not so different from the narcissistic individual in terms of his need for focused attentiveness; it is possible to relate this to the infant's reliance on his mother's focused attentiveness for his emotional regulatory process. Assuming that the infant lacks a sense of the self, he would vicariously regard his reflection in his mother as himself. This reflection occurs as a result of the manner in which his mother dote on him with her every being. Through her empathic regard while softly singing or talking to him as she changes his diaper or offers him the nipple, she offers him a window into a kind of reality.

His mother, the selfobject, is then able to assure him of his intactness as well as serving as a major source of transference input for him. In psychoanalysis, transference was described by Sigmund Freud as the patient's feelings and behavior toward the analyst that are based on infantile wishes the patient has toward parents or parental figures. In this work, I favor the use of the broader criterion for transference used in general psychiatry for designating the patient's feelings and behavior whether rational or irrational distortions arising from unconscious strivings. In this all encompassing sense, it may be appropriate to refer to transference as a relationship. In analyzing contemporary perspective on transference, Ellman writes that Charles Brenner "has extended the concept of transference to all avenues of a person's life. Transference is to be encountered not only in an analyst's office but in virtually every human interaction" (1991, p.86).

During infancy, the infant has very little ability to hold within the sense of who he is and what he is and how he should feel. Acting like a mirror, also known as mirroring transference, his mother has the power to regulate how he should feel about himself. Even though this may not be the reality, it is sufficient to hold him through to a time when he can be more independent in determining how he will experience his inner life. Mirroring allows the mother to participate in the infant's subjective experience as well as consolidating this experience (Mahler et al. 1975; Kohut 1977).

In idealizing transference, the infant holds absolute the belief that his mother will make him feel whole. With idealizing and mirroring transference, the infant is able to obtain adequate input to hold the self together despite lacking a true ability to self modulate emotions. Meares referred to the famous experiment by Sorce and Emde in which the infant was confronted by the visual cliff. The infant looked toward the mother seeking some sort of meaning to a strange situation. At this point, the mother's expression gave shape to the child's reality. "This experiment suggests that when the other fails to make adequate responses to the experiences of the child, the child will be left with a diminished sense of the reality and meaning of his or her existence. This deficit is sometimes the central presenting feature in those who have suffered a disruption in the evolution of self (Meares 1993, p. 143-144)." Similarly, the borderline patient can vicariously acquire a better state of function through mirroring and idealizing transference with his therapist. Like the infant's reliance on his mother to form his rudimentary sense of the self, the borderline patient may have to look to his therapist and other selfobjects for temporary sustenance.

In my view, the evolving emotional stability of the infant would then allow him to make a projection of the "valued" parts of himself as adaptive projective identification. In this manner, the mother and child are indeed involved in mutual reciprocal influence. In a later chapter, I would refer to this as the emotional satiation of a metaphorical cup by which adaptive or positive projection can take place. Vise versa, a near empty cup is one in which negative projection is exercised, causing the object to respond in anger and rejection. The consequence of negative projective identification will be further discussed and case example rendered in chapter 9.

The critical points to consider here is the bi-directional interaction between the infant and the mother using idealizing and mirroring transference as well as adaptive and negative projective identification. In some ways, the "valued" parts of the infant's self, the positive regard or transference that is a gift from his mother, is nothing more than the reflection he sees of himself in his mother. In this symbiotic state, what he is able to receive from his mother is given back in return for the perpetuation of this cycle through the mechanism of positive projective identification. Naturally, if his mother is unable to provide for healthy mirroring and idealizing transference, the infant would not be able to operate optimally and negative rather than positive projection takes place from the infant which destroys any opportunity for mirroring or idealizing transference with the mother. Subsequently, the introjection of the maternal selfobject becomes less efficient.

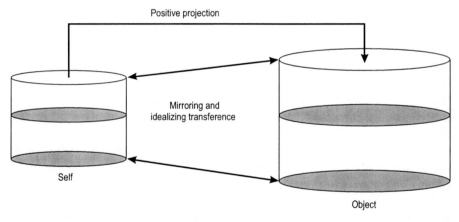

Fig. 2.2 *Mirroring and idealizing transference serve as temporary survival tools for the infant by helping to modulate content for an early cup. Having a sense of content, the infant is then able to reciprocate by projecting the valued, positive parts of the self toward the mother.*

In this chapter, the genesis of the pathology of the self can be understood through the myriad of frustrations that confronts the infant and the toddler. Despite the evident resilience of the human organism, some individuals can be more vulnerable to experiencing misattunement and original anger. Viewed through the scope of early development, one can now better comprehend the mechanism by which innate frustrations can contribute to the pathology of the self. Understanding this early dynamic allows one to truly appreciate the vicissitude of character pathology encountered in the clinical arena.

·III·
ASSESSING TREATMENT ISSUES

"The biggest disease today is not leprosy or tuberculosis,
but rather the feeling of being unwanted."
-Mother Theresa

A General Clinical Picture

When the patient with BPD becomes acutely decompensated, the patient and his outpatient provider turns to the psychiatric inpatient setting with hopes of quick stabilization and positive contribution to long term work. It is now up to the institutional setting to produce a way to stabilize this very challenging patient. The psychiatric provider in the inpatient setting will generally review this patient's medication history to determine if there is any medication treatment regimen that has not been explored. Just as there is a paucity of methodology in the treatment of BPD in the outpatient arena, there is a paucity of appropriate psychotherapeutic program of treatment in the inpatient setting. Inpatient treatment facilities generally cobble together bits and pieces of treatment modalities without sufficient cohesiveness. Many psychiatric inpatient programs try to put together a program from the best of available information but little attention is generally given to the patient's chronic feelings of emptiness. Without emphasis of emptiness as a central feature to the pathology of many who seeks treatment, there can be notable inconsistency and lack of efficacy in inpatient work.

The complexities of the treatment of borderline personality disorder is so challenging that few therapists see themselves as totally devoted to working with this type of disorder in their practice. This work brings fourth some of the most challenging situations that we face in the daily struggle to help our patients make forward strides in their quest to be more independent and content in life. Individuals with BPD face each day with great uncertainty. He or she is often highly dependent on family, friends and significant others yet he is unable to feel a sense of belonging anywhere in his world. His daily life is filled with the tensions from the push and pull with each and every relationship. There is rarely any calm in relationships. Quite often, his therapist comes to experience the transference frustration that is a recapitulation of the patient's existence.

With respect to his relationship with other, the borderline patient can appear quite stable in the inpatient setting for an extended period of time. Quite often, this quiescence becomes interpreted by the treatment providers as a sign of improvement only to find out, perhaps, months later in the case of residential treatment settings, that the patient can still revert to very poor functioning when stressed. The keen follower of this discussion will no doubt understand that a hospital setting can easily fulfill the internal emotional needs of the patient in a non-therapeutic manner; indiscriminate emotional filling of others do not constitute treatment in the home environment nor the inpatient milieu.

Regardless of his environment, he tends to jump into relationships impulsively and exit the relationship just as quickly. Most often, he can appear to be too trusting in relationships but at the slightest alarm that others may not meet his very high and demanding expectations in a relationship, he takes flight with an intense sense of betrayal. He lacks the ability to see the more global picture of life, unable to learn from previous mistakes or to observe patterns of his own behavior, and would repeatedly enter into destructive relationships. A woman with BPD may repeatedly enter into similar abusive relationships or return to abusive husbands or boyfriends. At times, she makes the trade off for someone who she believes to provide some sort of emotional filling and may then tolerate the abuse.

For one 15 year old patient, his inability to attend school has been a confounding mystery to everyone of concern. There were no obvious abuses in his middle class upbringing in an intact family of origin. He is a rather large boy but his size has not been an issue of teasing but likely intimidated would be bullies. In fact, he denies actual academic difficulties and has never reported of incidence of bullying. He insist that he has some friends but family moved often. He complains of feeling anxious about school and feels that he has a difficult time making friends. Careful probing would reveal an individual with a strong pervasive sense of aversive inner tension that he would eventually identify as akin to emptiness.

Although diagnosed with anxiety disorder or perhaps, panic disorder with agoraphobia, this is really a patient suffering from the pathology of emptiness. It is all too convenient for him to interpret his internal emotional pain as a discomfort that attacks him from the outside world. With this view, he would naturally experience many others, including that of school in general, as perpetrator of aggression somehow. Despite his intense discomfort about school, he was unable to explain the specifics of his anxiety; he seems comfortable anywhere else, including the hospital milieu. This is an example of the unconscious underlying pain of emotional emptiness that can contribute to severe debilitating illness through the dynamics of projective identification.

When asked about what upset triggered an episode of acting out, one patient could only recall vague generalization without the details. This would of course preclude him from any successful analysis or learning from a life event. Upon closer examination in therapy, it would appear that he tends to make very hasty, impulsive and often inaccurate judgment of a situation. Despite such repeated experiences, it would seem that it is very difficult for him to learn from past experiences. He continues to misjudge and misinterpret interpersonal issues.

Life is a tremendous storm for this individual. His "self" is prone to fragmentation. He has difficulties soothing and sustaining his "self". If he happens to have some insight about his internal turmoil, he may already have noted a tremendous sense of numbness or lack of aliveness that pervades his being and invades any semblance of joy left in his life. Possibly, despite intense therapy, he continues to live a tumultuous existence that is marked by frequent close calls with death. His despair is deep and painful beyond description and at times, he feels the only way out of such depth of depression is to take his own life. Some individuals attempt suicide and others surrender themselves to the grizzly acts of self-mutilation.

As chair legs and debris flew, followed by loud pounding, slamming of doors and deafening screams, staff stood with utter abhorrence at the unfolding of a scene of such magnitude that any intervention would surely risk injury to someone. Here is witnessed another apparent cycle of extreme outburst occurring at about one week interval for this patient. Due to his propensity for such violence, not much can be demanded of him in the milieu. Interestingly, as if in a post-ictal state, he is at his calmest and most quiescent in the days following such outburst; then the cycle would begin again with the gradual escalation of agitation. In the days leading up to another episode, staff often comment that he seems to "hate" everything about himself. Curiously, he rarely complains about being wronged by others, but rather, he mostly expresses an intense dislike for the self. Is this a cyclic venting of accumulated stress, an episode of mania or the result of gradual emptying of some important material of emotional sustenance?

Referring to figure 3.1, this individual is able to describe a nebulous sense of unwell that he simply states as an intolerable feeling that consistently precedes each episode of extreme acting out. He reports that this is followed by a brief period of quiescence that he equates to better mood and awareness of calm. He, like many borderline patients, is also conscious of the brevity of this state. He is often quite prepared to act out once again to seek some type of subjective calm.

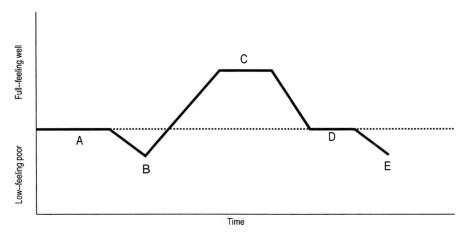

Fig 3.1 *This graph depicts mood as a cycle manipulated through acting out behaviors. **A** is base line. **B** is point of low mood and start of acting out behavior. **C** is achievement of improved feeling through overt or covert acting out. **D** is on return to baseline. **E** is encounter of another episode of low mood.*

People in his life, including his own therapist, are often left to just watch helplessly at the sideline. It would be fortunate if he still has a therapist after much frustrations in treatment and many therapists later. This is because he is prone to dismissing his therapist when he senses the slightest hint of betrayal consistent with interpersonal disappointment. In the case of the aggressive young inpatient, his seemingly unpredictable and violent behavior generally relegates his existence to one of isolation and loneliness. Whether in an out-patient or inpatient setting, developing an effective treatment approach for a patient with such a wide spectrum of issues and myriad of resistance to treatment can be highly challenging.

The Broad Spectrum of the Borderline Condition

I will use the pronoun, he, to denote the individual with BPD although the literature suggests that more females are diagnosed with this condition than males. The theoretical constructs behind DSA would suggest that the developmental issues related to the self would likely apply to many human conditions beyond the classical description for BPD and likely affect both sexes equally. Many issues in life are set upon a continuum that bears upon the affected individual through the extent to one side or the other that the symptoms lean. This is to say that, come what may, the fundamental pathology for multiple illnesses of development could arise out of the same roots but the expression of symptoms depends on the individual genetics as well as the severity of the external insult.

It is my belief that the classic writers of object relations school held the understanding that the pathology of the self is far more pervasive than has been accepted in practice today. In a medically driven health care world that we live in today, practitioners push to categorize illnesses in neat categories and distinct individual labels; this tendency has caused us to be blind to mental health issues that are perhaps on a continuum. The all inclusive male pronoun is used here for the purpose of reminding the reader that the pathology of the self can be very broad and clinically pervasive in many of the most common ills that one encounters in society and the therapy office.

A 2005 study using Structural Interview for DSM-IV Personality found that personality disorders are among the most frequent disorders treated by psychiatrists. About one-third of the patients in this study were diagnosed with one of 10 official DSM-IV personality disorder and this figure increases to 45.5% when personality disorder not otherwise specified were included (Zimmerman 2005). Borderline personality disorder was much less frequently diagnosed with unstructured clinical evaluation until treating clinicians are presented with information from semi-structured interview (Zimmerman 1999).

Having explored the developmental genesis to the pathology of the self in the previous chapter, this opens up the notion of the many faces of BPD. The borderline individual may be an unhappy housewife, the extremely driven executive, the footloose thrill seeker, the young man seeking meaning through a deadly cause or the ever troubled media starlet. What I hope to instill in the reader is the awareness to recognizing borderline pathology in all walks of life. It is through this encompassing view that the clinical providers can best serve the wide patient base of the community and hospital. As has been mentioned earlier, I strongly believe that this clinical approach allows for an effective treatment formulation for a multitude of mental health issues.

Control and Dependence in Narcissism

Case 2.1: Stephen is 22 years old and having difficulties deciding what he should do in life for the next few years. He has not been able to concentrate on schooling but works hard to please his boss. He has discovered that by working long hours and be at the beck and call of his boss, who he looks up to with jealous admiration for the man's success, is just about the only way that he feels any sense of aliveness and worthiness in life. As he talked about his work, he had an air of confidence about him that bordered on arrogance. He had little or no respect for his co-workers and minded his boss only because he felt constantly insecure about his employment.

He made it quite clear that he holds great contempt for most of the world. Interpersonally, his life with others has been an even greater sham. He has had a string of relationships but none has been satisfactory to him because he is quickly tired of the relationships and usually comes to feel that he has been the one to carry the relationship. He then explains that the others in these relationships are not his intellectual equal. Despite these disappointments, he is practically never without a girlfriend.

On the occasion of our meeting, he was just released from an intensive care unit after having shot himself with a gun, although he missed any vital anatomy, he is left with a disfiguring scar on his face. He has been feeling depressed for some time and his moods are often quite labile. In session, he has been talking about feeling increasingly angry, bored and lonely in life. He talks about being extremely unforgiving with the people in his life. He says, "Once someone upsets me, I will not talk to them again." Now he finds that he has practically no one that he could really count on in his life. On that fateful day, he just wanted to find someone to spend time with but no one called him back; on impulse, he attempted to end his life.

Yet, it is not as if he has many horrible life stories in which he was seriously hurt in relationships. His family and friends seem fairly supportive in a general sense. If anything, he is probably more likely to alienate himself from others or to terminate a relationship. "People are always walking on eggshells around me." In the milieu, he can present himself as intelligent, friendly, likable and charismatic. He can easily gain the trust of staff and seems to enjoy a special status amongst his peers and staff. With his native intelligence and skillful social ways, he manages to earn special privileges and trust from others. At times, he can be extremely cordial and personable as to appear surreal. In the milieu, he seemed needy of caretaking by his peers while concurrently tormenting a few individuals, both peers and staff, on a daily basis. He would make a point of humiliating and belittling them publicly but always back away just in time to not get into real trouble for himself.

One day, on a particularly less guarded moment in his life, he admits to feeling a profound sense of emptiness within. However, this was not a door he allowed open for long and shut it immediately. Acting as if no such discussion took place, he moved on to talk about how staff could better run the activities. Despite having declared that he has a subservient girlfriend waiting for him back home, he used every available moment flirting with his female peers; naturally, he paid little attention to treatment. When confronted about his use of caretaking and emotional rescue by his peers, he became outraged that staff would dare to limit his social contact with "friends" at such a time of crisis for him. He was determined to have constant access to his peers and when this was prohibited, he demanded discharge.

In preparation for discharge, he made arrangements for his girlfriend to quit her job and move in with him and his parents to take care of him full time. He was insistent that her undivided attention will keep him safe and uplift his spirit. He left the hospital artificially buoyed by the intense interpersonal experiences on the unit as well as having been on the receiving end of a tremendous amount of attention from a family terrified by his recent deeds.

Discussion:
Stephen, like many individuals with the pathology of the self, seems unable to tolerate the imperfections of human relationships. He frequently waves his high IQ score in front of others and complains that no one can keep up with him intellectually. He is highly critical of the world around

him and sees himself as a victim of other's lack of enlightenment. He has an exquisite need for his friends and family to be emotionally supportive of him at a very high level. He scrutinizes these relationships closely. He seems to invest heavily in a relationship, at least in the beginning, in the name of helping the other but it always turns out that this is not so altruistic because he is looking for a strong return on his emotional investment.

Any faltering would cause him to immediately terminate the relationship and reiterate his feeling that others are just not worthy of his love. He glorifies those in envious positions but secretly jealous and holds open contempt for them at the same time. As a result, he is often left feeling abandoned and highly angry. Projective identification is a rampant part of his interpersonal world. He feels abandoned although he is usually the one to sever the relationship. His intense need for others can turn into just as intense of anger when his needs are not met. He will surround himself with a group of "ideal" supporters because he has no time to cope with people who are not so perfectly supportive and understanding. He is highly dependent on others; yet, he can not depend on anyone. When his world is fairly intact and he is able to exert sufficient control, he is better able to function; he is often blinded to the fleeting nature of his happiness by his narcissistic characteristics. Of course, when there is any crisis, his world can easily spin out of control and he could exhibit every bit of severity of symptoms suggestive of BPD.

Inpatient Challenge

The psychiatric inpatient milieu presents a very unique set of challenges in itself. Just as group therapy can be viewed as a "microcosm" of the larger world, the inpatient milieu, made up of multiple therapeutic groups, can certainly be viewed as a microcosm of the outside world (Yalom 1985, p. 30). In such a restrictive environment, the dynamics of interpersonal interaction is bound to be intense and behavioral patterns of an individual would likely be replicated. Often, people talk about the "honeymoon" period when an individual arrives on the hospital milieu. However, the intense interpersonal needs of the borderline patient will soon surface along with his repertoire of acting out behaviors.

Splitting

Case 2.2: Janice is a 15-year-old who has been in and out of the hospital many times for acute crisis related to suicide gestures and attempts. Each time she blows onto the unit like a hurricane. Her arrival is often marked by anxious anticipation by hospital staff members who know her from past hospitalizations. At times she comes in under involuntary treatment orders. Even though she may resist hospitalization at times, she can acclimate quickly and actually resist leaving the traditional inpatient milieus. Whether her resistance is in coming to the hospital or leaving the hospital, it is emblematic of her constant state of confusion in life. Although she can storm in like a hurricane, she also has a very personable side that endears her to many staff.

Shortly after arrival on the unit, she began to exercise a number of demands and if she does not get her way, she would work her way through any available staff who will listen. She can actually be quite skillful socially in a manipulative sense. With sweetness and charm, she can make friends easily and there is never a lack of compassionate staff willing to be of help. However, her demands are strong and fast as if she is being swept along her own emotional river. If she can not maneuver sufficiently to get her way, she would call her parents and get them involved. She is intelligent and articulate and can argue like the best. Pretty soon, she has taken an event or issue and spins it to such proportion that few can recognize its original form.

A most familiar scenario ensues as she began to vent her dissatisfaction with staff. In this victim stance, she was able to garner the sympathies of numerous other patients and rally their support in protest of what is perceived as the staff's lack of compassion. Many group sessions had to be devoted to untangling the collective angst of the treacherous anger of group tension. Perhaps powered by their own guilt, her parents got pulled into this dynamic out of their concerns for an acutely ill child. Furthermore, some staff began to operate out of their own uneasiness and took side in this caldron of emotions.

Soon after, everyone around her began to feel lied to and manipulated. If arguments fail to align an issue in her direction, all those around her should brace themselves for a tremendous emotional meltdown, in another word, a temper tantrum. She would repeatedly surprise everyone by how minute the issues of contention that could cause her such outburst. It seems that the magnitude of her despair is often incongruent with the disappointment experienced. Very often, the inherent message that she communicates at such moment is that of feeling overwhelmingly disappointed by others and the unbearable anger of betrayal.

Even more unpredictable are those moments when she would suddenly start to kick at the door, bang the wall and began to yell and scream for no apparent reason. When asked, she would explain that she just had a painful or difficult thought of some sort that brought on a welling up of emotions. At other time, she is just at a loss as to why she had the sudden outburst; from an observer's point of view, it looked simply as if she was just looking for a fight. Many people in her life have questioned whether she is "antisocial or psychopathic."

Discussion:

Splitting is one of the most common dynamic the inpatient treatment team faces. Splitting can essentially be viewed as an indication of the tremendous need for support, protection and alignment with others. In a world where the borderline individual may feel that others are predominantly "bad", splitting can be a psychological mechanism that allows him to be able to experience some people as "good". He hangs on to this thread of hope that there can be good objects out there so that not all is lost in his world.

Many mental health providers come from the background of wanting to be in a profession that gives help and being empathic and understanding is seen as a virtue. As a result, one can easily succumb to our own countertransferential feelings as well as the projective identification by a patient. Countertransference is the powerful dynamic that causes us to respond to a patient as if he or she was an important figure from our past. This same countertransferential issue can bring positive feelings toward a patient or negative feelings toward a patient. Depending on one's relationship with this patient at that moment, one can come to feel positive or negative toward this individual. Therefore, it is easy to imagine how some staff may tend to interact with her in one way and other staff may interact with her in very different ways. As a result, she gets her "favorite" staff to make special concessions for her which can often bring about a stern rebuttal from the staff who "does not understand." Once the parents enter into this ongoing turmoil under these circumstances, agendas became skewed and distrust is brewed between family and provider. When this occurs, there can be little effective treatment that can take place.

Otto Kernberg summed up splitting the following way: "Splitting is the division of external object into "all good" ones and "all bad" ones, with the concomitant possibility of complete, abrupt shift of an object from one extreme compartment to the other; that is, sudden and complete reversals of all feelings and conceptualization about a particular person." Kernberg also added that splitting is often coupled with what he termed *primitive idealization* (Kernberg 1985, p.29-30). This is the tendency to see an external object as totally good and cannot be contaminated, spoiled or destroyed by one's own aggression, in order to make sure that they can protect one against the "bad" objects. Kernberg sees the borderline individual as projecting a great deal of "bad" onto others surrounding him and the manifestation is that of a primitive, protective fantasy structure in which there is no authentic regard for the ideal object, but a simple need for it as a protection against a surrounding world of dangerous objects.

Beyond the classic understanding of splitting, which is quite cumbersome when one tries to convey this concept to the patient, I use DSA to help the patient understand his or her role in the dynamic of splitting. If we view splitting as arising out of a person's fundamental need for support, protection and alignment with others, then we can further understand the purpose of primitive idealization as a way to fill this need. With this approach, the patient can more easily comprehend and accept his behavior because no blame is attributed; only individual responsibility encouraged. For example, rather than experiencing the patient's attempt at splitting as a distasteful method of manipulation to seek superficial personal gain, through DSA, one can come to appreciate his desperate need to seek intense alliance with those around him in order to experience emotional equilibrium. With this approach, it would be far easier for the therapist to feel compassion for this individual and therefore, accomplish therapeutic relationship while maintaining healthy therapeutic boundary.

Treatment as Usual

Case 2.3: Tina is a 16-year-old with a great smile and the face of such innocence that only a person so young could posses. Her eyes tend to dart about and never seem to make actual contact. At first glance, she appears no different from the teens around her in this group therapy setting in the hospital milieu. Then she rolls up her sleeves revealing a multitude of cuts to her arms. Some of the cuts are superficial and others appear repeatedly aggravated and some have received new suturing. She tells the group about the fresh cuts on her arm that she made last night when she could not sleep. She rationalized that she was upset and fearful because the night staff seemed to take no interest in her sudden sense of feeling "unsafe." She relished in this discussion when a number of her peers joined in to vent their frustration at the lack of greater display of empathy by the staff.

The group leader then asks her to cover her arms but instead, she got increasingly defiant in words and behavior. Very soon, she expressed feeling that everyone was against her and she stormed out of the room. One could hear the screaming and the profanity as she headed down the hallway. Another staff approached and she unleashed her anger at him and postured threateningly. She was then escorted to the quiet room so that she could be monitored safely. While in the quiet room, she starts to pull apart a recent suture to one of her deeper cuts. Having done this, she became more calm and controlled. Showing concerns about this patient's self-harm, a staff entered the room and tried to process with her and she was able to engage in this conversation and talked about the profound sense of despair that she suddenly felt in group on this day. This staff then diligently guided the patient through some cognitive behavioral coping skills that the patient has been exposed to recently in one of the skills training groups. Eventually, she fell into a deep sleep for a good long time.

Discussion:

This patient started the group session in an upbeat mood but one can not help but feel that she seems to be monopolizing the session and enjoying the attention that she was receiving. The group leader's requests appear to be quite reasonable in response to the issues at hand. Group members are concerned about the existence of sharp objects in the milieu and her notably scarred arms are drawing far too much attention in this session. In the hallway, another staff had to deal with the fallout from group. Repeatedly, this patient seems to decompensate to the point of needing constant supervision to keep from severely injuring herself.

Would any amount of processing during and after such an act of self-mutilation help to improve the long-term outlook for this patient? Some therapy convention would dictate the need for confronting the patient about such acting out while other methods advocate intense dialogue or to examine the event based on transference conversation and interpretation. In this case, soon after this patient acted out in group and proceeded to self-mutilate in follow-up, a staff approached her and attempted to process with her regarding what had just happened. Frequently, processing at such a moment has the undertone of a reprimand from staff, which is difficult to avoid given the possible countertransference from staff. At times, the processing can take on a tone of overt empathy and perhaps, anxiety on the part of the staff. At other times, staff may question this patient as to his failure to utilize coping strategies at the moment of crisis.

The patient could then engage the staff in a discussion about the pros and cons as well as all of the specifics about why the strategies did not work or that the situation did not allow him an opportunity to use his skills. Even though the staff urged her to use some coping skills, is such an interpersonal contact at that moment necessarily therapeutic?

Often, after such an extended processing and discussion, the staff would inevitably walk away form this conversation feeling that the patient gained something from the talk but what was gained was unlikely therapeutic. Behavioral intervention based on consequences to deter future acting out is unlikely to be of long term value given the severity and chronic nature of her illness. Of concern though is the possibility that interventions at inopportune times would only reinforce the patient's dependence on the therapist/staff. Whether intervening to keep a patient safe in the inpatient milieu or working with a patient to prevent a hospitalization, a therapist has to carefully consider the script of treatment. What is considered conventional therapeutic intervention may be highly counterproductive in working with an individual with pathology of the self. In our discussion, I want to introduce the reader to an effective method of intervention in dealing with this most challenging of clinical scenarios without reinforcing negative behavior or secondary gain.

Several unique dynamics about the individual with BPD can be played out intensely in the inpatient setting. Of great concern is the tendency for borderline patients to experience "reinforcement" for his dependent behavior toward others and for this behavior to be magnified by inpatient hospitalization. This concern is indisputable but as I will discuss elsewhere in this work, the use of hospitalization is at times unavoidable and perhaps even advantageous when DSA is implemented as a part of treatment.

For the individual with BPD, the traditional inpatient environment can be highly stimulating and emotionally intense. In a smaller inpatient setting than the larger world beyond the hospital walls, the close proximity to other people such as other patients and staff on the unit can bring about a great sense of comfort for this patient. There is the constant availability of people to talk with and interact with or just to be next to. The staff on the unit is scheduled by shift and this offers a constantly fresh set of crew on the unit for interpersonal interactions. Most experienced mental health workers in fact do a nice job of setting good limit and boundary on their interaction with a patient so as not to encourage the patient's excessive reliance on staff. When one shift is exhausted, there is always another set of staff coming onboard. This can offer a never-ending set of available staff to meet the emotional needs of the patients.

Patients often feel that the inpatient setting is the only place where their needs can be met, but this perception is not totally accurate. Although hospital workers get to go home after a shift, they do return again and again. Staff frequently comment, "Seemed like this patient needed someone to talk to but after spending an hour together, as I get up to return to my neglected duties, I get this nagging feeling that, as soon as I turn around, this patient is going to do poorly and act out." After a period of time, staff too can get quite exhausted from the demands of this patient and feel discouraged at not being able to meet his needs. When this occurs, this patient is likely to feel ignored, avoided and marginalized. His sense of emptiness and loneliness will seem more intense and he could struggle even harder to meet his interpersonal needs or he could elect to act out in other ways.

On the inpatient unit, the borderline individual is exposed to many other patients and this opens up the opportunity for one person to capitalize on this chance to indiscriminately meet his own emotional needs. Other patients on the unit may be oblivious of the uneven interpersonal dynamics at play and become an unwitting accomplice in care-giving to his emotionally painful internal world. One can witness such a drama when the borderline patient marshals his peers to devote their full attention to him and care take him. When the peer feels powerless to further satisfy his needs, in one case, the peer brought out his secretly stashed razorblade and offered it to him as a gesture of understanding and support. As pathological as this act appears, it is likely done without malice. It is more likely an act of validation between two individuals suffering a common ill.

Addressing behaviors that interferes with treatment as well as behaviors that place the safety of the individual and others in jeopardy is the cornerstone of treatment requirement on most inpatient units. Many institutions invest greatly on the details of how best to closely monitor patients and provide physical containment. Although important, these are not the efforts that bring about productive change. In the current health care atmosphere, individual therapy and family therapy work are practically foreign concepts in most acute inpatient settings. As a result, inpatient settings are more or less an opportunity for a temporary change of environment that would hopefully modify the patient's current outlook. At times, this is highly useful as a life saving measure but contributes little to the quality of life of the patient.

Many of the strategic concerns about the use of inpatient care for the borderline patient can be addressed by the use of DSA as an integral part of inpatient treatment. Through this approach, the patient is encouraged to function as independently as possible; boundary issues are foremost in this work and the patient is reinforced for his use of positive, independent, coping skills. When he has utilized his treatment, he will find his feelings appropriately validated by his peers and staff, and he will find that others are so much more welcoming of the time spent with him. In this way, in the very controlled environment of the inpatient milieu, he is able to quickly find success and motivation to continue the work on an outpatient basis.

Therapeutic Relationship

The fundamental platform for psychotherapy is the power of interpersonal connection. It is through this relationship that the beneficial transformation through psychotherapy takes shape. This beneficial transformation is hopefully the changes that occur in an individual that promote greater sense of self and an improvement in overall function. How the therapeutic relationship develops is actually the core substance of treatment and there are of course many ways of achieving this result. The therapist as a professional, sage, authority figure, parental figure or as a trusted selfobject, plays a critical role in the 3-steps in DSA.

It can be said that regardless of the method of treatment, without a therapeutic relationship, there can be no real treatment. This is a truism spanning from psychoanalysis to the most fundamental of behavioral management style of treatment. Sigmund Freud felt so strongly about the issue of transference that he expressed feeling that only individuals capable of transference neurosis could be analyzed and that the greater the narcissism the less likely the possibility for successful analysis (1916/1917) However, contemporary views of analysis and other modalities of treatment take a more encouraging approach to treatment of the self. Charles Brenner maintains that therapeutic alliance should best be looked upon as transference and interpreted in the process of analysis (1979). Merton Gill theorized that the collaborative exploration of the transference experience and the beneficial transference experience with the therapist constitutes the "corrective emotional experience" in therapy work (Ellman 1991, p. 90).

The 3-steps is akin to dealing with transference issues without explicitly delving into the patient's transference behaviors directly but rather, to begin to make for a "corrective emotional experience" from the first moment of therapy. People enter into treatment with a variety of psychopathology and variations in severity. Within this continuum, an effective treatment modality must promote the healthy development of therapeutic rapport. This is especially critical in working with narcissistic individuals who tend to be highly resistant to developing adequate therapeutic alliance. In most modalities of therapy, it is often difficult to discern the difference between what is the benefit of the psychotherapy and what is the benefit of the intense interpersonal relationship that develops in the setting of treatment. No doubt, the therapeutic relationship can be a powerful dynamic in helping many who enter into treatment. DSA takes into consideration the eventual transference relationship and through the 3-steps, places a healthy structure around each therapeutic interaction.

Managing transference in the therapeutic relationship is challenging. As a therapist, I often find that the subtle nuances of psychotherapy completely escapes the attention of my patient who is just living from one crisis moment to another crisis moment. To the patient, nothing matters much while he is in the throes of an emotional crisis, the fragmentation of the self. At such times, the therapist could barely maintain rational balance and may have to forego interpretation of transference. The attention of the therapist is more likely to be centered on rescuing the patient from the crisis. Even the most stouthearted would have a hard time maintaining sufficient treatment boundary when faced with a patient in crisis.

The therapist is often confronted with the conflict of being seen as cold and aloof or overly involved and enmeshed. Without any better solutions at hand, many therapists make themselves available by phone, email or appointment at anytime. The therapist then abandons any objectivity and becomes just the "coach" and support to the daily upheavals in the patient's life. The therapist can become a reluctant partner in this interplay with the knowledge that this act of help is not necessary a productive approach to treatment and long term improvement for the patient. "Coaching" may be appropriate at times but it can not be effective when it becomes the exclusive domain in this treatment. Once this occurs, the therapist and the patient then engage in a dance of sort with a dramatic score that engulfs everyone within. The patient who may already be lacking the ability to soothe himself will then become even more reliant on the therapist. At the end, this type of intense interpersonal interaction can only play a role in bringing about temporary stability. It would be wrong to assume that such intense interpersonal support constitutes psychotherapy. I feel that a note of caution is needed here in terms of complete reliance on the "therapeutic relationship". After mentioning that the therapeutic relationship can be very instrumental in bringing about changes, I would also like to add that the "relationship" alone may not be sufficient for long term change. In response to a child patient who jumps on his lap after a particularly moving play session, her therapist reflected later that "I know that no amount of holding, though feeling good for the moment, could make up for what she had missed getting from her blood mother, nor could it neutralize the trauma she'd experienced." There were also strong concerns that when the painful impetus to therapy was defused that she would "lose the immediate incentive to explore and grieve her painful longings, and leave therapy neither wiser nor stronger than when she came" (Bromfield 1992, p.77).

One has to be cautious about what constitutes a "therapeutic relationship" or is it just the intense giving of attention? It is understood that the therapeutic relationship and exploration should lead to long term changes; but many individuals with BPD ride the crest of such interpersonal support but their tendency is to retreat from this "treatment relationship" when it could no longer meet his very deep emotional needs. Sometimes the "on" periods of treatment are shorter than the "off" periods of treatment. This could make treatment even more challenging and less productive.

Within the framework of treatment of BPD, the therapeutic relationship is critical but the therapist must encourage the patient toward greater independent function. The pathology of emptiness often leads patients to develop an unhealthy dependence on others at a cost to the authentic self. At a more in-depth subjective level, treatment work should have the goal of helping the patient discern the difference between the true self from the false self. This is a central issue that has shaped my development of DSA in the treatment of BPD. In this approach, *even a small modicum of independence is valued and encouraged*. Greater independent function fosters the development of the self. I would like the reader to pay attention to how this is played out in the work of the 3-steps to be described here.

Role of Self-observation in Therapy

Whatever may be the issues touched on in therapy and whichever the modalities of therapy work, the patient's ability to make self-observations and engage in reflections are important to his therapeutic success. The patient's complete awareness of his internal emotional pain is one of the keystones of the treatment work with DSA. Unconsciously or consciously, many individuals spend a lifetime trying to avoid being engulfed by emotional emptiness. The natural consequence of this behavior is to become an unwitting slave of this rogue emotion and seek relief from all of the wrong places.

DSA places emphasis on patient's self-observation which lends itself to encouraging the patient to do well in a variety of psychotherapeutic modalities. Through self-observation, the patient can then become more aware of the existence of an internal emotional life. An individual who is capable of self-observation is more likely to become someone who is more self-reflective and open to therapist interpretation. Self-observation is encouraged from the moment of starting work with DSA. The precise nature of "emptiness" is not so critical since this is a state that could be uniquely different in each of us but this process brings the work of self-observation into sharp focus. These are the qualities that make an individual more psychologically minded and able to benefit from psychotherapy. As a result of the focus on self-observation, DSA can play a complimentary role in the treatment combination with traditional psychotherapy.

Daily Practice Work to Enrich Therapy

Psychotherapy is most effective when it is practiced in everyday life. It is my belief that insight development and working through of transference can be helpful although such exploration without daily practice with significant people in our life is unlikely to contribute to healing of deeper wounds and bring about actual change. Consistent with the understanding of the concept of corrective emotional experience, one would predict that healing comes from repeated positive outcome with as many selfobject figures as possible.

The lack of daily mindfulness about the work of therapy is a common dilemma for those undergoing psychotherapy. Many therapists recognize the limitations of insight development but neglect to reinforce learning through high repetition. Other therapists incorporate some cognitive behavioral work along side of the more traditional exploratory work of therapy to encourage frequent practice. Thus, patients are often given "homework" to take away from the therapist's office. DSA encourage the daily application and practice of treatment work with significant selfobjects to improve internalization of psychotherapeutic learning.

Therapist in the Selfobject Role

Modification of the projected self or object representation onto the therapist is a classic illustration of the role of the therapist in treatment. When the "bad" selfobject is projected onto the therapist, it is through the recognition of projective identification that the therapist can then contain and modify the projected bad object, which is then re-introjected by the patient and assimilated (Gabbard 1990, p.33-35). In case 8.1, a teenage girl negotiated her interpersonal relationship with staff by using projective identification to place outwardly her experience of vulnerability and sexuality. As a result, her staff/therapist will have to be vigilant and to respond with good boundary. In so doing, her projection is contained and modified for re-introjection by the patient.

The cup, as described in DSA, is a metaphor for the mutable nature of the self in any given instance in time and its reliance on the external selfobjects for the maintenance of the self. In the context of psychotherapy, the transference that naturally takes place puts the therapist in the position of being that external input to the cup that helps to maintain cohesion. When the therapist is able to be fairly successful in helping the patient to achieve sufficient self-cohesion through mirroring and idealizing transference, he or she can then be internalized by the patient to become a more permanent part of the patient's self. "Although the therapist relates the present situation to the patient's past whenever such interpretation is possible, the therapist also encourages the patient to make full use of the therapeutic relationship in satisfying his need to have a more successful transaction than he was able to have with his father. In a very real sense the therapist gives the patient an opportunity to fulfill a childhood wish" (Basch 1980, p.45). Possibly more than a wish fulfilled, this transaction may serve as a transference input. Even though the therapist can fulfill the patient's self needs, this process of cohesion is seen as temporary in DSA and further therapeutic work is required to truly make for repair.

When viewed as a continuum, object relations theory and self psychology are appealing for their value to the therapist. Self psychology describes the reliance of an individual on external relationships to help maintain self-esteem and self-cohesion. Object relations, on the other hand, exemplify the internalized relationships between representations of self and object. In so doing, the therapist plays a selfobject role that is no different from the parental role as described in object relations theory. Part of the therapeutic effect relies on the corrective emotional experience derived from reworking of past issues through the consistency of trust and validation in treatment.

Meares described the therapeutic relationship elegantly as one in which both the patient and the therapist are gazing at a metaphorical play space that allows the patient to feel ownership of the experience while turning to the therapist for approval and value. "The aim is not the delivery of insight. Rather, it is to further the kind of mental activity that underpins the play of the preoperational child" (Meares 1993, p.171). To me, this is a most elegant conveyance of the role of the therapist in the context of self psychology and object relations therapy. In our work, the attempt is to integrate this essential healing principle into a consistent pattern of relating to one another.

Allowing for True Self in Therapy

The dynamics of therapy naturally means that, very often, the therapist is regarded with respect and experienced as an authority figure by the patient. Added in to this mix is the therapist's attempt to validate the patient's feelings as well as the empathy and the compassion shown by the therapist, it is unavoidable that the patient should view the therapist as an authority figure. Most often, this regard for an authoritative selfobject translates to a submissive stance toward the therapist or an inpatient staff.

Whether this patient has a positive or negative transference toward authority, this passive stance toward a selfobject is bound to cause the patient to put his true self on hold while attempting to align with what he perceives to be a favorable position in relations to the object. This disregard for what is true to the self is being unauthentic. This is an individual who will put his feelings on hold in order to avoid the wrath or the criticism of the object or parental figures. An example is the individual who seems to feel that he or she has to be sexual and seductive in order to gain the attention of certain object figures. In this case, he or she has to put aside their sense of true self in order to experience the relationship with the object of his or her desire. An unauthentic stance is one in which the individual is seeking rescue and reaching for temporary fulfillment through acting out behaviors. It is conceivable that true self can not be consistently present as long as one seeks fulfillment through unhealthy channels. Issues regarding the true self will be further discussed in chapter 7.

It is important to be mindful of the therapist's role as an authoritative object. In doing treatment, it can be all too easy for the patient to slip directly into his comfortable role of being passive by presenting a false self toward pleasing the therapist. When this occurs, he is going to harbor a festering undertone of resentment and frustration that will bring treatment to a halt. He may start to miss appointments or forget to be mindful of the coping skills taught him during recent sessions with his therapist.

When such resistance in treatment occurs, it is difficult for him to make good use of even the most logical dialectical skills. It would be most difficult for him to see how he could get his needs met when he could not be authentic. He may "behave well" but he will certainly realize that he has not diverged from his usual passive and unauthentic way of interaction or that he has been covert and manipulative in control. He will have trouble accepting himself when he could not be true to self. It could be difficult for him to validate himself when he does not see and feel the validation from others. When he resorts to the use of the false self interpersonally, he will not be able to feel any true validation from others due to the false front that he has utilized. In the company of splitting and projective identification, which he tends to invoke, it would be difficult for him to develop a real therapeutic relationship with his therapist. He does not feel attuned to; therefore, he tunes out and maintains a false self in treatment.

DSA addresses this issue by prescribing a strategy based on the empowerment of the self. The therapist is experienced as a guide but not as a coach. Ideally, like all selfobject figures, the therapist play the role of consistent others. The patient then starts the healing process by a structured learning experience of self initiation rather than the motivation to respond to or please the therapist. In this treatment, his therapist will help him to understand the true purpose of his coming to therapy. With the insight about this internal pathology, he can better direct his energy toward more independent function that reveals his true self. In this fashion, he does not have to experience the self as polarized into good or bad, but more integrated and true to the self. Here, the therapist operates by a structure defined by the 3-steps and as long as the boundaries in this work is respected, the patient can feel more free and at ease to be his true self. Hence, healing begins by revealing the true self rather than being stifled by the desire to indiscriminately please others.

Choice of Empathy or Compassion in Therapy

I would like to take this opportunity to say something about empathy and compassion. Empathy is important in the work of psychotherapy of any type. Empathy is broadly defined as the capacity to share or participate in the feelings or ideas of another. Empathy carries with it the connotation of one human being attempting to understand the pain of another and to comprehend his needs and feelings. This is precisely what the therapist attempts to achieve in the therapeutic relationship. "Perhaps the most striking evidence of successful empathy is the occurrence in our bodies of sensations that the patient has described in his or hers" (Havens 1979). If successful, this can be a powerful dynamic to strengthen the work of therapy.

However, this ideal is not so easily achieved even in the case of the most progressive concept of projective identification. In the course of therapy, the greatest challenge for the therapist is the ability to maintain empathy regardless of the issues and behaviors that transpire in sessions. This is especially true in the context of inpatient staff in constant and extended contact with patients in the hospital milieu. In this setting, the staff members are privy to the words, emotions and actions of the patients mostly without much censorship; in daily life, one does not have the luxury of picking and choosing just what one will be exposed to. The therapist or staff member is then subjected to the extreme display of emotional words and behavior that come from the unfiltered and uncensored interaction with another human being.

In Piagetian developmental terms, the child moves from a pre-operational phase (age 2-7) of egocentrism to that of the operational phase (age 7-11) with the ability to appreciate that others have an independent existence. The developmental stasis in the phase of egocentrism is thought to be the reason that many borderline patients suffer the deficiency in the area of empathy (Meares 1993, p.156).

The therapist's ability to maintain a steady and consistent sense of empathy about a patient may be very subjective to our countertransference as well as the impact of projective identification upon a relationship based on focused attempt to relate to one another. This makes it difficult for the therapist to maintain consistent empathy when empathy comes from the emotional source of one person trying to share in the feelings of another. There must be times when a therapist will genuinely be challenged due to the incredibly extreme behaviors that one can witness in the context of working with a borderline or narcissistic patient. At such times, it is highly likely that many therapists will be stretched in terms of any reasonable way to share in or relate to what the patient is truly going through.

In the course of therapy as well as in the daily interaction with our patients, there can be times when the therapist fails to establish sufficient empathic reserve; this can easily lead us to feel as if we have failed miserably as a provider of mental health when it is merely a natural course of human interaction. One view of empathy through self psychology suggest, "perhaps one has experienced similar affects oneself—but one is not experiencing them now beyond "picking up on" what the other is feeling, and one is not sharing the other's suffering" (Wolf 1988, p.38). Whether sharing or not sharing in the suffering of another, call it sympathy or empathy, the fundamental issue of how best to establish a solid therapeutic connection with the patient is always central to effective treatment. The therapist's sense of a lack of empathy can be highly discouraging in a therapeutic setting which can further contribute to the development of negative countertransference. For this reason, I would argue that a reliance on empathy in treatment is often not tenable and not reliable.

On the other hand, in the Oxford dictionary, compassion is defined as "sympathetic pity and concern for the sufferings of others." Even with this definition, compassion imparts a more reachable concept of relatedness that does not require a deeper personal or psychological understanding of another individual. "Compassion can be roughly defined in terms of a state of mind that is nonviolent, nonharming, and nonaggressive. It is a mental attitude based on the wish for others to be free of their suffering and is associated with a sense of commitment, responsibility, and respect towards the others" (His Holiness The Dalai Lama, Cutler et al. 1998). Compassion is about placing all living being on an equal platform and treating them with parity. Compassion should be further differentiated from sympathy. Sympathy involves personal identification which has little value in treatment and can cause the recipient of such comment to feel a sense of obligation to concur and therefore feel entrapped. When treatment is rendered through the scope of compassion, human misconduct become more comprehensible; in turn, it allows the therapist to continue to function without blame or anger.

Not to quibble over the definition of words that perhaps have essentially the same meaning and common usage that is often seen as interchangeable; my attempt here is to emphasize the importance of approaching a patient with an openness and respect that goes beyond our personal understanding of this individual. Although it is useful to understand the developmental basis of ego-centrism, I prefer to view the borderline patient's lack of empathy as resulting from the desperation of the emptiness within. In so doing, it is less likely that one will be disillusioned by the words and actions of others in the context of treatment. It is my hope that the model of treatment introduced in this work helps us all to develop better access to our compassion for another human being.

Aristotle on Happiness

Greek philosophers such as Plato and Aristotle had a great deal to say about mental health. Through their deliberation on the issues of virtue and excellence, they provided us with some very important guidance for happiness. In Nicomachean Ethics, Aristotle stated, "that happiness is not a characteristic; if it were, a person who passes his whole life in sleep, vegetating like a plant, or someone who experiences the greatest of misfortunes could possess it" (Ostwald 1962). He further expounds, "There is no pleasure without activity, and every activity is completed by pleasure." Of course, he is speaking of an activity with virtue and excellence. He clarifies by declaring that activities contributing to happiness do not consist in amusement. About happiness,

"It is a life which involves effort and is not spent in amusement" (Ostwald 1962).

Aristotle places great emphasis on the importance of achieving excellence in one's chosen area of expertise. To him, it is the activities of excellence, in conformity with virtue, that will ultimately bring about happiness. In DSA, one is encouraged to strive towards the use of certain productive and useful activities in the 3-steps that is to form the pathway to emotional healing. If at all possible, one might consider the development of activities with excellence and virtue in mind. A musician playing an instrument in a crisis of emptiness is able to use his skills to self soothe; while the playing of good music also serve to bring the world closer together through a common language of peace and harmony.

Encouragement versus Praise

Addressing the issue of validation, many experts advocate the use of encouragements over praise. Although subtle, there are clearly some clinical issues worthy of consideration. Just as I feel that there is a distinctive difference in display of compassion over the conveying of empathy in the initial phase of treatment, I feel that it is important to distinguish between encouragements over praise. Whether viewed from a parenting, cognitive behavioral, psychodynamic, psychoanalytic or victim perspective, how the therapist could best convey a positive regard about the patient's treatment progress is an important consideration. "Many parents believe they are encouraging children when they praise them. They don't realize that praise can be discouraging." "Praise, like punishment, is a method of social control." "Praise is an attempt to motivate children with external rewards. Encouragement, on the other hand, is given for effort or for improvement, however slight" (Dinkmeyer and McKay 1989).

Very frequently, the child who is used to praise will continue to work for praise but stop when praise is no longer forthcoming. This individual may grow up to feel that his self-worth is based on the opinions of others or pleasing others. There are those who seek to control or manipulate another individual in an abusive manner through the use of praise. To the victim of abuse, the sound of praise in therapy can be a reminder of past trauma or contributes to the surfacing of the false self. There are times and situations in which praise is quite appropriate but the excessive or the exclusive use of praise can interfere with genuine empathy and validation for another.

In accordance with the awareness of the state of emptiness as central to our design on treatment, as shall be discussed in detail in the following chapters, one must consider the potential for ordinary praise to be emotionally toxic if not at least invalidating. Even an innocuous utterance of, "Isn't it great that you enjoyed our outing today" can convey a disconnect with the borderline patient's state of constant inner tension. Upon the rare moment in which the borderline patient may have a smile on his face, it is common for someone to comment that, "I am glad that you are feeling better today." When even the most casual interpersonal exchange can bring about the stinging reminder of his persistent loneliness, any praise or lighthearted banter could escalate his sense of despair. The counterintuitive nature of the borderline patient's experience of daily life can befuddle the best of intentions by others but the empathic awareness of this very important dynamic will encourage better therapeutic rapport.

Addressing Independence from the Start

To me, the achievement of independence is possibly one of the most important goals of any type of mental health treatment. Independence can of course mean different things to different people. Independence can mean that one comes to be free of the symptoms of a major mental illness and one can then regain most or all of one's previous functioning. Independence can mean the achievement of freedom from the infantile and primitive ego structure from which we all spring. Independence can mean the achievement of freedom from a malformation of the self. This latter dynamic is the one in which we will concern ourselves in this exploration of the treatment for BPD.

One can argue that the achievement of independence is the eventual goal of any type of therapy modality for BPD. Often, the intense therapeutic interpersonal interaction itself contributes to greater interdependence with the therapist. It is difficult to imagine how such intense interpersonal interaction could lend itself to easy extrication when it is time for greater independence. However, rather than hope for improved functioning before attempt at independence, the patient should be encouraged to experience autonomy in every step of treatment. *There is no better time for independence than right now, even if independence can only be experienced for a few moments at a time.*

The human tendency is strongly programmed for a great deal of independent function. This is how a young child learns to cope with the world and this natural inclination to try things by oneself is strength to be encouraged and not stifled. For this reason, I would often encourage my patients to experience independence as often as feasible, even if such forays into independence lasts for only a few minutes at first. For the infant, the maternal selfobject is not always available. There are inevitable moments when the infant would have to fend for his emotional security by himself. The infant is then forced to contend with his vulnerability but as a result, he discovers that he is indeed able to successfully soothe himself. Then his mother appears once again to confirm for him that she is consistently available and she validates his feelings and existence. In some ways, DSA strives to replay and reinforce the learning through this mother and child dyad. DSA is a method of treatment that seeks to strengthen the self and promote independence through greater patient self-help.

Codependence and the False Self

The discussion of any topic relating to emotional emptiness should of course touch upon the term codependency. Understanding codependency can help us grasp the importance of independence and why, perhaps, the achievement of independence is such a vital life long issue. Codependency has been defined as an addiction to people, behaviors or things. Codependency is the fallacy of trying to control interior feelings by controlling people, things and events externally. They struggle relentlessly to fill the great emotional vacuum within themselves (Hemfelt et al. 1989). However, their whole being seems to light up when they talk about that special something that they do to an excess or make heroic sacrifice for the good of another. It is at such moments that the codependent individual is able to distant himself from the painful feeling of the emptiness within.

In the traditional definition and discussion of codependency, one can easily come to the conclusion that problematic family of origin is often to blame through neglect or abuse. As is frequently inferred, the codependent individual is unable to see the destructive and unhealthy patterns in his family of origin. The codependent individual may inherit some very negative messages from his family of origin; this "baggage" or historical scenes of shame then contributes to his low self esteem and prejudiced view of life as a teen or an adult. However, I would caution that this view would be too narrow and not taking into consideration the wide variety of possible causes for such conditions as codependency and BPD.

In the theoretical understanding that underpins DSA, we will make the assumption that outright abuse and neglect are not the only conditions under which the dynamics of the pathology of the self develops. Codependency and perhaps, in more severe cases, BPD, likely arise out of conditions in life in which one is deprived of the opportunity to experience the self as true and real to one's natural predispositions. However, many unfortunate circumstances can happen in life that can take away the ideal setting for the real self to grow and mature. In short, whether it is family tragedy, natural disaster, manmade disaster or war, as well as innocent insensitivities of life, one can shun the realities by coping through a false sense of the self. In this manner of coping, one can come to develop codependence as a matter of routine survival. What happens is not necessary related to an individual becoming a victim of evil or wrong doing, it may just be life circumstances. It is quite possible that the majority of such personality pathology develops under a much more subtle environmental and emotional setting. Nevertheless, given the important role of the family in the development of the child, problematic family dynamic will require consideration and exploration.

Codependency can come into being when an individual faces the harshness of his world through the denial of his true feelings. He may be someone who has had to take care of his younger siblings because his father was never home and his mother was inebriated nightly. The urgency of caring for his younger siblings takes precedent over his own feelings of anxiety. He has no time to feel and no time to cry; he has to be brave because his younger siblings depend on him. His mother may also depend on him for all of the chores and maintenance of this household. He may not know of any other life than this as he continues to toil in this setting but the lack of adequate support for his self is going to become the central issue going forward in his life.

Given he has never known any other way of life, he may come to think that his role in this family is what is normal and think nothing of the hard work and sacrifice that he is making to assure the survival of this clan. Yet, the external hardship of his life has another very important dimension; the lack of recognition of his needs can contribute to the development of the underlying anger and frustration that could lead to complications in the healthy development of the self. In the life of this individual, there is no place for frequent anger and frustration, which could easily lead to even more intolerable fear, anxiety and guilt. To avoid these intolerable feelings, defenses such as splitting comes into play but in so doing, this individual can no longer experience his true self; later in life, he is likely to experience this as the pathology of emptiness.

His fortitude in raising his younger siblings credits him with some degree of maturity and resourcefulness but is not an indication of the state of health of his internal emotional being. It is quite possible that in later years, he will come to discover that a sense of emotional wellbeing is difficult for him to maintain unless he finds himself in the care-giving role. Altruism may be the last thing on his mind this time given his need for control. It is only through this excessive need for control that he could manage to achieve temporary sense of wholeness but the price of such exquisite control is to take up battle with the world. He can become easily angered and frustrated with his spouse and children through his "codependent" state and turn to alcohol to soothe the disquiet within. As he goes down this path, he is recreating the horror of his own childhood and playing it out with his children.

In a different scenario, one might find a timid young child who is highly observant of his surroundings. He is the expert at picking up the most subtle of emotions from those around him, especially the mood of his parents. His parents seem never at peace with each other and rarely content with themselves. From early in life, he came to be aware of the influence he has upon them. His behavior and even his feelings can have dramatic impact on his parents. His misbehavior, or at least the behavior that causes his parents to be very displeased, can bring about great outburst of anger from his parents. When he feels hurt, they seem quite lost and perturbed with him. They appear unable to empathize with his feelings or tell him that he is a big boy and should not cry; he usually scuttles to a corner and licks his own wounds.

He came to discover that he has to play down his own feelings and keep his thoughts to himself or he could bring great distress to his parents; his parents already appear emotionally fragile and stressed. As he got older, he is now a master of control of sort. He is totally focused on taking care of those around him but has no sense of how he really feels. He often experiences the hollow feeling at his core and suffers from depression. He is never quite sure what he needs or what he wants because he has spent so much of his time and energy on figuring out what other people need.

The codependent feels strongly that his happiness is based on others but he also feels powerfully responsible for others. Since he is dealing with such a painful void within, it is not difficult to imagine how his taking of responsibility for others is not as altruistic as it first appears. Often, he expects a return of some sort for his caretaking of another. This is not because he is so selfish, although it would appear thus; he may simply be in a survival mode in dealing with his own emptiness within. In DSA, we understand this as the pathological filling of our emotional cup. As a result, he is very extreme in his emotional reactions to the world around him. When things don't go his way, his anger is like a switch turned on.

Codependents frequently reach beyond relationships and draw upon such things as work, food, extreme risk, control, sexual acting out as well as alcohol and drug use. (Sex, drugs and rock and roll) The reader may ask at this point as to what is the difference between codependency and BPD? I do not view these two terms as separate entities but really the two sides of the same coin with BPD as a formal DSM IV diagnosis. There is the risk of grouping multiple conditions into the same basket and not giving each the individualized treatment that it deserves. However, the core pathology in each case may be similar but perhaps symptom manifestation and acuity are different. In comparison, the symptoms described in codependency may not appear as acute; the self-destructive nature of these individuals and the suffering involved is no less severe. These are all individuals who are struggling with a profound sense of emptiness within and would go to great extent to neutralize this tremendous pain through rescue seeking and/or acting out behaviors.

Understanding and studying codependency allows us to gain another angle of view towards symptoms of the pathology of the self. Regardless of what one would call it, we can now see how pervasive these symptoms can be and how subtle the symptoms. At times, the symptoms of codependency can be subtle and covert because the codependent feels that he or she is simply acting in accordance to what is expected of them or that they are simply trying to help. Years can go by or perhaps someone finally points the problems out before the codependent may be aware that his unhappiness has some profound roots.

Shame as a Central Feature

When viewed through the scope of the types of developmental frustrations likely to afflict an individual, shame can be a natural precursor of the false self. As will be discussed further in this work, false self then contributes to the damage of the emotional system, the "cup" in particular. Shame is a focus on the global self; guilt is about a specific behavior or acts. Studying from a psychoanalytic perspective, Helen B. Lewis views guilt as a result of identifying with the threatening parent with the consequent experience of an internalized threat, whereas, "identification with the beloved or admired ego-ideal stirs pride and triumphant feelings; failure to live up to this internalized admired imago stirs shame" (Lewis 1971). As has been suggested by Erik Erikson (1950), the stage of autonomy versus shame and doubt is at work even as early as age one to three years. "Though terror speaks to life and death and distress makes the world a vale of tears, yet shame strikes deepest into the heart of man" (Tomkin 1963, p. 118).

Through the various sources of shame in the human life cycle, "The affect of shame becomes both internalized and magnified, thereby shaping and ultimately dominating the emergent personality" (Kaufman 1989, p.27). Being sentient of the insidious shame within from the earliest consciousness would undoubtedly contribute to the seething undertone of anger and frustration that might already accompany original anger. Later in life, ever so vigilant about their surroundings and slow to trust anyone, the borderline patient is easily offended and shamed by the most exquisite of gestures and expressions. Such perceptions of affront can come from one's parents or from one's culture. Mary Pipher (1994) addresses the issues of the adolescent self in relating to the social pressure that forces these young people to put aside their authentic selves to be someone they are not. Whether regarding intelligence, career path, appearance, popularity, temperament, independence, family role or sex role, shame and un-authenticity exact a toll on the development of the self.

Indeed, scenes of shame reverberate within the depth of emptiness and cause us to respond defensively. Clinically, shame appears central to persons with borderline personality disorder (Lieb 2004). A 2007 study confirms that women with borderline personality disorder score higher in shame and shame-proness. Shame may be an especially debilitating emotion in that it was associated with low self-esteem, low quality of life and high anger-hostility. There appears to be a correlation that shame-proness may contribute to anger and hostility, which are common in BPD (Rüsch 2007).

It would seem sensible to look at treatment solutions for individuals with anger and hostility by trending back to the individual's awareness of shame, an issue of developmental importance, to his awareness of the numbness of living with a sense of the false self while grappling with a looming sense of fluctuating emptiness. Hypothetically, shame and the false self may be fairly consistent over time but the experience of the core self may fluctuate with our external experiences of the moment. False self just might be described as our perception of how one presents oneself under the dictate of circumstances as well as self representation as a result of our mirroring and idealizing transference. Shame, if left unresolved from the earliest of time would likely remain fairly stable as well. Beginning with original anger, add in shame and doubt, then usher in the false self and the foundation to the healthy development of the core self is truly impaired. In DSA, the core self is represented by the metaphoric cup; it is here that the reparative process takes shape.

Pathological Narcissism in Treatment

Narcissism is an interesting topic in the overall discussion of the disorder of the self partly because it is so difficult to determine where to draw the line as to when narcissism becomes pathological. In our discussion here, every person has a leakiness to the core self, including the higher functioning narcissistic individual. Therefore, emotional emptiness is also of concern to the narcissist. As viewed through self psychology, narcissistic personality disorders consist of individuals whose damage to the self is less severe and temporary restorable through expressed attempt to force the environment to yield the needed selfobject experience via interpersonal maneuvers or acting out behavior. These individuals are highly dependent on the tribute of others or their own grandiose fantasy. They often idolize people who are perceived as useful in narcissistic supplies and deprecate those seen as of less value. Many luminaries of industry, politics, academics, arts, as well as many in the field of mental health function to a degree in the narcissistic spectrum. It would seem plausible to consider narcissism as a continuum to which we all belong.

"What distinguishes many of the patients with narcissistic personalities from the usual borderline patient is their relatively good social functioning, their better impulse control, and what may be described as a 'pseudosublimatory' potential, namely, the capacity for active, consistent work in some areas which permits them partially to fulfill their ambitions of greatness and of obtaining admiration from others" (Kernberg 1988, p.229). At first glance, the narcissistic individual appears to function quite well in the society at large. He may have fought his way to a highly respected position on the corporate ladder or tendered an academic tenure while earning a reputation as an arrogant professor. His conversations are usually peppered with a degree of self-reference as he seeks tributes from others with very grandiose self promotions. When he suffers physical illness, he seeks out only the most famous and respected physician with whom he feels a kindred spirit while simultaneously wishing his own worth to be recognized by such an esteemed individual. At work, he is merciless toward those he sees as worthless and defenseless; he is especially cruel toward people he has no use for in his world.

Through achievements of various sorts, the narcissistic individual is able to obtain a degree of interpersonal and work stability. However, the price of such functioning is steep because this existence is based on neglecting the emptiness within. While he is able to engineer a world that caters to his needs, he is scarcely able to pay proper attention to the aversive inner tension; of which, he generally knows intimately but refuses to acknowledge. Because he built his world to escape emptiness, he has a weak foundation to withstand the tremors of a serious assault to his personal integrity. At which point, even the narcissistic individual can become suicidal. In DSA view, this individual has no self love (narcissism is really a misnomer), he despises what he is aware within and works to fill his emptiness with the admiration of others or turn to overt or covert acting out to maintain tenuous function.

The root of narcissism has been described as a lack of empathy through exploitation by a mother who is unable to support the child's real self. Psychotherapeutic measures often focus on repeated analysis of the source of such vulnerability as related to the maternal failure to acknowledge and support the real self (Masterson, Klein 1989, pp. 70-89). In object relations understanding, he is unable to depend on internalized good object. "They need to devalue whatever they receive in order to prevent themselves from experiencing envy" (Kernberg 1989, p.237). The narcissistic individual may not present as clinically ill as the borderline individual, but the narcissist is also more recalcitrant to change given that it is in his nature to deflect personal responsibility for his behavior and focus on the faults of the outside world.

In addition, the narcissist may recall memories of being attacked, devalued, and disparaged as a child. The narcissist's world revolve around power, fame, money and status and his need for idealization, mirroring or merger generally means that he is intolerant of the slightest of wounds and confrontation can mobilize further distancing, defense and therapeutic stalemate. Such are the challenges that the therapist is faced with in the treatment of a narcissistic patient. Therapy then becomes a highly delicate dance between the therapist's desire to bring insight to this patient and the patient's intolerance of confrontation. Without the successful usage of confrontation, the therapeutic work of interpretation is also limited and the treatment can easily come to an impasse.

DSA attempts to help the narcissistic patient understand the source of his internal pain without causing him to take flight from treatment and without fragmentation. Developmentally, it is sufficient to recognize the similarity between the early deficits of the narcissistic individual to that of the borderline individual. Lack of attunement and respect for the budding self can be viewed as the fundamental etiology to pathologic narcissism. As in the borderline condition, the inability to hold steady the transferential content of the self, as represented by the metaphor of the leaky cup, is seen as the pathology leading to narcissism. Familiarizing the patient with his internal emotional world through an easy to understand and less interpersonally confrontational fashion is the thesis of DSA. This treatment model offers the patient a way of understanding his past, present and the future. He can use this model to understand the impact of past frustrations, the resulting emotional state he has to contend with today and how he can be the master of his future without the constant manipulations of his world.

Addressing Control Issues

In many ways, the individual with BPD is a challenge to work with in any setting. For the therapist, it can seem as if the patient spends all of his spare time contemplating obstacles to treatment at every turn. We call this resistance. At times, he wants to shape treatment to his own liking even when it could be detrimental to his care. He wants to dictate the minutest of details in our way of working or he wants to limit what could be addressed and when certain issues could be addressed. When that is not enough, he wants to dictate what medication he would take and mode of delivery of his medications. Of course, he is quite a veteran when it comes to the psychotropic medications and he has no qualms about throwing this knowledge around.

Exertion of excessive control can be the means of defense when feeling helpless or it can be an expression of a false sense of what is needed for the self to feel he is deserving of love and care. Self talk in this situation may sound like, "I have to be strong, brave and in control or my father will think that I am a wimp and not deserving of his love." For most therapists, this is where countertransference can easily arise and if not addressed, it could easily affect the course and outcome of treatment.

There are many reasons that "control" is such an important issue in treatment. Every human being tries to exert as much control over his life as possible, even for people who seem fairly easy going. Passivity is in itself a form of control for some. Depending on our sense of self, we cling to "control" over how much "power" we deem necessary. The powerful Fortune 500 CEO who gets hospitalized for congestive heart failure may pose a tremendous challenge for the doctors and nurses because his illness has now caused him to feel powerless and impotent; therefore, he is fighting for his life to regain "control". On discussing such an example, healthcare providers invariably ask how they can handle this issue. Clinically, it is advisable to obtaining a psychiatric consultation since the mismanagement of this "control" issue is likely to lead to the patient's poor compliance with treatment. Frequently, narcissism is at the core of individuals with fame, fortune and/or power. Being sick and laying helplessly in bed is a dynamic that can invoke some strong narcissistic defense responses; which can often complicate treatment.

Control issues can be encountered with individuals suffering from many other maladies. The individual with BPD enters into the hospital setting repeatedly because he is unable to exert sufficient control over his world and now he feels even more powerless in the inpatient setting. In this context, it is not surprising that he should be so controlling about his interpersonal interactions and his treatment. It is important to disengage from this power struggle and allow this patient to experience a degree of control without sabotaging treatment. This is not easy to accomplish given that in most treatment settings, there is generally a "professional and client" relationship that set things up in an uneven power structure. However, this hierarchy can be helpful in the case of a narcissistic individual by appealing to his needs to be seen as special and therefore, people who work with him and help him should also be special. It is also natural for the patient to experience transference, splitting and projective identification toward the authority figure. The inpatient hospital setting is especially prone to such transference issues. A skilled therapist will recognize these defenses and navigate deftly through these time consuming issues with patience and working through of transference; this then paves the way for further treatment in a medical or psychiatric setting.

In the language of DSA, the behavior of excessive control is viewed both as detrimental to the experiences of the real self and as acting out behavior with the very specific function to fill a deep emotional void. Control of the selfobject through projective identification is a way to control the bad self (Gabbard 1990, p.35). This type of control is counterproductive toward one's natural and real self because it is driven by the pain of emptiness which can lead to severe anxiety of abandonment, anger and frustration. This desperate need for control causes us to engage in an external battle while neglecting the true needs of the core self.

Fear of Being Unloved

Case 2.4: Diana is a young woman on a psychiatric ward. She is 14 years old but looks no more than 9. She weighed a total of 70 lbs. She looks pale and frail but struggles to keep up a peppy facade to keep people from reminding her (once again) that she is weak from not eating enough. Peering from behind her glasses, her eyes look larger than expected probably because her face is so thin. She suffers from amenorrhea; her menstrual period has not begun. As soon as she started to speak, one is instantly aware of her keen wit and sharp intelligence. She comes from a large family with a number of siblings. She was sexually abused at a very young age although she probably has no recall of that trauma. Of course, in the case of such early trauma, it is the developmental damage and the assault to the self that is of ultimate concern.

In this single parent household, she has already seen a number of mother's significant others come and go; some might suggest that she has had a hand in this. She has systematically created havoc at home by making sure that, if her family made her angry, they will experience such unpleasant behavior from her that they will think twice before challenging her again. Her behaviors were so repetitive and bizarre that some thought that she suffered from obsessive compulsive disorder. Of course, her "compulsions" were only steadfast as long as they were still sufficiently punishing for her family. Although her behavior has gotten more aggressive over time, most of her behaviors up to this point consist of struggles for control. As such, she dictates what her mother should cook, in the name of good nutrition, but the cooking is never good enough, so she never wants to eat much of it. Given her exceedingly low weight, one could make the assumption that she must have some issue with her body image but she denies that she is trying to lose weight.   S h e persistently refused to work with any of the therapists that her mother has tried to get her to connect with. Finally, worn-out from their daily battle over how the household should function; her mother forced a hospitalization through the court when Diana got overly aggressive with one of her siblings. On admission, she refused to sign a release of information to allow the hospital to communicate with anyone. This became an issue of contention between Diana and everyone she worked with in the hospital. She stubbornly held fast to this position through the course of the hospitalization while everyone watched with dumbfounded amazement.

In the milieu, she was never outright oppositional but she was never fully cooperative either. She was eating and drinking just enough to keep from knocking her electrolytes into the abyss but annoyed staff with her dainty feeding. In session, she generally directed the course of the conversation toward blaming her mother for all of her woes. Without a release of information to communicate with family and the frustration from her resistance in therapy, the treatment team felt completely upstaged by a tiny girl. She was giving the treatment team so little information that it was not even possible to make a psychiatric diagnosis. The treatment team asked for psychological testing but she refused to cooperate.

On observation, however, she seemed sad and lonely. On a blind conjecture, her therapist commented that her self esteem seems very low. Surprisingly, she answered that she indeed feels poorly about her appearance. "I am ugly and gross." One look and most people would probably think that she is delusional. But, she still would not admit that she has any concerns about her weight. On further processing, she started to reveal a life traumatized by a father who was highly critical of her and never valued her as a person. He was not overtly abusive but he was rarely physically available and emotionally distant. Following the parent's divorce, he has not shown much of an interest in her despite her quiet longing for his approval and acceptance. He has since gotten remarried and has two other children in that marriage. Diana is too proud to pick up the phone and call him. He has now drifted too far away for her to reach him. This much she would share about her feelings toward her father but she would shut down before talking about how all of this affected her relationship with her mother.

In further discussion, the treatment team decided to treat her excessive struggle for control as a high intensity acting out behavior as discussed in DSA. This had a profound impact on how the team viewed her behavior. Everyone started to be more empathic and compassionate with her; staff members were also less likely to engage her in power struggles. She continued to be a very challenging patient in the milieu because her treatment could not be fully implemented without the involvement of her existing family; yet, she steadfastly refused to sign consent for the release of information. At this time in her life, relinquishing control is a greater terror than the prospect of continuing to live with the pain of emptiness. The most challenging patients are those who enter into treatment with eyes closed, ears plugged while loudly expounding on how they suffer.

Discussion:
The powerful struggle for control as exhibited by this patient reveals a great deal about the pathology of this patient's self. Whether young or old, it is understandable that an individual will fight fiercely for what he or she feels to be the last semblance of control. After all, having a sense of control is critical in one's general sense of well being. For the individual with pathology of the self, she will be even more demanding of a strong sense of control. Observation of this individual will show that this control is directly linked to the dynamics of splitting and primitive idealization.

Diana wants to make sure that at least a few of the people in her life see her as a good person who deserves to be loved and respected. During the past few years of her life, she has come to experience a high degree of loathing for herself. If she could verbalize it, she would probably say that she is fundamentally a good person and deserve the care and respect from others. On the other hand, through her past, she has somehow internalized the idea that she is "bad" and undeserving of any love. So it would appear that she is at least not thinking of herself as in just one form but she also has tremendous difficulty in being able to hold in mind the idea that she could be composed of both the good self and the bad self. From the point of view of developmental psychology, Diana is fearful that the "bad self" in her could contaminate the "good object" around her; therefore, using control, she tries to separate the world into the good and the bad so as to make sure that there are sufficient number of the good objects around to be accessed to fill her profound emptiness.

In her case, no one individual in her world is labeled as continuously good or bad; instead everyone in her life is essentially reverberating between good and bad although these two states never seems to occupy the same space at the same time. From her perspective, people will either love her or destroy her. Her treatment providers on the unit represent just such a picture for her. They at once symbolize all that is wrong in her life in which others are trying to rule over her without regard for her feelings, as well as all the people that she longs to connect with and embrace in life. She experiences anger toward these people while still wanting to keep them sheltered from finding out just what sort of a "bad" person that she thinks she is. She is unable to hold the co-existence of the "good" and the "bad" within her; she is unable to hold the co-existence of the "good" and the "bad" in others. What appears to be the manipulation and control by a young girl turns out to be an epic battle between the good and the bad self and the good and the bad object.

If her treatment team had been given an opportunity to further work with her, what method of work could bring about rapid engagement of the patient in the milieu and validate the dichotomous state of her internal world? To say that her emotional world is "dysregulated" is like reminding the enraged person that he is angry; it does not point to the source of her tendency toward such emotional display. In DSA, object relations and self psychology theories are presented in a manner that helps the patient to cognitively internalize the cause of her pain.

Collapse of Resilience

The desperateness for extreme control can best be understood through DSA for reasons that will become clearer for the reader in the later chapters. Extreme control is viewed as acting out behavior in DSA. The defense mechanisms of splitting and projective identification as well as co-dependence and control issues are viewed in terms of an individual's fundamental need to reach emotional equilibrium. *Emotional equilibrium* will simply be defined as a state of calm, content, satiation for the sake of our discussion. The "cup" will be used to illustrate this equilibrium or the lack of equilibrium (the void) in a later chapter. The assumption is that this individual knows that he is unable to achieve emotional equilibrium in an un-enhanced fashion (meeting his needs through normal and everyday interactions) and will work single mindedly to achieve this equilibrium by many other means; most of which contributes to his dependency and addiction. In the process, he will utilize co-dependence, control, splitting or any number of pathological methods to fill his needs.

Most people will agree that, by looking at the human organism, the human child is a very resilient being. In 1965, Winnicott coined the term the good enough mother to characterize the minimum environmental or selfobject requirement needed by the infant for normal development. In one study, children of depressed mothers exhibited lower rates of disorder in homes in which a psychiatrically healthy father was present (Conrad 1989). Conversely, beyond the variance accounted for by mothers' depression score, fathers' score on a measure of depression added to the prediction of emotional or behavioral problems in their children (Thomas 1991). Furthermore, "a youth with either a depressed mother or an antisocial father is at risk of both major depression and conduct disorder." Exacerbating an already troubling situation, depressed mothers tended to partner with antisocial fathers (Marmorstein 2004). Despite natural resilience, a lack of certain fundamental stability in a child's life can bring about the development of a disorder.

Studies now suggest a markedly higher risk of developing borderline, narcissistic, obsessive-compulsive, and paranoid personality disorders related to maternal verbal abuse and in combination with physical abuse and neglect, produce the direst outcome (Johnson 2001, Ney 1987, Ney 1994). While physical and sexual abuse have garnered the intense attention of child protective service agencies as well as come under scrutiny as psychiatric risk factors, emotional maltreatment may be a more elusive and insidious problem. Looking at "limbic irritability", depression, anxiety, and anger-hostility, one study found that parental verbal aggression was a potent form of maltreatment (Teicher 2006). Children who suffer frequent verbal aggression by parents exhibited higher rates of physical aggression, delinquency, and interpersonal problems than other children. This study found 63% of American parents reported one or more instances of verbal aggression, such as swearing at and insulting their child (Vissing 1991).

How some children survive cruelty, abuse and disasters in life is testament to the will of survival that is somehow built into our early self. On the other hand, this survival has a price that is paid for by the concealment of the true self. Through years of fostering the false self, the beautiful resilience of the child is no longer recognizable. Hence, grappling with a false sense of self, the child would have to fight the feelings of emptiness through the use of extreme control, pathologic dependence as well as severe acting out behaviors that ultimately leaves the individual broken, defeated and without a trace of resilience.

Experiential versus Exploratory Therapy Work

Individual psychotherapy and family therapy, couples therapy, and most variations of cognitive behavioral therapy can all take place within the context of DSA. Any issues appropriate to the treatment goals of greater independence and strengthening the self can be addressed. Abuse and trauma issues can be an integral part of treatment as tolerated. Most importantly, the therapist has to help the patient to come to awareness of the existence of emptiness. From the DSA perspective, appropriate psychotherapeutic exploration should not be ignored but that DSA can help to bring about sufficient clinical stability in preparation for further psychotherapeutic work. It is my clinical experience that most patients are quite tolerant of the here and now exploration of the feelings of emptiness while still resistant to touching on traumatic and interpersonal issues.

Patients who are emotionally fragile and unstable may not be able to tolerate the exploratory nature of psychotherapy. These patients may have suffered severe trauma, abuse and neglect; the recall of such memory can be too intense emotionally to handle and he may lack the skills to deal with the pain. Even just a cursory survey of a historical time frame that corresponds to a period of abuse or trauma can evoke such intense and unbearable feelings in the borderline patient that he can rapidly decompensate to the point of severe acting out or regression. Perhaps such forays into the past could bring back memories of events and experiences that are coupled with painful feelings of unfulfilled needs. Recalling the emotional pain of unfulfilled needs, whether due to abuse, neglect or the autistic inability to connect (to be further discussed in chapter 9), can bring about anxiety and guilt; he may turn to acting out behavior to distract and seek some respite.

The recall of emotional pain could be more intense than at the actual time of abuse. The way to understand this is related to the concept that splitting is a coping and defense mechanism and with the successful use of splitting, this individual should actually feel and function slightly better than the pre-split state. Through the predominant use of splitting or primitive dissociation, the narcissistic individual is able to tolerate the co-existence of haughty grandiosity with shyness and feelings of inferiority (Kernberg 1985, p.331). It has been thought that without the use of splitting, the other option is to fuse with the object, which leads to psychotic identification. Splitting likely occurred slightly later in life and the recall of memory prior to this period can potentially be highly painful and raw without the presence of splitting as a defense. Psychotherapeutic exploration to divert around this defense mechanism can potentially induce intolerable underlying angst. In this work, defense mechanism such as splitting is addressed by fortifying ego functioning achieved through the 3-steps.

Given that he is likely to already experience a great deal of the pain of the emptiness in the present, the recall of past anger and frustration could exacerbate his current pain. DSA takes into account that the patient's decompensation will be characterized by severe acting out behaviors as a form of temporary remedy for psychological pain. Whether he acts out by self-mutilation or regression to a more infantile stage of operation, he is acting to address the profound emptiness. Such regression places him back in time to the point where he is at the mercy of his care taker to soothe and provide for him. At that moment, the regression can be seen as delusion of fulfillment. He could well be in a dissociative like state; a place where he could experience what he believes to be the presence of the all giving and all loving maternal object. It is not uncommon for this individual to regress to the point of experiencing hallucinations of the borderline type. Reports of visual and auditory hallucinations are common. This acting out behavior or regression is of course not conducive to the work of treatment.

The prevailing wisdom may assume that this patient just needs to get through this difficult phase and come through better on the other end. "-some postanalytic patients who were well "analyzed" but not cured: They had achieved wide and deep knowledge about the dynamics of their conscious and unconscious mental functioning but had not benefited to any significant extent from a lasting amelioration of their psychological pain nor from any meaningful improvement in their unhappy relationship with others" (Wolf 1988, p.91). More productively, Wolf points out that the mutative experience in therapy is based on transference feelings about the therapist that is associated to events involving significant others in the patient's early life, and that "no blame is attached to either patient or therapist for the painful interactions that are taking place" (Wolf 1988, 100-101). In this classical approach to affect change in therapy, the value of this work is not so much the exploration of factual truth but an experience of transference.

If exploratory work can not be performed, what type of work, if any, should be undertaken? Experiential work can be highly valuable and effective. Irving Yalom wrote about the experiencing of the *here* and *now* for his psychotherapy group members (Yalom 1985, p. 135-198). This type of work is based on the immediate or in the very recent past and can be powerful in helping the patient examine his tendency in interpersonal interaction as well as developing an awareness of the existence of an internal emotional life. Here, in the work using DSA, an emphasis is placed on creating a therapeutic setting based on fundamental experiences with reliable object figures.

By the repeated experiencing of a particular interpersonal dynamic, the individual can then learn valuable lessons about his interpersonal effectiveness. This repetition teaches him to accept a new form of positive interpersonal dynamic and also reinforces his learning of the corrective behavior. In most cases, giving him feedback in the context of the here and now would not be so emotionally charged because this experience is still far removed from the direct recall of past events although current issues can evoke past memories. For example, I could say to the patient, "It has occurred to me that every time Jack (the staff) asks you to wait your turn in group that you would then wear an expression of annoyance and belittle him in return." At the next group, I might add, "Are you aware that you verbally attacked him once again after he told you to wait your turn?" This is *experiential learning* based on the here and now and this could be done without much in depth exploratory work.

Of course, in the hands of an experienced therapist working with a fairly stable patient, this work can be extrapolated to the exploration of more detailed interpersonal history. This population of patients is likely to be continually fragile for an extended period of time but they are also highly in need of treatment intervention. If in need of challenging exploratory work, a DSA therapist would engage the patient in the pre 3-steps exercise followed by the 3-steps to allow the patient a method of self soothing along with mirroring and idealizing transference in the journey to greater insight. This treatment approach should provide the flexibility needed in assisting those in need of acute stabilization or those who are ready for further exploratory therapy.

In summary, therapeutic relationship, dependence issues, and control issues have to coalesce with experiential learning in order to have long term developmental impact. In a challenging treatment setting, DSA helps to set up an effective treatment expectation that involves both the patient and the therapist. DSA places an emphasis on a balanced involvement of patient and therapist as well as the patient and his world. Within this framework, the patient has to come to a deep level of understanding of emotional emptiness in order to truly integrate this work into his life. In so doing, DSA enhances the experiential learning that is at the core of emotional healing. Some of the complexities of working with the individual with BPD have been discussed in this chapter; in the following chapters, I will take us through a discussion and some case examples on how DSA might offer some solutions to addressing these concerns in treatment.

·IV·
DIAGNOSING AND SELECTING THE PATIENT FOR TREATMENT

"If it is to be, it is up to me."

-William H. Johnson

Differential Diagnosis

To begin our discussion of the acute treatment of individuals with disorder of the self, we need to make sure that we are all in agreement of the types of patient under discussion. I will rely on the DSM IV-TR for the diagnostic criteria in our discussion. If there is a purpose to the use of a diagnostic label, our topic of discussion is one that certainly can benefit from the use of such a label. As always, labels are only useful as a keyword to our collective knowledge about a particular disorder. This is useful for our purpose here to make sure that we are, first of all, referring to the same disorder when we discuss treatment options.

There are a number of clinical conditions that can mimic or overlap with symptoms of BPD. Patients with BPD can suffer co-morbid conditions such as depression and anxiety disorders. Psychiatric conditions such as major depression, bipolar disorder, anxiety disorder and even some psychotic disorders for example can present similarly to BPD. There have been instances in which a patient given the diagnosis of schizophrenia reveals over a period of time the symptoms consistent with BPD instead. Alternately, therapists can become overly zealous in diagnosing BPD and this diagnosis then becomes overly utilized; this can lead to the consequences of the risk of overlooking important differential diagnosis. Although I do advocate a broader recognition of the condition of emptiness, it is prudent for the psychiatric practitioner to weigh carefully the usage of the term BPD.

When an Axis I diagnosis is identified, it is crucial to take every measure to address it directly and perhaps, aggressively. In some individuals, the symptoms of depression can bring about such irritability and destructive acting out that mimics a picture of borderline symptoms. In this case, it is important to be certain about a diagnosis of depression and offer adequate treatment in terms of medication treatment as well psychotherapeutic treatment. For young people, irritability and acting out behavior can be all that is displayed externally when depressed. Without identification of mental health issues, these individuals can get into serious trouble with family, the law and in relationships.

Examples abound in clinical settings in which an individual's acting out calms greatly when his mood symptoms are finally treated. Vice versa, it is just as crucial to recognize BPD underneath the symptoms of other major psychiatric conditions. Too often, patients undergo aggressive and long-term treatment for depression with psychotherapy and medications only to be frustrated by the lack of any lasting improvement. It may turn out that this individual also suffers from the borderline condition and the underlying symptoms hindered progress for the treatment of illnesses such as major depression. Conceivably, many therapists avoid making the diagnosis of BPD due to the generally accepted sense about the poor prognosis of this condition

Patients who display a great deal of "mood swings" and "acting out" behavior may end up receiving intensive treatment for bipolar disorder. Although bipolar disorder, specifically type I, has a fairly precise set of diagnostic criteria in DSM IV-TR, this is a disorder that has met with much ambiguity in use. Currently, its criteria have been loosely utilized to encompass a wide variety of symptom descriptions; the consequence of this is easily apparent, and the risk of missing important differential diagnosis is high as well as making an error of specificity in over diagnosis. However, there is the concern that mania can worsen through the "kindling" effect of simmering symptoms if not treated in a timely fashion. There are many issues of safety and suffering that accompanies a disease that is not identified and treated.

A wise colleague once cogently described the intensity in which the bipolar manic patient experiences the vicissitude of life. His point is well taken; mania can present differently in different people. It is important to recognize mania in order to render the important treatment required. Nonetheless, once a diagnostic label is given, it can remain stubbornly stuck through time as well as even a change of provider. Authors have warned against the growing tendency to view borderline personality disorder as "really" examples of bipolar disorder (usually, bipolar II) and often omitting the personality disorder altogether. Treatment for bipolar disorder is very distinctive and specific; once down this road for treatment, the patient can be exposed to many medication trials and simultaneously neglecting the psychosocial interventions critical to the treatment of BPD (Stone 2006). One study concluded that there was only a "modest association" between borderline personality disorder and bipolar disorder (Gunderson 2006).

A common clinical scenario is the steadfast pursuit of a medication solution for a disorder such as depression or bipolar disorder when the more severe underlying condition is that of the psychodynamics a patient's life or perhaps the dynamics of BPD. The patient then risk being overly medicated while not receiving proper treatment for borderline symptoms. At times, a patient may undergo treatment with antipsychotic medications due to what appears to be psychotic symptoms when in fact he is exhibiting borderline psychosis, a detachment from reality that is distinctly different from the functional psychosis of schizophrenia. In this case, antipsychotic medications may be helpful in alleviating some of the intensities of borderline symptoms, such as anxiety, but it would not address the underlying etiology.

Diagnostically, beyond the obvious need to differentiate between any number of mood and anxiety disorders as well as psychotic symptoms, it is important to recognize the co-existence of borderline features. Many patients with commonly recognized psychiatric conditions such as obsessive compulsive disorder, eating disorder and even autistic spectrum of disorders can perhaps suffer co-morbid symptoms consistent with BPD. Rather than to rule out Axis I disorders for treatment using DSA and run the risk of not effectively covering important underlying dynamics of the pathology of the self, DSA suggest that the treatment of these conditions should be covered from a number of fronts. A patient diagnosed with bipolar disorder can have a co-morbid condition of BPD and both disorders will require attention and treatment. Depression may even be secondary to BPD and both conditions will need to be addressed.

A Wide Range of Patients for DSA

Are all patients diagnosed with BPD suitable for treatment with DSA? This is a clinical judgment that each individual clinician needs to determine for his or her patient. I will touch on this issue further in the section on resistant patients. I have found that, beyond patients suffering from BPD, patients with a variety of "acting out" behaviors and patients who are of lower cognitive functioning also do well on this treatment regimen. The DSA treatment program can be titrated to meet the needs of a number of different types of patients. When necessary, portions of the method can be down played and other sections can be emphasized. Please refer to case number 8.2 for further illustration.

On Paving the Foundation to Therapy

Case 4.1: Kayla is 26 years old. She has been recently married and also landed a good job as an accountant. She came to treatment when her anxiety about death became an all consuming preoccupation in her life. She could recall that for all of her life, she has always needed repeated reassurance from her heterozygotic twin sister. This means calling her sister multiple times a day, sometimes every hour, in order to ask her sister for words of reassurance. She assumed that by getting married she would "grow up" and be more independent from her sister. In actuality, she enjoyed the attention from her husband but never gave up her reliance on this sister.

After starting her first job as an accountant, she began to experience an increase in her anxiety and in addition, she started to suffer from serious symptoms of depression as well. Soon, she was unable to continue with her job although her boss and co-workers were very understanding and supportive of her. Aggressive use of medications was followed by several episodes of inpatient hospitalization. When she finally pulled out of the acute phase of her illness, she was more stable in her depression but still not feeling well. She continued to call her sister constantly and at times, demanded that her sister drop everything she is doing in life to come to her bedside.

Through all this, she was generally highly compliant with medications and worked hard in cognitive behavioral therapy. As she was unable to reach further progress in her treatment, she was becoming frustrated and disheartened about treatment. Subsequently, she turned to increased use of alcohol to numb some of her emotional pain. In time, she brought up the topic of feeling somehow empty and lonely. She admits that this may be why she has to call her sister so much; her sister is the one person who can soothe her more than anyone else in the world.

As Kayla decompensated further into the depth of depression and increased alcohol use, her sister felt torn between the desire to come and rescue Kayla once more or remain at a distance and implement "tough love." Kayla understood the idea that her sister should not "enable" her further. However, she reacted angrily each time she feels her sister seem unsupportive of her. As her conflict with her sister escalates, her use of alcohol became even more prominent. Finally, she conceded that her alcohol use is indeed pathological and consented to enter into inpatient alcohol treatment. Upon discharge, although sober, she continued to have very angry feelings toward her sister for not being more available. Kayla was at once fearful of losing her independence if she moved closer to her sister but needed more reassurance from her sister than ever before. Attention from her husband lacks certain substance and the marriage became non-existent. In her frustration, Kayla turned to superficial relationships with other men. At the same time, she started to reduce her involvement in AA. Now her sister could only watch painfully from afar her acting out behavior and question whether Kayla can remain sober for long.

At this point, Kayla switched to a DSA therapist and an invitation was extended to her sister, husband and close relative to attend a family session to discuss treatment and develop some understanding around her emotional dynamics. In this model of treatment, her therapist used the metaphoric cup to represent an emotional system with both input and output. "Given our previous conversations about feelings of emptiness, do you feel that you can relate this to the cup?" asked her therapist. The answer was affirmative and her therapist was able to smoothly broach the subject of treatment. The patient and her family listened attentively and seemed to accept this model without reservation. This patient and her family were made to understand how the near constant access of her sister could only delay her ultimate healing. She also came to understand that her relationships have been overly codependent. She even came to see how her use of alcohol can temporarily fill the emotional void within and recognize how quickly it leaks right out of the bottom of the metaphorical cup.

In the next few months, she diligently applied her treatment work using the 3-steps in a scripted fashion in every area of her personal life. Her parents and her sister joined in this daily work. She expressed feeling very encouraged by the family's enthusiastic involvement. Within a few months following the initial family session, it was notable that she no longer required frequent sessions and she was able to reduce her phone calls to her sister as well as return to her work.

Discussion:

Although this woman does not exhibit the typical symptoms of BPD, she was, nevertheless, suffering from the deficiency in being able to soothe her emptiness within. Most likely, her condition is related to her genetics of anxiety as well as subtleties of early frustrations, given that there was no history of abuse or trauma. On the surface, she seemed anxious and meets criteria for obsessive compulsive disorder. Subsequently, she showed much symptoms of depression with suicidal thinking. She also "self medicated" with alcohol when antidepressant in combination with antipsychotic medications may have helped with her depression but did not help with that "something that was still missing."

Traditional cognitive behavioral work seems to reduce some of her symptoms but worsened when she got depressed. Quite often, the patient's cognitive understanding of his or her illness may be limited to the awareness of distress or emotional dysregulation and the primary focus of treatment then involves exercises in cognitive countermeasures. For many patients, this style of work is insufficiently informative of the core emotions involved and tends to evoke in the patient the feelings of false self when real emptiness is not recognized. When we added DSA, this model of treatment offered more dimensions in the therapy work by providing a theoretical underpinning to her illness as well as clear and explicit instructions in the work of healing. It gave her a direct sense of understanding regarding what she is trying to accomplish in the therapy given that traditional work did not bring about timely result.

Like the experience of many people in therapy, she was becoming disenchanted about her progress after years in treatment. DSA allowed her to finally bring all the pieces that she has learned in treatment together and comprehend the CBT work. She was taught the skills to contain her behavior and to check her own reaction and cognitive interpretation of her feelings at a time of crisis, and she was asked to manage all this on her own. Her friends and family were made to understand the risk of becoming paralyzed in their concerns about her wellbeing as well as becoming obstructive in their attempts to help. Once she is able to contain and let time pass, she would then meet with her therapist at the designated time and place to process these events and her own skills at coping. Beyond the periodic sessions with her therapist to review her use of the 3-steps, she was also able to make good use of her relationship with her sister in the work of therapy. Her sister and her husband were taught to play a role in the 3-steps protocol and this allowed them to interact in a fashion that is respectful of boundary as well as allowing for developmental healing.

When she was introduced to DSA, she was given a developmental perspective for her work and she had a more concrete picture of what she had to accomplish. She can then own her picture of pathology and can readily see that it is her leaky cup that has to be repaired and ceased to place blame or to relinquish her life to bad circumstances. She was still using the skills that she had acquired in CBT but she is now aware of what types of behavior might distract her from the work and what constitutes acting out behavior that detracts from the work. All her years of therapy work can now come together in a cohesive whole.

Borderline symptoms may be seen as being on a continuum. Some individuals appear to exhibit just portions of the clinical criteria or show a lesser degree of severity of symptoms or suffer the symptoms for a shorter period of time. Officially, one should not make a diagnosis of BPD unless the symptoms are consistent with DSM IV-TR. However, when a patient of any age presents clinically with symptoms suggestive of BPD, how to make a diagnosis may be more of an academic question, treatment still has to be rendered. Often borderline symptoms are observed in conjunction with symptoms of depression or other psychiatric diagnosis. At times, borderline like symptoms resolve following treatment of the concurrent illness. Whether or not the borderline symptoms are a temporary presentation or signs of borderline personality organization, in the treatment consideration with DSA, the model of illness is viewed similarly and the treatment rendered in the same way. In effect, many patients with varying Axis I pathology would ultimately benefit from incorporating a form of treatment that addresses the pathology of the self.

The Resistant Patient

Every clinician has stories about patients who seem bent on self destruction and openly proclaim that they do not want any help. If the clinician does work in a psychiatric ward with involuntary patients, he or she will be familiar with the dilemma of trying to help a patient who is highly self-destructive and at risk for death yet refusing to receive help. People refuse help for several reasons. The most obvious of such a case is when the patient is psychotic or delusional and therefore not able to understand or accept help. In this case, general supportive measures would be given while the patient is treated for underlying cause of the psychosis. Medications can often play a vital role in stabilizing such a patient before other modalities of therapy can be implemented. Ethical and legal issues should be considered in treating a patient who is unable to give consent.

Here, I will limit our discussion to the treatment resistant patient who meets criteria for BPD. Feeling a lack of trust in the therapist, feeling unable to connect with the work of therapy, and lack of therapeutic rapport are some of the common reasons that patients develop resistance to treatment. Anger and transference issues can of course interfere with treatment. It is going to be difficult for the patient to perceive the dynamics in treatment accurately when anger issues are played out or transference issues cloud the reality. Narcissistic individuals and those who are prone to negative transference can often be highly resistant to treatment. Often, this individual exercises his rather formidable ability to manipulate relationships to meet his needs or carry on a narcissistic rage that fill an internal void and distract from the internal tension.

We all tend to define the world according to our needs. The world can be a friendly place when our basic necessities of life are being met. The world is a hostile place when we feel our needs are not being met. As our needs increase, whether emotional or material, we form more intense and more rigid views of our world. We then become less accepting of the world around us and would accept nothing less than the concept that has now become concrete in our own minds. For example: "I feel good when I eat, therefore, anything or anyone that suggest otherwise is to be pushed aside." This then leads to: "The world is a hostile place because no one understands what I need to do." Indeed, most initial discussions about treatment sounds like attempts to take away his only ways of coping without replacing it with anything else. Knowing the pain that will result from letting go of his old ways of coping, of course, he is not going to allow for any changes. Holding this conviction in mind is natural human behavior; it's a matter of survival. In this fashion, people become resistant to changes. The reason behind such resistance is often because of fear; fear that our most basic needs will not be fulfilled. The borderline individual may base the value of a relationship on how his needs are being met. This single-minded pursuit of meeting basic needs may mean strong resistance to any change that can be perceived as interfering with basic survival.

As has always been my practice, I look toward understanding the patient's sense of emptiness to comprehend his resistance to treatment. Viewing emptiness as the ultimate expression of past hurt and searching for current expression of this pain allows the therapist to grasp the challenges in treatment. One extremely angry and aggressive young man explained that "I don't want to give up feeling angry." The irony of this picture is that he does not at all look like someone who harbors any fear at all given his general presentation of toughness on the outside. In reality, he suffers from near constant discomfort of inordinate inner tension; "I feel empty. Anger helps me to feel alive" and "fighting" brings about temporary ego cohesion.

In a later chapter, I will further discuss the issue of projective identification and give some examples of how this defense mechanism impact treatment. Here, I will mention that this is a powerful dynamic that can frequently interfere with the patient's ability to properly engage in treatment. Most often, an individual's internal experiences of anger is projected toward others and the people around him can inadvertently react to this projection in return. When this occurs, the patient can become highly resistant to treatment feeling that the others are against him.

When I am confronted with a patient who is highly resistant, I feel that I have essentially three choices: One, delay introduction of DSA as an intervention and hope that there will be a better window of opportunity to engage the patient in treatment. The decision to withhold a form of treatment that one firmly believes to be critical to the patient's wellbeing is both a moral/ethical as well as medical/legal dilemma. In the case of a highly resistant patient, forcing a treatment on this patient could further damage therapeutic rapport and trust. Worse, it could set up a power struggle between the therapist and the patient that could irretrievably damage the treatment relationship.

I firmly believe that the patient has to be at a degree of insight to recognize that his way of life and way of coping is not a solution and is ready to at least explore the possibilities for treatment. I do not ask the patient to readily relinquish his negative methods of coping in order to begin treatment, but I do want him to indicate that he wants help. Most often, even without implementing the DSA protocol, I would continue to observe and work with the individual on developing better insight about his illness and if possible, help him to recognize and describe his sense of emptiness within. Upon the improvement of therapeutic alliance, the patient gains some insight and becomes more receptive of treatment. At that point, DSA can then be introduced.

Two, continue and invite the patient and his family in for a session to introduce DSA and hope that in the process of this discussion that I can engage the patient toward some type of commitment to treatment. On the occasions in which a highly acute patient has little or no insight about the need for treatment, the treatment team may elect to proceed with the introduction of DSA. As one experienced nurse once said, "If we can just plant the seed..."

My team understands that this work is in fact geared for working with just such an acute and highly resistant patient. We have had good success in such cases. DSA addresses the fact that such a patient can be highly self destructive and therefore, the risk of death is increased. DSA addresses the need for interpersonal boundary issues to be clear, especially with a very acute patient. DSA is very descriptive of how staff and family could best interact with the patient when everyone is under stress due to the patient's acuity. Therefore, even if the patient is not receptive of his treatment, all others can still go about their daily life around him in a compassionate fashion without reinforcing his poor coping behavior and perhaps, act in concert to encourage him to comply with treatment. Clinically, the strict therapeutic boundary as advocated through the 3-steps, even if applied without direct patient involvement, can contribute to introjection of the selfobject.

Three, this option is to withhold DSA but the patient would still receive general management in the milieu. Our hospital program happens to also offer a variety of interventions based on some degrees of cognitive behavioral therapy, interpersonal/supportive therapy and behavioral management with level system for rewards. This is probably very similar to what is offered at most inpatient facilities across the country.

No New Leaks, Just Healing Old Wounds

Case 4.2: Mary is a 16-year-old with a history of severe neglect and abuse in her past. She was profoundly depressed but has not received much treatment. In the hospital milieu, she often looked disheveled and with disregard for her appearance. She remarked that she hates her physical appearance and does little to maintain minimal hygiene and grooming. Her way of living with her emotional pain and very poor self-esteem was to keep much to herself especially on those days when she appears visibly distressed. She tends to be quiet and asked very little of peers or staff.

Most people would not describe her as attention seeking or manipulative. In fact, most staff would have to approach her to check on her since she rarely approached others to ask for help. Often, she is found curled up next to her bed and covered by a blanket, crying or just staring at the floor. At these times, she is prone to superficially cut on her arms if she could find something sharp to use. If she does not self-mutilate, she would still report that her urge to cut is quite intense. She continued in this state of daily distress for nearly three weeks despite the exposure to treatment as usual in the inpatient milieu. The treatment team decided to proceed with the introduction to DSA.

She was quite resistant to the treatment with DSA at first. However, she was usually cooperative in exploration of her past as long as it is kept at a superficial level. She was polite but resistive and guarded in issues especially related to the abuse she received from her family. She was willing to share a limited facet of her life history but only on her terms and mostly on her timing. She continued to act out with self-injurious behaviors in private. She would quietly listen to the discussions about how to utilize the treatment with DSA but would do little to implement the skills in treatment.

I maintained consistent scheduled visits with her regardless of her lack of full participation. In so doing, I would try to give her credit for any semblance of treatment. Despite strong resistance from this patient, the team felt that she is unlikely to respond well to the treatment as usual offered in the milieu but persistence in the work of DSA seemed to offer some hope. Given any fresh act of self-mutilation, I would keep our daily contacts simple and brief but attempts to convey genuine compassion. These are also opportunities to clarify treatment issues or questions about the implementation of treatment. With compassion as the wind behind our sail, each member of the team devised a manner to briefly check in with her in a routine fashion while remaining vigilant for periods of time when this patient shows rudimentary attempts at treatment.

In this introductory phase of treatment, I looked for opportunities to engage her in setting up some short term, intermediate and long term goals. She stated that talking about some of the conflicts and losses in her life might be within the horizon of our work but to ease her anxiety about that discussion, I turned the discussion to that of more immediate goal of getting to know her emotional pain and aversive inner tension. She gave a look of inquisitive surprise and indicated that this was of interest to her. I asked her to picture an orange in her mind and place such feelings as anger, jealousy, guilt, shame and sadness on the surface of this orange. (Orange peel and orange core of inner life will be further discussed in the next chapter.) We then explored feelings at the core; she was able to start to identify a set of feelings that seems quite different from those at the superficial level of the peel. On the occasion in which the subject of emptiness was broached, she looked up through a tangle of hair and a glimmer of light shone through her eyes as if to say, "Did you just ask me about that intolerable feeling inside?" At this point, she began to better comprehend the role that emptiness plays in her emotional pain. This understanding opened up her motivation for treatment.

On a rare occasion in the initial phase of treatment, she suddenly related of her distrust of others. "I think people are always poking holes in my cup" says Mary. "This is why I don't want to be around people any-more" she reiterated. Once privy to this patient's concern, the treatment team immediately got into action to correct this very serious misconception about the timeline of developmental hurt. Having the understanding that the emotional hurt of today resulted from early developmental frustrations often frees patients to better focus on treatment at hand. This treatment approach tries to invoke a sense of self preservation to harness the energy for self motivation.

Gradually, the completion of the treatment steps became a more purposeful act on her part rather than a chance happening that occurred from time to time. She began to embrace the treatment concepts in DSA and exercising its use on a daily basis. Soon, she reported of feeling more encouraged by her success and showed more interest in this treatment. She was also more engaged with peers and staff. By the end of her stay in the hospital one-month later, she was feeling less depressed and more optimistic about life and family. She no longer engaged in self-mutilation in this milieu.

Discussion:
Very often, the patient with borderline symptoms can be quiet, isolative and possibly a bit regressed as opposed to someone who is actively acting out and demanding attention. This patient may present with the attitude that "I don't need anything. I don't want anything." She makes little re-quest of others as if no one really has anything to offer her anyway. This may be the result of very poor self-esteem and/or perhaps she feels that her needs are never truly getting met. All the years of neglect and abuse from her past, together with a broken family preoccupied with their own issues in life, would of course leave her feeling very disheartened that anyone cares to help.

She was in great pain yet she felt absolutely helpless and hopeless that anyone is going to help ease her pain. During treatment, she was able to come into some insight about a sense of emptiness within and shared that she has become weary of interpersonal conflicts that seems to multiply the pain that she experiences internally; every rejection only served to remind her of the depth of emptiness within. Although there is no doubt that people from her early life have indeed been abusive in their roles in her life, she continues to view most of her current relationships in life as hostile and abusive. The most likely explanation for such ongoing tribulation could only be understood through the defense mechanisms of transference and projective identification.

Through the subtle nuances of words, gestures, behaviors, expressions and emotions, she has managed to project her own anger and frustration toward others. This resulted in selfobjects experiencing her anger as if it is their own. Inadvertently, people around her feel anger toward her and react accordingly. This could contribute to her further withdraw from the world. Thus the fear of getting her cup further "punctuated" is likely unfounded but can certainly be attributed to her disappointment at others for not filling the deep emptiness.

Through my own clinical work, I am persuaded to the belief that the primary treatment concerns for the borderline patient resides in the resolution of early hurt and rarely the issues of sustaining current damage. Certainly, the fragile state of the borderline patient seems to offer a picture of ongoing susceptibility to constant psychic injury; but, most of these crises bore the hallmark of original anger. The significance of this issue plays out in treatment through a focus on making repair to past damage as opposed to being overly concerned about fending off current attacks. It is more important to be mindful of the repair to past holes in the cup than to be preoccupied about getting new holes punched into the cup.

Engaging her in treatment meant not being pushy but being persistent. She was highly skeptical of doing this work but she at least humored us by her passive participation. She never actually made any promises but none was asked for. Over a few weeks, she gradually came around to embracing the work and came forward to engage staff as is encouraged in this treatment. Involvement in this work means that she is now capable of self-soothing and exhibits safer behaviors overall.

Although she ceased much of her acting out behaviors in the hospital milieu, one could certainly question the longevity of this change. Gauging the effectiveness of a modality of therapy work is exceedingly challenging. Often, individuals do appear to improve, as determined by the reduction of acting out, while in the inpatient milieu or in the intensive outpatient management. However, if this result is achieved through extensive use of interpersonal coaching and high frequency of emotional rescue, it is likely to have very little residual impact once this type of interaction is somehow reduced. Whether the modality of work is cognitive-behavioral or psychoanalytic in nature, the patient has to incorporate insight development with that of a self assuredness that could only come from interpersonal practices based on compassion.

·V·
PREPARATION FOR TREATMENT

"Winning is about how you play your bad card."

-A poker player

Initial Engagement in Treatment

After careful assessment of the patient and a thorough review of the history, the therapist is now ready to introduce the patient to DSA. Before starting this process, one has to make sure that at least a rudimentary treatment relationship is present. As in any type of treatment, therapeutic relationship is of overarching importance. This therapeutic relationship generally arrives from the trust and empathy that comes from genuine caring and concern for the patient. The therapeutic relationship and rapport with an individual with BPD is especially difficult and tumultuous at times. As we have discussed in previous chapters, this is related to some of the characteristics of this condition, which may in turn have its roots in the possible abuse and other relationship difficulties in this individual's history. Treatment rapport may be particularly difficult to achieve due to the manner in which this patient is likely to use relationships to fill a deep void within. With the drive of the emptiness as motivation, the quality of his relationships may be based heavily on what others are willing to give him. With such a rather self centered approach to relationships, it is not difficult to comprehend that his therapeutic relationships are often superficial.

In one case, a young man with an extensive history of abuse and neglect presented initially as highly threatening to his peers and staff. Due to his aggressive posturing, his peers and staff naturally kept a good distance from him. He even fittingly commented that he feels people do not want to spend time with him; as a consequence, he is unable to make lasting connections with anyone. When people come close, he tends to take advantage of the relationship. He would monopolize and manipulate the relationship to the extent that others feel drained and betrayed. As a result, he has no working relationship with any of the staff and vise versa. When the treatment team needed to implement a specific treatment program with him, the team found itself in the position of a lack of therapeutic rapport with him. This can be a common scenario in the treatment of borderline individuals. In this case, he was becoming increasingly assaultive toward others and action had to be taken. He admits to feeling painfully empty within and his inability to adequately connect with others also meant that his emptiness could not be soothed. Consequently, he turned to severe provocation and violence to meet his needs.

Despite the lack of therapeutic connection, the team continued on and activated the DSA treatment protocol with this patient. The team made sure that he did not feel totally blamed for his conduct and accorded him full compassion which allowed him to be open to hearing the presentation of DSA. He was highly receptive to the presentation and was able to get in touch with his feelings of emptiness. The team was concerned about the likelihood that this patient can still possess the potential to be highly assaultive. In my consultation to the team, I shared the concern that it may be reassuring to develop a management program with sufficient external containment to discourage his acting out, but any such deterrent would not have longevity as compared to motivating the patient to head off potential escalation on his own. DSA will help him picture his internal emotional turmoil and pain; it would put the ball back on his court.

It helps to have therapeutic rapport and it helps to feel empathy for the patient but, in this initial phase in treatment, one may have to rely on simple compassion as well as an identifiable goal such as that of a reduction of pain to set the stage for treatment. In this early stage, skilled therapists would often instinctively provide a bit of ego lending or minimal care-giving to develop a rudimentary relationship. Granted that this is not ideal but if there is at least a combination of a small degree of trust, a small degree of compassion, and a small degree of mutual understanding about emptiness, then the therapist can at least attempt at developing a treatment contract with the patient. Without this engagement, the patient is likely to remain highly guarded and resistive to treatment. Without feeling understood and validated about his great sense of emptiness within, he is resigned to cope with his world as he has always done, with fixation toward instant emotional gratification. This underscores the importance of helping the patient fully identify and comprehend his acute internal emotional pain before proceeding toward the introduction to treatment.

An analogy I often use is one describing a person who is experiencing an uncomfortable tightness in his chest. As he is experiencing the physical discomfort and pain, he interprets this discomfort as annoying and irritating. Soon, this annoyance is now causing him to feel angry and agitated. At that moment, people came around and tried to help him. Surprisingly, in response to this internal pain, he starts to strike out at everyone in a blind rage. It seemed that he equated the pain to danger and this triggered anger and rage which put him in a highly defensive mode. He could also equate the pain to some sort of a negative mood and respond as if he just had a really bad day.

Although most people may not react in this manner to obvious medical emergency, the challenge here is to get this individual to understand that his pain is real and for a purpose. He is not having a bad day; he is in need of help. Similarly, the borderline individual can suffer greatly without realizing that his pain is real and help is available. Without recognizing this internal emotional pain, the borderline patient reacts to the pain of emptiness in ways that are not always predictable or self preserving. The borderline patient may strike out in anger to a mysterious internal pain without recognizing that the pain is within his body, just like the individual who was not aware that his chest pain could be a warning sign for ischemic heart disease.

Even prior to development of therapeutic trust, DSA can still help turn the borderline patient's attention to the internal emotional hurt and therefore, direct him toward addressing the most critical issue of seeking help for healing of the wound. Although challenging, I do believe that, in most cases, a therapeutic rapport and relationship can be developed. Correctly calling attention to and validating the condition of the emptiness within can be a very important step in treatment to overcome an impasse to therapeutic rapport. Often, the process of just doing the work, as directed by DSA, allows for the blossoming of a rudimentary therapeutic relationship between the borderline individual and his treatment providers.

News Flash: Emptiness is Universal

Very early on in my clinical work with borderline patients, it was their profound description of what is akin to emptiness that got my attention. While descriptions about the borderline behaviors abound in clinical literature, it was the nefarious and haunting descriptions regarding emptiness that seemed to hold the mystique about this highly disruptive condition. Because emptiness is such a personal state, it is not easy or perhaps possible, to convey the sense of it from person to person.

I believe that a sentience of emptiness is intrinsically a condition that can exists, to a degree, in all people. Throughout history, many prominent philosophers, writers and thinkers have commented about the vicissitudes of human pursuits that would ultimately end with the realization of the emptiness of uninspired human existence. Buddhism, as a way of life, emphasizes the emptiness of being as central issue leading to the pragmatic search for the purpose of life. Takamori and colleagues (2006) presented an intriguing collection of stories that paints a sobering picture of the depth of human suffering through a blind pursuit of meaningless acting out behaviors in life. I suspect that man's salvation as viewed through the scope of many of the major world religions is a survey of the vulnerability, impermanence and most of all, the emptiness of existence. There may be a common thread between the emptiness of the soul with that of the tension of emotional emptiness.

In DSA, emptiness is viewed on a continuum. Therefore, the work of healing this "emptiness" is work that we all have to do. Given this assumption for emptiness, this hypothetical fulcrum makes it feasible for our treatment to proceed with the confidence of addressing a universally present human condition. Unlike the diagnosis of depression, bipolar disorder or other psychiatric entities in which differential diagnosis is critical to the very individualized medication treatment, the treatment of the emptiness within is work that most people could embrace regardless of diagnosis.

The implementation of DSA does not require prolonged inquiry into the symptoms of "emptiness" given that, one way or another; it is a condition of all mankind. The assumption here is that emptiness is a matter of degree and that each of us has to contend with the fluctuating level of emptiness within ourselves. In its most severe state, emptiness is the opposite of being; as such, the self has no shape. In DSA, emptiness does not necessarily denote pathology; although "perfect" anything is perhaps rare. It would in fact be quite the narcissistic individual to insist that occasional emptiness could not be a part of all of our daily existence. Accepting this hypothesis of emptiness allows DSA to be useful in the treatment of a broad range of individuals with various discomforts in living with the self.

Recognizing Emptiness

In preparation for treatment, I begin by sitting down with my patient in individual sessions and review some of his recent difficulties. We would talk about how he came to be hospitalized or about his most recent episode of crisis. This is also an opportunity to appraise the frequencies of such sentinel events. These are of course just a review of the facts that we both are aware. Before starting treatment with DSA, the therapist and the patient should both be completely cognizant of the patient's issues with emptiness. *The most valuable use of treatment time and effort could well be that of spending sufficient time with the patient to adequately develop his awareness of the emotional emptiness within.* This can generally be accomplished through a careful catalogue of feelings. Each therapist must develop his or her own style of broaching the subject of emptiness in a compassionate fashion.

Not surprisingly, many patients do not connect an internal sense of emptiness with their acting out behavior or suicidal behavior. Naturally, it is easier for him to attribute his acting out behavior to anger, anxiety, depression, the faults of others, etc. Yet, when pointedly asked if he could identify and describe his "baseline" state of feeling, something beyond the cyclic occurrence of anger and extreme "mood-swings", like most others, he is probably able to recognize a sentience of internal emptiness. I am persuaded that many patients are keenly aware of the difference between their anxiety symptoms and the neurovegetative symptoms and signs of depression from that of a sense of emptiness within.

It is scarcely sensible to expect patients to talk openly about the emptiness within when such emotions could not be easily identified through facial expressions or words. Consider the poster of facial expressions of emotions that are often presented to patients to elicit recognition of feelings. Many patients stare blankly at this chart with a strong sense of loss and invalidation because he is unable to match his inner feelings of emptiness to that of a recognizable expression illustrated. Hence, it is therapeutic to help the patient acknowledge the presence of emptiness within.

If such terms as "nothingness", "emptiness" and "loneliness" were already in use in our previous conversations, a quick review of these terms and feelings should be sufficient. If this vocabulary were not available to this individual, I would try to see if he could name some of these feelings on his own; usually, this is not very difficult for him to do. To help elicit some thinking around the issue of emptiness, I would use the following lines of questioning to direct this exploration. If possible, I generally refrain from the use of the term "emptiness", preferring that the patient arrives at this description by himself. This makes for greater therapeutic impact when we talk about the need for treatment.

An example would be, "When you are able to put your reactions to the external world aside, what would you notice about the deeper feelings that exist within?" These are feelings that do not vary much over time. For someone who sees himself as generally embroiled in conflict with others, I might say, "On a day when no one is saying or doing anything to upset you, I wonder what you could be feeling on such a day." Furthermore, a question such as, "Do you feel that people understand you?" can elicit further discussions about his internal state. Often his answer would be, "No one understands me, not even my friends." To further trigger his thinking and clarify the question, one could say, "Do you feel full, complete, content and emotionally comfortable during an average moment by yourself?" The response is often, "No, it's just the opposite of all that." Often, patients describe that good feelings from interpersonal interactions do not last long after the end of each episode of contact. "When I am alone.....can't get motivated to do anything." After a particularly ineffective interpersonal moment, "Suddenly, all the energy just drained out of me....." Having secured the attention of a boy, a character in the film *Sisterhood of the Traveling Pants* laments, "How can something that is suppose to make you feel so complete, leave you feeling so empty?"

Many individuals falsely attribute their feelings which then results in profound lack of insights to ongoing problems. Feeling "tired", "floating", "dreamy" and "bland" are common feelings that most people can identify with.

One young man said that he often feels tired in conjunction with a non-specific sense of feeling "dreadful." Such ephemeral states usually do not garner any notion of psychiatric acuity. This is the case with one young woman describing her inner world as "blah and blank" on a particular day. She argued that she feels "fine" and that her inpatient staff should not be concerned about it. She denied that she has ever felt suicidal and has never intentionally self-mutilated. She did admit that these feelings frequently occur and that they are indeed unpleasant. They make her feel un-alive and "With feeling like this, if I was outside (of the hospital), I would definitely be partying and doing drugs." Her drug use was extreme by any standard; combined with her pervasive feelings of nagging disquiet, it is indicative of severe pathology of the self.

Virtually all individuals with BPD are aware that something like "emptiness" resides within but they may call it by a different name. Some will call it "anxiety" although there appears to be few of the usual characteristic descriptions of anxiety. He may not be able to identify any concrete worries. It is unlikely that he would report of physical symptoms common in anxiety disorder or panic attacks. He does not have the usual symptoms of shortness of breath, palpitation, diaphoresis or impending doom. He may even have the insight that his sense of difficulty in breathing is due to an emotional factor other than anxiety or panic episodes.

On perfunctory examination, one may note that some borderline patients seem to present as predominantly in a state of intense arousal. Anxiety is a state of intense arousal often triggered by identifiable stress. Panic attacks are a state of intense arousal without apparent identifiable stressor. The borderline's intense arousal has a very different quality as well as being a part of a broader symptom description more consistent with personality disorder. As in alexithymia, the individual is unable to or has difficulty in describing or being aware of one's emotions or moods. These individuals may describe the internal emotional unrest as some form of anxiety, but this arousal could have a quality more consistent with emptiness. It is as if he feels the state of emptiness intensely.

One young woman stated emphatically that this feeling inside is clearly different from the symptoms of depression, which she also suffers. She described depression as feeling overwhelmed, low in energy, lethargic and wanting to sleep excessively but all these feelings are distinct from "the void, the emptiness, the dark spot that won't go away." It is remarkable how many borderline patients make the comment that they can better deal with depression than the emptiness within. This is not to suggest that individuals with BPD can not possibly experience actual anxiety or panic symptoms as co-morbidity. However, the issue here is to differentiate the report of "anxiety" from that of "emptiness."

Some individuals describe an intense internal emotional pain and tension as some kind of profound "boredom." One individual said it is a feeling of "purposelessness and pointlessness." Others may describe it as "like I don't care about anything", "nothing matters", "left out", "suffocating", "don't belong", "blank", "hollow", "block of emotions", "emotionally exhausted", "feeling like nothing left" and "I feel apathetic." A young teen described her ongoing internal pain as "mad, sad and frustrated." One individual shared with me this very striking description; "It is like crying inside and no one can hear you." Some describe it as a physical pressure that builds up within. Another described it as a "light pressure on my face and my upper chest like a net is pulling me back."

Someone once said to me, "it is like if your emotions can ache." One young man said, "It's like I don't feel alive." One young woman said, "I feel dead inside." Another teen, struggling to produce a description of her internal pain, instantly embraced the terms emptiness and loneliness and added, "life is like an elaborate dream and I am waiting to wake up." Furthermore, "It feels like I need something but can't find it." In general, these individuals describe some sort of profound sense of unwell that can be so palpable as to seem as if one can almost touch such darkness and void. An interesting articulation of this darkness as described by one individual, "It is like a terrible itch deep inside my body but I am unable to reach it to scratch." Interestingly, a separate individual gave a similar analogy, "It is like being stung by a gigantic mosquito but on the inside."

I recall a 14 year old girl who was severely teased at school for being in special education and called an "idiot" by her peers. When we started talking, she appeared to me to have a particular sparkle about her that suggest a hidden intelligence behind her low self-esteem. In discussion about her "emptiness", I felt both pleased and proud of her when she used the word "indifferent" to describe her internal turmoil. I find this description a very fitting addition to all the other terms used but this word gives this discussion an additional dimension. Initially, she was not certain that "indifferent" is such a terrible feeling state. After some further exploration, it turns out that this feeling state is indeed highly unpleasant and can be the driving force behind much of her troubled behavior in daily life.

Many times, my patient will use words such as "nothingness", "emptiness", and "loneliness", without having discussed it previously. One heart felt description from a streetwise teen state, "It's like half my heart is empty. It will stay that way until I find my mother." Sometime people write about these feelings in letters, journals, songs and poems. I am always fascinated by how willing and how quickly individuals with BPD will use such descriptions. These descriptions are of course a major cornerstone to the criteria for BPD as described in DSM IV-TR.

When the Self is Full of Negativity

There are always outliers in every discussion. In her first session with me, one young woman was relentless in her sharing about how much hatred she has for herself. For her, any sense of internal discomfort has long been interpreted as an anxiety, panic, negative self image and of course, self hatred. In this case, she does, perhaps, experience symptoms of anxiety and panic, but on closer examination, her descriptions did not meet classic criteria for such disorders. Instead, hers were the crisis of internal pain of emptiness.

Interestingly, on cursory survey, one may miss her description of emptiness and dismiss her complaints as rather pedantic and unremarkable examples of anxiety or even, panic. One could also count this as a form of existential angst, but this would make the treatment far more complex and prolonged. In fact, she has undergone multiple medication trials for anxiety and panic disorders to no avail. Her condition continues to deteriorate with constant thoughts of suicide and the urge to self-mutilate. Hence, recognizing her statements as describing an intolerable emotional pain assures that the treatment would be relevant and effective.

The usual method of inquiring about the state of emptiness may yield some misleading results and wrong impression that could cause the treatment to come to an impasse or at least a detour. This patient does not recognize her internal state as emptiness. If anything, she describes it as being very full; it is full of everything negative. Intuitively, one may find this to be quite the opposite of our purpose here to discover emptiness. However, this state of negativity can be very closely related to our understanding of emptiness, if not the flipside of the same coin. The experienced practitioner should have little trouble in discerning the many nuances of describing the state of emptiness. As is often the case, symptoms of emptiness should only be considered if all other differential diagnosis has been considered.

I will refer to projective identification (discussed in chapter 3 and 9) for some clues to the negative state she conveys. In DSA, projective identification is equated with the unresolved early frustration and anger that then leaves a layer of residue at the bottom of the metaphorical cup. In a cup that is to hold the ideally positive transference that is exchanged interpersonally, there is actually a layer of sludge that is covered most times by this transference material. Naturally, when the cup runs dry and the residue is exposed, this borderline patient comes to experience a strong sense of fullness of everything negative; this bottom layer is the result of all the accumulated frustration, original anger and unresolved death instinct from the beginning of life.

With the focused attention of a high school linebacker, one very stout young man described his baseline feeling as "anger all the time." Yet, he denies that this feeling comes with any of the familiar sensations of the adrenaline charged physical experience before he gets into a physical altercation. Looking uncomfortable about the apparent contradiction in his description, he added, "that angry feeling is subtle"- with a puzzled expression on his face.

He was then asked, "What if you peeled away that layer of anger?"

"Well, then there would be nothing" Dennis answered.

"Nothing, you mean there are no other feelings?" asked the therapist.

"Yeah, nothing else" he responded, still in deep contemplation about these questions.

"So, how does nothing feel?"

"Nothing is a very bad feeling" he replied.

"This nothing feeling never goes away. I try to do things to distract from it but it is always there."

He went on to admit that it is the bubbling over of such a feeling state that could cause him to act in ways that gets him into trouble.

Often, the language pertaining to emptiness can be as varied as the number of people interviewed. Furthermore, the difference in description can be due to cultural, age and sex bias. Men might relate to the internal void as an anger or boredom while women might relate to it more as numbness and loneliness. In addition, there can be much confusion about being "full of negativity" as well as the "emptiness" that constitutes nothingness. It seems that this is all about experiencing the opposite of happiness although not just relegated to times of depression.

In order for the message regarding an internal emotional life to reverberate with the patient, it is paramount to help him relate through his daily experiences. In essence, out initial work involves the task of helping the patient to recognize the vicissitude of feeling intensely fulfilled one moment and exhaustively empty the next.

"Dennis, let's take this another step further. I wonder if you have noticed that there are times when you feel very positive, upbeat and very satisfied with how things are going in life; and then suddenly, something minor happens and you feel as if your world has just collapsed?"

"Yes. It just takes a comment from someone that indicates to me that they don't understand what I am going through. Sometimes I am able to feel fairly content and happy for a moment but I just know that the nothing feeling is waiting for me."

"Later on, we are going to use a paper cup to describe emotionally feeling full or empty. Do you think this analogy would fit with what you are saying about feeling full and then going empty?" said the therapist.

"It could be a little like that." replied Dennis.

Every human being harbors the secret desire to be understood from a very empathic level. Despite the fact that people generally have great trouble describing an internal emptiness with much finesse, most still expect to be understood and validated. For the therapist to miss or discount the meaning of boredom and anger, this can constitute such a major empathic failure that the work of therapy may not recover from this egregious act.

To differentiate normal boredom and situational anger from the pain of emptiness, the therapist has to rely on past, recent and current history of the patient to pinpoint a developmental understanding of this individual. A familiarity with the developmental pathology of the self is important in our understanding of the causative relationship with the state of emptiness. Hence, prepared with the patient's developmental history, the therapist can better make sense of the patient's utterances of mundane terms like boredom and anger.

Unrecognized Emptiness

Most often, when an individual is able to describe feeling empty, he or she is probably ready to admit that it is indeed an unpleasant state of being and that something should be done about it. After extensive exploration of the feelings of emptiness, one young man came to ready recognition that much of his acting out behavior could be directly connected to it. He realized that the pain of emptiness can be so intense that he would do practically anything to get rid of it or distract from it.

Just as often, there is the individual who will insist that he experiences no such emptiness. He claims to act out for the sake of acting out. I distinctly recall a discussion with some colleagues about a teen boy who insist that he wants to be seen as a "bad-ass" and would do anything to gain that reputation. This reminded me of an article in the newspaper about a 97 year old man who died in prison after a string of bank robberies that he committed at age 85. At the time of arrest, he revealed that he had discovered that each robbery job left him feeling highly emotionally fulfilled for days afterward. His acting out behavior was apparently not motivated by money. Is the boy and the old man just acting out for the sake of acting out? Have they acted out aggressively to experience the physiological response to the thrill or is it something more?

There are occasions in which one is witness to an individual who repeatedly pick fights with peers and staff on an inpatient ward to the point of requiring physical containment for his safety as well as others. One can easily get the impression that this individual did not always escalate because of an actual conflict or anger toward others, but that the end goal of such provocation appears to be the experiencing of the *intense stimulation* of such a physical confrontation. My instinct tells me that the fight or flight physiological response from such thrill and danger would not necessarily be a pleasant experience. Even the thrill of having survived a frightening rollercoaster ride is probably short lived. The endorphin ride of the long distance runner is just as temporary and the need to replenish the endorphin pulse is likely the result of physiological withdraw. Such physiology can not account for the underlying motivation of this type of extreme behavior.

The anticipation of a thrill such as a roller coaster ride is one issue, but, could something more primal and basic be involved in the motivation to repeatedly seek out such stimulations? It would seem that there is something else at play here that is more than an adrenal-rush or an endorphin pulse. On this occasion, my colleagues and I talked about the work of convincing the boy that his acting out can only lead to dire consequences and to accept the need for change. Most times, this dialogue would only lead to a debate with the patient about the reality and severity of consequences. Frequently, like most teens with a feeling of omnipotence, this individual may just yield a flippant comment that consequences do not matter and that his actions make him feel good.

I proposed that we should ask him how he might otherwise feel if he did not act out on such a routine basis. One might ask, "It seems to me that if you feel greatly better after an act of aggression, then on the other hand, there could be a great deal of bad feelings that is often there when you are not acting out and that you may want to find ways to get rid of the bad feelings." Another way to approach this young man, if this was someone that I know better, would be to say, "It seems that you often encounter very poor feelings inside. I wonder if this is why you seek to get rid of it by acting out so aggressively on a regular basis." The 85 year old man did not rob banks for the money or for the thrill. He likely conducted the robberies to experience a sense of aliveness that he could not easily achieve in the emptiness of his everyday life. Sure, one can certainly argue that some crimes are acted out of pure antisocial basis and some acting out truly has the flavor of thrill seeking no different from a rollercoaster ride, but most people only seek such thrills on occasion.

When considering those that society condemns as villains, whether someone committed serial crime against others, instigated genocide against humanity or brought global terrorism, future studies may reveal the pathology of the self as a common denominator in these individuals. In the criminal world, some act out due to opportunity, poverty, greed, lust, ambition, revenge or even religion. In the studies of the self, one may be inclined to view original anger, unresolved death instinct and emptiness all on a continuum that includes those who offend against others. Just as the young boy and the old man, the two are poorly informed about their false self and would be highly resistant to change. There is a lesson here for many of the ills of our highly acting out world.

Not all acting out behavior belongs in our discussion about the emptiness within. Understanding antisocial behavior is bound to be a fascinating and challenging issue in the years to come. However, for the purpose of our discussion, I would make the assumption that chronic acting out may have its basis in the pathology of the self. My treatment attempt would be to get the boy and the old man to see the less glamorous side of their acting out behavior by pointing out that they were acting out to address the pain within. This way, they could be shown a way to be motivated to make changes rather than to just accept their crime as mere glory, cause and machismo or out of actual necessity.

DSA can be a highly effective method of confronting the patient regarding his cognitive distortions by removing the glamour and mystique in his acting out behavior. In so doing, he and the world around him would have to take a new look at his behavior and view it as the pathology of the self as opposed to the vanity of his acting out. There are many vignettes that require the clinician to think out of the box to overcome resistance and identify emptiness; otherwise, most cases would slip from our fingers.

The Uncertain Terror of Emptiness

Tapping into the depth of emptiness to explore the extent of this pain may not be a familiar part of daily life or treatment repertoire for the borderline patient. However, probing the depth of emptiness is necessarily a requirement to starting in treatment and the lack of this step could contribute to the unauthentic investment in treatment. Entering into therapy without comprehending the depth of one's emptiness is comparable to buying a shirt without an idea of one's proportions; the hazy ideas of two sleeves and some panels of cloth may not be sufficient. Many borderline patients are vaguely aware of a sense of emptiness but few have truly plumbed the depth of this discomfort.

"What if I faced my total emptiness and it caused me to become insane?" asked one patient. This particularly astute individual made the observation that his reluctance to fully embrace treatment has to do with his fear of the potential unknown of his emptiness. The fear of being engulfed by this pain can easily be triggered by the rudimentary awareness of such pain. Being unable to fathom the depth of this pain can contribute to wild fantasies about its destructive possibilities. As a consequence, many patients are driven away from true investment in treatment due to the fears of confronting this terrifying state.

One young man, experiencing the confounding upset of auditory hallucinations, related that his "voices being a personification of my feelings." Confronted by the bizarre experience of hearing "voices", he naturally concluded that his feelings must be beyond tolerability. As a result, he became highly resistant in treatment. Besides, without true awareness of his emptiness, his work in this treatment was probably quite superficial and he was very aware of this dilemma.

Finally, while in the inpatient milieu, he went on to request that he be housed in the acute care area of the hospital in order that he could confront the depth of his emptiness in what he hoped would be sufficient containment for the unknown outcome. Taking command of his fears, utilizing the pre-3-steps skills, he voluntarily spent a solitary night in a stark white safe room and emerged the next day feeling rather victorious at having conquered this one great uncertainty and apprehension. He did not go "insane". He recognized that this emotional pain will be with him for sometime into the future but he is now confident that he can tolerate the most acute sense of this pain of emptiness.

Hence, he proceeded to further embrace this work despite the need to radically accept this emptiness in every round of treatment work.

Orange Peel and Orange Core of Inner Life

Commonly, there are patients who have never stopped to think about their inner life. These individuals may require a bit more work in the exploration of the emptiness within. Attempts should be made to distinguish the difference between what could well be a concurrent state of depression that may superimpose on a more baseline state of emptiness or aversive inner tension. This is a most difficult distinction to make.

Often, however, this individual has already been treated for disorders such as depression and anxiety. Many are frustrated by what appears to be aggressive pharmacologic and psychotherapeutic interventions for depression, while still wanting greater easing of the internal emotional pain. At this point, it may be helpful for this patient to then further explore this internal pain of emptiness as a separate entity from that of depression; he can then truly devote his attention to psychotherapy in conjunction to pharmacotherapy.

The metaphoric cup is used in this work to represent the core self. This core is viewed as the crucible of our character as well as our emotional experiences. The view of life problems through the core issues is the fulcrum that gives treatment the focused leverage in DSA as well as in most accepted modalities of psychotherapy.

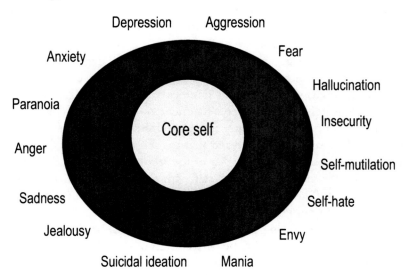

Figure 5.1 *The external layer of the orange represents the more superficial feelings and behaviors that are observable and expressed externally. The core is where the self resides (the metaphoric cup) and is at the heart of the pathology of the self.*

Sometimes it is helpful to develop a mental image of a particular problem one is trying to solve since language can be a limiting factor. I like to use the analogy of an orange or an onion in illustrating the layers with which we wrap around our emotional core. The surface layers or peel can be seen as superficial symptoms and feelings that are connected to external events. Most people are readily able to relate to this description and are able to separate out surface symptoms such as anxiety and depression from that of the deeper core issues such as emotional emptiness. Individuals who have not considered the existence of the state of emptiness will now easily recognize this internal emotional pain and identify it as a distinct entity from situational feeling states and mood disorder.

Fragmentation

Self psychology can be helpful in our understanding of the concept of emptiness. Heinz Kohut described the self as reliant on the objects such as people, symbols and others for the emergence, maintenance and completion of the self. When objects are used to sustain the self, Kohut tended to include human as well as non-human objects, it is termed the *selfobject experience*. "Maintenance of the self as a psychological structure depends on the continuing presence of an evoking-sustaining-responding matrix of selfobject experiences" (Wolf 1988, p.28). The mother's ability to bring calm to the infant, the special pen that brings creativity to the writer, the focused attention of the audiences that bring confidence to the speaker, are all examples of selfobject experience at work. Hence, any interruption and disruption of this selfobject experience can theoretically cause the self to fragment; the self is no longer experienced as coordinated or fitting together and depending on the degree of fragmentation, one's experience can range from mild anxiety to total loss of self structure.

In the language of DSA, this fragmentation of the self is equivalent to a crisis of emptiness. Kohut presents fragmentation as the result of faulty self and object experience but also imply that the self is a structure that is fairly stable over time. However, he recognized that the self clearly fluctuates according to the presence, absence or the quality of the selfobject experience. DSA attempts to describe the vicissitude of the self with the metaphor of the cup. In this model, the self fluctuates in accordance to a variety of input as well as the self sustaining ability of the cup.

The acts of mirroring and idealizing transference between the mother and child dyad could not possibly be perfect even in the most ideal circumstances; while others suffer even greater disjunction of transference due to emotional, physical and sexual abuse. When the transference with significant selfobjects becomes dysregulated, the contrast in the fluctuation of the core self/cup brings about insurmountable uneasiness. This tension can be released through the use of various defense mechanisms or acting out behaviors. The alternative solution is the reliance on some degree of input from others or the dependence on some type of symbolic representation of the subjective selfobjects, without which, we stand a high chance of fragmentation when our emotional cup is empty. In DSA, one wants to make the distinction between what is avoidance of fragmentation and action that constitutes healing.

It can be said that everything we do to experience reward, whether it is to play sports, play music, create a painting, write a novel or engage in a religious experience, are all infused with a high degree of selfobject representation. It has been argued that many artists express their creativity through a vague sentience of important past selfobjects (Miller 1997). Perhaps, the majority of our activities are infused with a subconscious awareness of our present and past selfobject representation. We seem completely dependent on the selfobject experience to keep from fragmentation or emptiness but the degree to which we suffer can be ameliorated through improved independence which is the aim of this work.

A Contract for Treatment

"Following his initial assessment, the therapist's next task is to summarize the impressions he has formed and make some recommendation to the person who has sought his help." "The psychotherapeutic process is facilitated if the treatment contract includes an explicit agreement between patient and therapist on the objective of their work together and on the procedures they will follow in attempting to reach these objectives" (Weiner 1975, p. 74-87). In the following session with the patient and his important others, the pathology of his emotional pain will be clearly identified and treatment strategy formulated, thus, laying the groundwork for his commitment to this model of treatment.

With respect to the treatment contract, I say to the patient, "I appreciate that you have allowed me to better understand the exquisite emotional pain that you suffer on a daily basis. It seems to me that it is this internal pain that could be the source of much of your difficulties in everyday life. This pain is also related to your seeking help here in the hospital. You have helped me to understand that you are suffering from more than just depression; your sense of feeling empty appears to cause you even greater pain. You have obviously tried to cope with this pain the best you could but you continue to suffer. Do you want to reduce this pain?" At this point, my concern is mainly that of helping the patient to acknowledge the existence of "emptiness" and to accept the need for treatment.

It is imperative that the therapist makes it clear to the patient that this treatment requires hard work and sincerity in seeking improvement. To underscore the importance of the treatment contract, I would generally allow the patient and his family a chance to reconsider their involvement in this work at the end of our initial family conference which serves as our first survey of DSA. By this time, they should understand that this treatment is based on the *emphasis of repetitive behavioral learning and healing through interpersonal dynamics.* They will then understand that the daily work of DSA is done through the involvement of reliable family members and significant others in his life, if they are available, as well as his therapy provider.

Due to the manner in which this method of treatment involves a number of people in his life, the consensual participation of the patient and those involved is integral to the successful outcome of his treatment. It may be advisable to assess the patient's commitment to this treatment following the initial recognition of emptiness and then again at the conclusion of the presentation of this methodology.

·VI·
THE FAMILY SESSION

*"All things, events, and phenomena are dynamic,
changing every moment; nothing remains static.
So, at any given moment, no matter how pleasant or
pleasurable your experience may be, it will not last."*
-His Holiness The Dalai Lama

Stopping the Blame

DSA is a paradigm in treatment that does not embrace any blame but encourage all involved to come to the treatment discussion with forgiveness. This session attempts to help the family members understand their own roles and perhaps, their sense of guilt and shame about their individual dynamic with this patient. If at all possible, the therapist should try to help the family make amends and draw upon the power of compassion to join in the work of treatment. It is important to note that, to a large extent, the success of this work hinges on the support of the family; the family can truly be an effective support only if they can step away from the possible anger, guilt and shame that engulf them through their history with this patient.

As emphasized here, treatment involvement by the family, relatives, significant others and all who plays a role in this individual's life, is critical. Frequently, parents may blame themselves for having somehow failing to parent or failing to protect this child. Siblings may be angry and highly resentful of the attention that the patient has monopolized in the family. Friends feel that they may have somehow let the patient down somewhere along the way. Grandparents express great sadness about feeling helpless in watching all of this drama unfolds in front of their eyes without being able to assist. If sexual abuse or some type of trauma was involved, then the complicated dynamic involved in a family grieving and angry over this atrocity may still fester in the undercurrent. The purpose of the initial work is to provide an inviting and safe environment for the selfobjects to participate in this patient's treatment.

"If people hold their parents or others responsible for their growing up, they may go through an entire lifetime faulting their parents and looking for someone who can finally give them what they have always 'needed.' If people relinquish the notion that parents were 'supposed' to have done it 'right,' they have many options for growing up themselves" (Kerr, Bowen 1988). The purpose of this family meeting is not to belabor troubles of past history; such background information would have been covered in previous sessions to elucidate an understanding of the family dynamic and the role each individual plays in the family system. The family history can then point us in a direction toward understanding how the family system can hinder or help in this individual's healing process.

Family system is to play a major role in the healing of this patient. Family and friends are to be praised for entering into a contract in the treatment of this patient. The purpose of this important family session is not to elucidate or hypothesize about the cause of this individual's borderline condition. The goal of this family session is to dislodge the family from a state of paralysis and anguished frustration over their sense of helplessness. One has to take this opportunity to get the family into a better functioning shape in order for them to be of help to the patient in this treatment. The therapist will try to get them to see how they can put guilt and shame aside and focus on the treatment at hand. When the family can lower their own sense of guilt about this patient, it would be far easier for them to step away from their usual frustrated and anguished view of this patient to experience a whole new understanding of his condition.

It may be worth noting the poor relationship many borderline patients have with their family of origin. This raises the issue of whether the patient and his family can work together therapeutically at this juncture or further family work will be required. "I don't trust my family, who can I work the 3-steps with?" DSA is designed to help improve such broken relationships while, at the same time, allowing the patient to begin his own healing of the self. It is a treatment approach that helps to build trust as long as all of the members are committed to renewing this relationship. *Trust is derived from action* and the call for consistent action is a hallmark of DSA. Family members who desire to vanquish their guilt for some sort of wayward past has the opportunity to recompense the patient through their commitment to treatment. One young girl boasted of how she has all but severed her connection with her family of origin to completely rely on quick friendships to meet her needs, tearfully admitted that the attention she wanted most is that of her imperfect family.

Another goal of the family conference is to develop improved interpersonal boundary of the family members toward the patient. It is often evident that family members can intentionally or inadvertently benefit from the patient's dependent relationship. In this case, the family or friends are actually filling their own "cup" at the expense of the patient. As I will discuss in a later section, each person has a "cup" to fill, and this makes for a delicate balance in the emotional ecosystem. Any imbalance can tilt the scale and the consequence is not beneficial to the system or individual. It is critical for the family or significant others involved to all be present and to have understanding of their own role in this delicate balance. It is only when this is achieved could the patient begin the path to healing and better independent function. However, the purpose of this initial family session is not to resolve all the enmeshed family issues in one session. Far from this, the goal of this session is only to set the groundwork for further discussion and elucidation of family dynamics that could be better understood through DSA.

Use Universal Issues to Preserve Confidentiality

Family sessions are a challenge due to the difficulty of respecting confidentiality while attempting to address relevant issues. The whole of this approach to treatment centers on placing no blame on the patient and his family. Hence, this invitation into treatment has to be handled delicately. The patient's apprehension about treatment has to be assuaged through trust and confidentiality.

DSA can be particularly amicable to engaging the patient and his family through the understanding of the disease condition. One of the keys to successful treatment without intruding on confidentiality is to focus on the common denominator in the psychopathology of the self. Whether the pathology involves substance use, sexual deviancy, aggression, anorexia, bulimia or gambling addiction, treatment discussion can take place without open confession in the family session. The metaphor of the cup can be representative of the most typical of interpersonal interactions and revealing of common problematic behaviors. This treatment work relies heavily on the mechanistic discussion of the pathology of the self to achieve a congruous understanding. Thus, confidentiality is preserved.

Repetition Compulsion in Multi-generation

Erikson, on explaining Freud's phenomenon of the "repetition compulsion", described it as the need to re-enact painful experiences in words or acts. Furthermore, "the individual unconsciously arranges for variations of an original theme which he has not learned either to overcome or to live with: he tries to master a situation which in its original form had been too much for him by meeting it repeatedly and of his own accord" (Erikson 1950, p.216). In one story, Freud interpreted a young boy's behavior with his toys as a manner of addressing abandonment fears through the play sphere by repeatedly making an item with a string attached disappear and then appear to mirror his mother's reappearance after being away for work (Erikson 1950, p.217). Beyond self mastery, repetition compulsion can have consequences that impact others in one's surrounding.

Many of us have forsaken our true self long ago. We have, instead, accumulated silent anger, aggression and frustration, for which, we have dealt with them through the use of splitting and projective identification since our childhood. It is possible that we have grown up in an environment in which children were viewed as insignificant being that "should only be heard when spoken to" or just the opposite, as the object of such focused attention from our parents that unattainable expectations were heaped upon us.

For some, the pain of growing up has to do with being admired for those things that they can do with great gift and talent; for others, this early pain comes from being exploited and sexually abused as children. Whether the suppression of our self, not to cry, not to feel, not to be a bother, came from our intuitive understanding that such behavior would negatively impact our caretaker or in fact, one was forced to keep all emotions locked inside in order to avoid severe physical punishment, the end result is a denial of the existence of the self (Miller 1997).

From abandonment to severe misattunement, such is the early anger and frustration that many suffer. As adults, the scar of such injury continues to plague us in the form of our continuing to search for the love that we deserve but never received. We may seek and accept love and admiration in ways that are not always appropriate or apparent to us. As adults, we may act out through humiliating others, play out bossy or authoritarian demands on those under our care or guidance and in so doing, derive a sense of control that we were rewarded for as children or indeed, reminded us of the pride of survival that control offered us as children.

Having thus denied our true self, we face a lifetime of feeling cheated, marginalized, disrespected, empty, loveless, resentful and bitter. Worse, without professional help, as adults, one wanders through life seeking what every child seeks and can only get from his or her own parents, frustrations are bound to follow. Not having been exposed to nurturing and proper attunement as children, we are also not able to share nurturing and attunement without adequate modeling. Frustrated and angry, it is very easy to victimize the most vulnerable population in society, our very own children.

Whether these are our biological children or children as members of our society, these children can become victimized in subtle or blatant fashions. If as adults, we are one of the children who grew up having to deny our true self, in the emptiness of this existence, one is at risk to victimize the next generation through the same acting out behaviors of the previous generation that caused us to deny our true self or traumatized us through outright abuse. A number of studies have found familial transmission of externalizing disorders (Conger 2003, Thornberry 2003)) several others have linked grandparental and parental major depressive disorder to that of psychopathology in the grandchildren (Olino 2008, Weissman 2005). Regardless of the mode of transmission, the compulsion to deal with one's own internal pain through ineffective coping can lead to a picture of multiple generations of sufferers in the same family.

Embracing Change

A brief note about the complexities of family dynamics is warranted at this point. Regardless of the tragedies that befall an individual or his family over the course of time, the occurrence of these events may be dependent on a great multiple of factors that can not be easily accounted for by cultural, social, religious or political context. It is too easy to place blame on the notion of the "mother" for the poor development of the self. One must not forget the bidirectional influence of the mother and child dyad.

From my own observation, certain temperaments in children are anything but passive and can reciprocally influence the parent by inducing in them various defensive mechanisms. One must keep in mind the propensity for splitting and projective identification to be roused in each of us as the result of facing overt frustration, isolation, loneliness and anger. Emptiness, resulting in fragmentation, is the bane of motherhood for those of fragile emotional self. While maternal attunement is ideal, for some, the demands of a young child can be overly stressful and reciprocal interpersonal interaction becomes fleeting. Interpersonal interaction is ongoing and fluid; this should dispel the notion that the hurt of development can be firmly attributed to any one person or entity. Change and challenge is expected and to be handled well.

The Buddhist acceptance of the "suffering of change" seems an appropriate place to further our understanding of the complexities of an individual's interaction with his family. Much of our unhappiness as an individual and as a family arises out of our aversion to seeing our own idea of happiness change without our input or control. "The acceptance of change can be an important factor in reducing a large measure of our self-created suffering. So often, for instance, we cause our own suffering by refusing to relinquish the past. If we define our self-image in terms of what we use to look like or in terms of what we used to be able to do and can't do now, it is a pretty safe bet that we don't grow happier as we grow older. Sometimes, the more we try to hold on, the more grotesque and distorted life becomes" (Cutler 1998).

In referring to our aversion to changes in life, Dr. Cutler cite an example of a married couple who have no enmity for each other but seeks a divorce due to a diminution of earlier passion in their relationship. "And more often than not, the first whisper of change in our relationship may create a sense of panic, a feeling that something is drastically wrong." Dr. Cutler correctly pointed out that our culture is one in which relationship experts are busy churning out books to help us regain or prolong our experiences of passion and flame of romance. If rekindling the original passion fails, many would then consider the relationship ended. It is unfortunate that many relationships are terminated without realizing the long term growth and changes that takes place over time.

What is disconcerting about such a cultural tendency is our hesitancy to seek and accept change. Sometimes a family would demand that a member seek help only to express utter dismay when changes do take place and others start to feel displaced. Change is to be embraced; and in accepting it, one hopes to experience greater happiness. Status quo can be miserable but it can become all too comfortable. Making a commitment in a relationship, the birth of a child, coping with job change, adjusting to a move, experiencing retirement are examples of facing changes. Whether a condition in life happens to be good or bad, the resistance to change prevents us from marshalling all of our strength to overcome the challenge. Since change is ever present, the resistance to change can only bring about hardship and unhappiness.

From Forgiveness to Freedom to Enlightenment

This simple formula came out of one of my sessions with a brilliant but tortured individual that I had the fortune to work with in therapy. He always teaches me so much about life and therapy work in the course of our meetings. On this occasion, we were talking about his quest to find the self. As he traced his path in this exploration, he came to realize the importance of being able to put his past behind him. Without forgiveness for all, he was full of guilt and suffered from very poor self-esteem as a result. Once he began his journey of self-discovery, he realized that he had to live with quite a false self due to his inherent biological makeup as well as a product of his very unusual family system.

Like many, feeling different, neglected, isolated, teased and subjugated under powerful selfobjects, he survived by retreating into a world where he survived through being invisible; he never had a chance to develop a good sense of the self. He suffered anger and frustration from an early age and his *original anger* sat deeply at the core of everything about him. He felt empty and lonely and acted out through his behavior toward his family as well as through his compulsions. Through therapy and his own research about life, religion and the truth of science, he also discovered the importance of being able to forgive himself for all of the "sins" of his past. It seems that whether from the perspective of religion or mental health, forgiveness has to come from inside the self.

Once he found forgiveness for himself and others in his past, he discovered that he felt very free in some sense. He began to see his life in very different light and discovered how very "stuck" that his life has been for so many years. As a result of this newfound freedom, he no longer felt quite so compelled to stick with his old habits. He began to relate to his colleagues and his family differently as well. The status quo just was not sufficient anymore. He felt more creative and was ready to shake up his life a bit and take on some small risks that he would never have allowed himself in the past.

With respect to this progress, he could now enjoy a much broader horizon of both emotional and intellectual possibilities in life. Having found forgiveness, he experienced the freedom to question the past as well as the present and experienced torrents of ideas and feelings that he never felt before. As a result of this new freedom, he easily embraced the need to heal the self through acceptance of change. He had no difficulty in visualizing his trouble with the self through the concept of DSA and readily expanded upon the basic concepts in DSA to adapt it to his unique experience. He felt that he was no longer quite so "stuck" in his old ways; I would distinguish that as being on a path to enlightenment.

The Family System

System denotes an entity that is generally seen as dynamic. If it is not dynamic, it would only be components. Most people would accept that a family is not just made up of components. It has been argued that the human organism has evolved much the same way as any other organism on earth; the rules that govern its behavior is therefore little different from other organisms. Therefore, the family system of humans is really no different from other organic systems. It has been suggested by sociobiologists that Charles Darwin's theory of natural selection can indeed be consistent with the concept of family or group being a system that act on its members.

Darwin recognized that natural selection does not have to occur only in the context of the individual promoting his own survival. Sociobiology has since concurred with Darwin in this regard by citing examples of the cooperative nature of social organisms and how the altruistic characteristic of some of its members who do not get to procreate do actually have their genetics passed on due to the success of the group. It would then appear that the study of other organisms might yield understanding of the human social system given that nature probably does not vary a great deal from system to system. Family systems theory as proposed by Murray Bowen would take us further down this path by pointing out the difference between feeling system, intellectual system and emotional system.

Humans contribute feelings and intellect into a system. However, feelings and intellect came in rather late in the evolutionary process and seems to be mostly unique to humans. As such, it can be seen as the icing on the cake as far as the evolution of the system in the process of natural selection. It would seem that it is the basics of "emotion" that has been around all along and has been the essential tool of natural selection over eons. In systems theory, emotions and feelings are differentiated and this allows the term "emotional" to be applied to all living things.

Ants do not act in concert for survival due to feelings; ants act out of emotions. One would then expect that human evolution has been steeped in the influence of "emotion" just as all other organisms. "Over the course of evolution the emotional system became increasingly complex, but perhaps none of its basic features has been lost." "While all aspects of the human emotional system may not be in the monkey, probably most aspects of the monkey's emotional functioning are in the human." From this point of view, one can see how the understanding of the system in nature can contribute greatly to our understanding of the family system (Kerr, Bowen, 1988).

In particular, the purpose of this family session is to make inroad into the way this system affect the members of this family. Bowen described the human family as an emotional unit, also called an *emotional field* which is analogous to the gravitational field of the solar system. This field then results in individuals occupying different *functioning positions*. This functioning position has a significant influence on an individual's beliefs, values, attitudes, feelings and behavior. "Another important facet of functioning positions is that they operate in reciprocal relationship to one another. A younger child shapes the behavior of an older sibling as much as the older one shapes the behavior of the younger one. An 'overfunctioning' person shapes the attitudes, feelings and behavior of an 'underfunctioning' person as much as the underfunctioning one shapes the attitudes, feelings and behavior of the overfunctioning one." It is said that the healthier individuals in the family will try to function for the sicker individuals and as a result, a type of family stability develops that incorporates the chronic symptoms. "It is easier for the family members to make accommodations that make it possible to live with the symptom than it is to address the underlying relationship process that fosters the symptom in the first place" (Kerr, Bowen 1988). In other words, this is very much a picture of the resistance to change.

In formulating the basic belief system in DSA, I felt that, beyond the dynamics of infant and mother dyad as described by object relations theory, the maintenance of symptoms in the patient has to be related to the ongoing dynamic in the family as well as relationships in the near orbit. It would be naïve to think that the anger and frustrations in early life can somehow find enough fuel to continue the pathology into adulthood without further kindling along the way. Viewed another way, this original anger may require a fairly optimal environment for eventual resolution. Anyone who has spent time with young children can attest to the perception that a child is a very resilient being. Therefore, it is conceivable that some type of ineffective selfobject experience would have to take place to perpetuate the early symptoms of anger and frustration. This is not always apparent to casual observers and even seasoned professionals. The 3-steps attempts to put in place a structured interaction that reduces ongoing anger and frustration within the family system.

Family evaluation with family systems theory in mind can be instrumental in shedding light on the dynamic of pathology in the family and how such pathology is maintained. Regardless of the explanations for the transmission of risks within a family, numerous studies show that this is indeed the case. Offspring of sexually abused parents are significantly more likely to be sexually abused themselves, make at least one lifetime suicide attempt, suffer from post traumatic stress disorder and have higher levels of impulsivity (Brodsky 2008). Twin studies indicated that genetic factors account for about half of the variance (Statham 1998, Brent 2005) while environmental factors such as familial instability and childhood abuse contribute independently to the transmission of suicidal behavior (Gould 1996, Brand 1996). Emotion, as discussed in family systems theory, is differentiated from feelings and intellect. No one ever says that they are intentionally doing things that keep the family or the individuals in the family in an unhappy or miserable way. In most instances, a group of people somehow manages to maintain the pathology through their collective "emotions" possibly because this is a way to maintain some degree of family function.

This is like the ant colony performing at an "emotional" level to maintain functioning. At a fundamental level, the family system is functioning at an "emotional" manner in order to maintain some degree of "stability" in the system. Acting on emotion, a family system attempts to make any maneuver feasible toward the ultimate survival of the unit. This means that the system is willing to adapt and integrate to any pathology if this meant the survival of the unit. Consistent with natural selection, mankind is still reacting with "emotions" to assure the survival of the clan. Perhaps emotions are more powerful than feelings and intellect. Perhaps, at an intellectual level, members of a family realize the fundamental importance of providing greater support for its member but at an emotional level, it is getting swept along with the family's desire to survive in a society that is constantly changing.

An example would be the two wage earning family in which both parents spend a great deal of time working outside of the home. At an emotional level, this seems to be the way to maintain survival or keep up with the expectation of the society. On the other hand, the parents have come to realize that they are not actually making more money doing so and that their feelings tell them that they would rather spend more time with the young. Will their "emotion" win out or will their "intellect" and "feelings" win out? In any case, one can then picture how maintenance of pathology in the system is tolerated as long as it does not interfere with what appears to be a semblance of stability. Of course, as we shall examine, this stability is fragile. Additionally, the individual with the pathology continues to suffer, and becomes increasingly unhappy and discontent, threatening the stability of the whole system.

Functioning at an "emotional" level does not allow for intellect and feelings. The emotional functioning does not allow much room for change. For example, tolerating and accommodating to the functioning of an alcoholic member of the family operates at an emotional level which is highly resistant to change. Homeostasis is more suitable for lower organisms. Parenthetically, there are some similarities between the "emotions" of the ant and the emotional emptiness of our principal discussion in that both types of emotions are bourn out of a more primary primitive state that is more instinctual rather than intellectual or that of the feeling. A family system may tend to function at an emotional level like all other organisms and it does not allow for easy acceptance of individual change.

As discussed earlier, change is inevitable and the acceptance of change is important before any personal growth or healing. Original anger is a tremendous obstacle to change; the subconscious anxiety, fear and discomfort holds us all to a primitive stage of functioning at an emotional level. We split, we project and we try to organize our interpersonal orbit around our most intense primitive instincts and needs. The intricacies of the family system in conjunction with the natural tendency to resist change for the purpose of homeostasis can be one of the greatest challenges to the mental health of the individuals involved. One of the goals of this family session is to enlighten the members of this family to the ineffectiveness of clinging to status quo.

Bring Together a Supportive Team

The emotional state of a family system often operates more like a democracy than a meritocracy. This system often votes to maintain stable function for the whole rather than the optimal function for one. As a result, powerful forces may be at play to keep status quo; a state of function that may be very detrimental for some in the system. Democracy has its benefits as well; it offers a more reasonable voice at times of crisis and perhaps, brings a better focus on the long term. Thus, the inclusion of the family system is an attempt to harness the power of the emotional field to function positively in the borderline patient's treatment.

In this critical family conference, the initial task is to be certain of adequate participation from all involved. This is to include anyone who is in the *emotional field* of this individual. This may not be the first meeting that I have had with the family of this patient. At this special family conference, the invitation goes out to the immediate family members such as the parents and any sibling who is old enough to be involved in this individual's treatment. I generally do not invite any sibling who is under eighteen.

In terms of family, I would also invite any member of the extended family that the patient and his guardian are comfortable with. This could involve the grandparents, aunts and uncles and even cousins. Adult friends of the patient, neighbors or friends of the family who are directly involved could also be invited. Next, I would look at anyone involved with the individual from school, or even religious and other activities. Foremost, all invitations to this family conference should involve the permission of the patient.

Some parents of borderline patients view close emotional involvement with their adult children with an eye of leery reluctance not bourn of uncaring attitude but, rather, out of a sense of reservation about their own ability to intervene and help. Nevertheless, occasional parents intervene vigorously while others tend to take a more passive stance. Either way, many parents become ineffective bystanders in a world in which useful and productive involvement is at a premium. Maintaining a civilized yet distant relationship becomes all that is feasible in some families. For others, the insistent struggle to effect a change in the troubled child is often a lonely affair.

Sociologists have long studied the changing landscape of the American family. Many have wondered about the role of the family since the transition from an agrarian society to that of an urbanized industrial nation. Many sociologists have grappled with the question of whether our society is now based more on the isolated nuclear family or are we still in touch with our kin. Interestingly, in one study in Ireland, the modern upper middle class parents would prefer to leave their child with a friend or neighbor rather than a kin (Gordon 1977). Despite the appearance of greater distance between kin attendant upon industrialization and geographic mobility, "yet there is no current evidence to suggest that people were cut off from kin either metaphorically or literally" (Gordon 1978, p.41). "While the great majority of the couples live apart from their parents, they do live close by" (Klatzky 1962). Although the preponderance of adults has ready access to kin, few would consider involving their parents in a cooperative capacity in therapy. Many borderline patients do continue to access their parents in enmeshed and dependent fashion that causes great stress for both parties. It is my clinical experience that parents are eager for some direction as to how best to participate in their offspring's life without being over indulgent or respond through interpersonal rescue.

In the beginning of treatment, the borderline patient is often full of intense anger and frustration with many of his selfobjects. His display of splitting and projection could well be at full force. Of the many difficulties in the initial work, the patient's refusal to involve important family members can be one of the most challenging. Although lacking in this important component in starting treatment, having impressed upon the patient about the need to involve critical selfobjects, this work could proceed in the hope that, with some amount of initial work, the patient will allow for additional members of his family to be included in future family sessions. This is in fact how a good number of individuals had to begin life in treatment, lonely, rejecting but wanting.

Last but not least, I would ask the patient and family for permission to invite any treatment provider that he may currently be working with. In the context of a family conference that takes place in the inpatient setting, the outpatient therapist should be invited because he or she is likely someone with whom the family has developed trust and rapport. They have perhaps been working together for some time and the therapist is often the one who generated the referral to the hospital in hopes of obtaining a professional consultation about the management and treatment of this patient. Working effectively with the patient's ongoing outpatient therapist is critical for the continuity of care. At times, invitation to a caseworker representing the social service agency would be appropriate if the young patient happens to be a ward of the state. Sometimes, this caseworker may be all the "family" there is for this individual. Like anyone else in this patient's life, it is important for his state caseworker to be a part of the team approach to this treatment.

In a family conference in the inpatient setting, the hospital social worker or the case manager for this patient would also be involved. If possible, I would also invite one or two of the line staff who will be working closely with the patient in the milieu. A representative of the inpatient team is critical in that these are the people who will temporarily function as the patient's critical selfobjects in the milieu. They are to play an important role in the developmental issues in this patient's treatment. They will be responsible for creating a validating and supportive environment for this patient in the inpatient setting.

The family session is a very unique opportunity to work through the impasses in the patient's treatment. With such an earnest gathering of key people in the patient's life, this session can have an immense impact on the course of this patient's treatment. This session is so critical that I often view it as the pivotal point of how this patient would respond to the treatment with DSA. If I can bring the patient and his family on board of this treatment during this session, then I know that there is a very good chance of a positive outcome in treatment.

Beyond Countertransference

In seeking psychotherapy, a multitude of challenges face the patient at this juncture, one of which is therapist countertransference. The therapist's response to the patient as if he or she was an important figure from the therapist's past is the commonly accepted definition of countertransference. If not monitored closely, the therapist's feelings toward the patient can interfere with the therapist's effectiveness in this work. Countertransference should be carefully differentiated from one's culturally based and fundamentally human reaction to an act, event or an individual. A strong revolting feeling toward a heinous act of inhuman crime or terror attack should not be labeled as countertransference.

The therapeutic setting is clearly different from the everyday life. One may not necessarily refer to an interpersonal interaction in daily life as a countertransference. The sense of revulsion on watching someone spit gum on the sidewalk would not constitute countertransference. However, in the therapy office and in the inpatient milieu, the same drama should warrant further examination. Depending on the therapist or staff's response, much could be learned about the patient and his interpersonal interface. If the therapist has good psychological insight about himself or herself, this becomes an important tool in his work with the borderline patient. However, if the therapist reacts without sufficient insight about the dynamics at hand, he risks the danger of imposing his own psychological shortcoming on an already vulnerable patient.

Here, it is appropriate to make a brief comment about therapist's countertransference toward the family or the parents. Prior to this conference, it is not unusual for the therapist to have been privy to the family history and having formed some sort of judgment or feeling about the story. Whether out of empathy for our patient or simply the result of our human nature, one can easily develop a negative countertransferential feeling toward one or more member of the family. However, it is important to keep in mind the rare case in which one can determine with any great certainly the cause of a patient's personality pathology. While a history of chronic chaos, neglect or abuse can contribute to the patient's current suffering, it is also important to recognize the family's attempt to seek forgiveness and to help heal his wounds. Countertransferential feelings can also contribute to overt empathy and care-giving beyond reasonable boundaries. It is important to maintain therapeutic neutrality.

Sometimes, in the best of circumstances, one or both of the parents can be overly preoccupied by their own issues in life and failed to provide sufficient support and attunement for the child. In unfortunate accounts, a tragedy may befall the family while the patient was in his critical developmental years; this could cause the parents to become distracted from their tasks in parenting. There are certainly instances in which one or both of the parents have borderline characteristics and therefore, struggle in their own balance in life. In many instances, there is no discernable trauma, abuse or lack of parenting.

Human beings are fallible; children can be highly resilient. I hold these sentiments in mind as I try to understand the history of my patient. There is no excuse for abuse but I always try to understand the condition in which a parent might become abusive. Was the child's temperament a poor match for the parent? Was the child suffering from some type of medical illness or psychiatric condition that challenged the parent's ability to manage him? What could have caused the parents to become distracted from parenting? Was the birth of the child unexpected? Did the family face economic uncertainty? Was there a loss in the family? These are just a few of the questions that one might ask oneself as well as the patient in an evaluation in order to fully understand the circumstances under which the patient's developments could have come to be arrested or frustrated. As a therapist, it is our responsibility to search broadly for a way to understand these clinical circumstances with neutrality and compassion. At times, the patient's pathology can only be attributed to severe abuse and neglect.

It may be helpful to allay the family's anxiety about this session by assuring them that the purpose of this meeting is not to place blame. I may say something like, "My discussion today about treatment may be based on the developmental damage that perhaps started when he (the patient) was an infant, but like most diseases, this type of pathology usually has a genetic basis as well as environmental factors. When it comes to environmental factors, some things done in the name of good parenting can go wrong. I recently read an article in the paper about a new study that suggests that more than three glasses of milk a day can actually cause obesity in children as they grow older. How often have we, as parents, encouraged our kids to drink as many glasses of milk as possible?"

It is my belief that even if the parents were responsible in contributing to the development of this patient's psychopathology, much has probably changed during the timeline of this family. As in any good psychiatric assessment, one has to be certain that this patient is not currently at risk of suffering from reportable abuse from those that we involve in his treatment. At times, with a high index of suspicion, the family of a teen may be informed that it is our obligation to report potential abuse to the Child Protective Service. Interestingly, after such a report, most families remain very engaged in treatment.

Many times, I have parents and family coming to my session with a firm conviction to do all they can to help this patient. They may already feel guilty and sad about the complications in this patient's life. Perhaps the abusive individual or the perpetrator is no longer in the picture. Some parents I have worked with tell me that they have finally achieved a degree of sobriety and have also woken to the reality of life with a very troubled child who is still in great need of their involvement in his life. With tears in their eyes, they have to face the guilt and shame of their earlier missteps in life and realize the important role that they can still play in this patient's healing.

As a therapist, we have to keep an open mind and understand that we are neither the judge nor the jury but a guide for our patient. As a guide, we have to look compassionately at the broader global picture of this patient's life and realize that it's a therapist's job to help the patient pool his resources together despite his own tendency to act on his own transference issues. The patient may not see the need or the wisdom of working with his family. At such times, the therapist's recognition of the valuable role of family should be shared with the patient.

An understanding of projective identification in the context of DSA can be helpful to the borderline patient with an inexplicable anger toward current caretakers who were possibly uninvolved in his traumatic past. One very polite and likable young man held such vehement hatred for his grandparents, his legal guardian, that it had an insidious effect on those around him. Soon, he had convinced everyone that he was a victim of a duo who were somehow worse than evil. On closer exploration, he could not give any good reasons to justify his feelings. It turned out that he had exercised projective identification and that the anger and animosity he experienced were indeed his own projection of anger and frustration.

To do our job, we have to check our own countertransference. In the preceding example, the therapist could have easily sided with the young man; our own past could have interfered in this most common of scenario in the struggle for independence. It would be sophomoric for the therapist to impulsively validate the patient's anger through the therapist's countertransference issues without further elucidation of the source of this anger. Rather, the identification of the patient's own projective identification allowed the therapist to help this patient gain greater insight about this dynamic which could bring him closer to his family. I hope the work presented in this writing helps the therapist better develop a compassionate understanding of the patient's acting out behavior and a neutral understanding of the family dynamic that could contribute to the patient's pathology.

Beginning the Session

The focus of this phase of the work is to paint a stark reality of the condition of BPD. I begin the session with a review of any recent acuity that has brought matters to this juncture. For example, this could be the suicide attempt or the severe self mutilation that prompted the re-hospitalization. This sentinel event could also be a severe outburst at home that threatened property destruction as well as threatening the safety of others. Just as frequently, the hospitalization could be triggered by a psychotic episode related to alcohol or street substance use. Sometimes, the borderline patient presents as highly paranoid and may even report of experiencing hallucinations without apparent use of street substance or other organic etiology.

Usually, everyone in the room nod in agreement about how acute and frightening this recent episode has been for all involved. Because I am already familiar with the history of this patient, such as frequency of hospitalization, numbers of attempts at suicide, I would proceed to do a very quick survey of such history. Reviewing the patient's recent and past history in the presence of such a large group of his supporters can be a delicate endeavor. The therapist has to be a mediator and an ally to the patient in order to maintain trust. This should not be an open complaint session about the patient. This session should be very controlled and measured in providing an agenda that all can agree upon. A brief review of history and developing an understanding around the issue of emptiness helps everyone arrive on the same page regarding the purpose of this meeting.

I would usually take a very directive role in this particular family session. I run it more like a didactic class than a traditional family discussion. Hopefully, most everyone is in agreement with the picture being developed at this point. If necessary, spending just a few minutes to correct the facts would be good to make sure that there would not be contentious issues later in the discussion. The therapist needs to be well prepared and knowledgeable about the patient's history to help the family feel confident and comfortable in allowing the therapist to take the lead in this very important family session.

Next, I try to explore with the patient the feeling state that he may have experienced in this most recent episode. Since this is a discussion that he and I have had recently to put some language around his internal feelings, he is now quite ready to review this with me and name some of the emotional states such as "emptiness", "nothingness", "numbness" and "loneliness." Often, the patient may describe feeling "bored". However, without leading the patient, I might explore this term a little and usually the patient can come up with other terms such as "nothingness" or "numbness".

One very interesting young woman said that she has a peculiar sense of never feeling satiated after a meal. She could eat a large meal and feel extremely hungry right after she has finished. Frequently, this hunger pain can be so intense that she curls up on her bed in a fetal position and cry. A young man, who survived a hanging when the leather belt broke, talked about an intense perpetual boredom as a feeling state rather than a fleeting sense of inactivity. Clearly, there are many ways to describe the sense of aversive inner tension. In most cases, the family and others involved have not been aware of the intensity of these feeling states within the patient.

They may experience the patient as frequently making such statements as "bored" or "numb" without being aware of the significance of these words. I would then try to get my patient to elaborate on these states to further all of our understanding about these feelings. The point here is to help everyone understand just how painful "emptiness" can feel. At times, it is appropriate to lend the patient some assistance in conveying his feelings of emptiness. I might add that the English language is quite limited in how we can communicate this type of emotional pain but the metaphor of the cup that we shall embark upon can usually expound on this point. I would also add that it would be extremely difficult for most people to be able to relate to the tremendous psychic pain that can be the result of such profound feeling state of "emptiness and alienation". Using the concept of fragmentation from self psychology, the therapist could ask the family members to think of an instance in which they were faced with sharing an idea to an individual or a large group of people wherein their sense of confidence was shattered when the audience began to indicate disinterest. One can then experience a disconnected and uncomfortable state of feeling like one is "falling apart", a familiar encounter for most.

I want the family and friends involved to start developing a greater sense of empathy for this patient by understanding the tremendous and very real emotional pain that he has to live with each and every day. Other's lack of understanding and empathy for his very painful internal experiences can lead to his feeling even more alone in the world. I find that most families are quite riveted and enthralled by this conversation. Many times, you witness tears streaming down the faces of a few family members at this point. At the least, you see many heads bobbing up and down in agreement. They may have never considered the possibility that these feelings could exist in such a powerful way in this individual but perhaps through their love for this individual, they are usually quite ready to accept it.

Next, a brief discussion of the most common symptoms of BPD would take place to consolidate our understanding of the purpose of treatment. Depending on therapist personal preference as well as the particular case situation, one may opt to not use the term borderline personality disorder in the family session. As is common in treatment, many individuals have come across such terminology as BPD without proper understanding of the meaning of the various criteria. Others with a preliminary knowledge of BPD may find themselves outraged by the idea that the patient involved here could possibly suffer from this condition. Some may jump to the preconceived idea that this is a hopeless condition without good treatment outcome.

I am always concerned that this diagnostic label may serve more as a distraction at this particular family session and distract from the focus of the talk. One option at this point can be the attempt to have a discussion to correct any misconceptions or simply go around this issue and direct this discussion toward that of the symptoms involved rather than be preoccupied by the label involved. The therapist could say, "All in all, some sort of early developmental damage has occurred and I want to discuss with you how such damage can result in many of the symptoms we are discussing here." I do have to comment here that I believe diagnostic labels to be highly helpful in the communication of information about a condition. It does help to allow providers to instantly know what another provider is trying to convey about a given individual. A diagnostic label also helps to allow providers to be able to draw upon our collective knowledge about a given condition.

In this discussion of the symptoms of BPD, I often observe family members to be listening silently yet nodding their heads vigorously in agreement with the description. This is because the descriptions of BPD in DSM IV-TR would often mirror their own experiences with this individual. Because of the profound and constant sense of emptiness, he is very needy of attention but never seems to feel satisfied. What positive interpersonal relatedness that occurs may last only momentarily and he is back to feeling very empty emotionally once again. The instability of relationships is a hallmark of his personal world. One moment he is on good terms with you and the next moment you feel like strangers. One moment you are the best friend a person can have and the next moment you feel like a traitor. Family members often recall crisis moments vividly. They too feel the pain of the patient who can not find any stability and joy in life. Being in the life of the patient with BPD is like living in a storm.

The therapist can decide on how much of a description of this patient with BPD to detail here. You want to treat this description carefully so as to not cross the line of confidentiality. I find that a general description of the hallmark symptoms of BPD as described in the DSM-IV would be sufficient. Once again, family and friends in this session often agree vigorously about this description of their loved one. These are descriptions that they are so familiar with but never thought that it could be described so succinctly. Families often express a sense of great relief that their experiences are not unique and others experience the patient in such a similar way.

How is the patient handling this conversation thus far? Maintaining the strictest respect for confidentiality, the patient generally finds this conversation intriguing and of new territory for him. We are simply reviewing a collective set of symptoms that everyone is aware of. The patient has already given consent to share with everyone the existence of "emptiness." In most cases, the patient has already indicated that he is in such severe pain that he is now ready to explore some treatment options. Even though he is not fully aware of all that is involved in this discussion about DSA in his treatment, he may be quite pleased with this attempt to bring his family on board about his plight. This discussion often serves to help the patient communicate feelings that he has not been able to communicate before.

In fact, in most every case, the patient seems rather glad and relieved that such an effort is made to help everyone understand his emotional pains. This is an attempt to *super-validate* his experiences of the internal tension. It is conceivable that some parts of his dramatic self-mutilation or even suicidal gestures have been to try to convince the world of his desperate sense of existence. To have the symptoms of this condition conveyed in such a direct fashion by a professional and a person of authority, such as the therapist, makes it a very gratifying moment for the patient.

In this discussion, there is on occasion the borderline patient who may be inclined to feel rather exposed and vulnerable toward any thoughts regarding his secretive internal world. Despite the loneliness of his existence, he, nevertheless, feels more secure within the familiar pain. For some, the darkness of emptiness only reinforces the angst of adolescence. As such, the merest mentioning of this forbidden zone can be treading on confidentiality and privacy. The therapist has to be very skilled in traversing between the tasks of taking the patient and his family into the treatment arena from that of a break of trust.

High Risk of Death

Once we have covered the discussion about symptoms in this initial family session, we proceed to one of the most critical portion of our pre-treatment preparation. I want to remind the reader to keep in mind that I generally try to deliver this complete talk in one sitting with the patient and his family. Therefore, even though I separate this discussion into different sections, I try to finish in one extended session. This means that I would cover the family confer-ence and then go straight to the next two chapters in one extended session. I feel that this is important for the overall effect as well as, surprisingly, easier retention of the whole concept with the presentation of the complete picture.

This next topic is probably a discussion that is ventured by few therapists. This is probably because this topic feels so counterintuitive in the conventional work of therapy. Most mental health practitioners would much rather avoid talking about patient death, not to mention talking about the potential for patient death with the patient's own family. The risk of death is so prominent in treatment that many facilities have had to review best practice measures to prevent sentinel events. Suicide risk assessment, frequent patient visual checks, and careful inspection of hospital physical plants for potential risks are just some of the common cautions taken. One study looked at the method of briefly discharging a patient who threatens to engage in or engages in self-harm. While banned from the inpatient services, the patient could still gain access to outpatient care from relationship management therapy program and could then request readmission after 24 hours. Authors of this work recognized that this is a difficult protocol to justify in our litigious society. (Hoch 2006) Due to the high risk nature of undertaking borderline treatment, it is exceed-ingly critical to address the manner in which self-harm and suicidal threats will be handled before one can proceed to the next steps in the DSA treatment method. Dislodging the family and the therapeutic process from paralysis is the ultimate goal in this initial phase in treatment.

Once I bring everyone to the same page about the emotional pain and the common clinical picture this patient suffers routinely, I proceed to discuss the very real possibility that this individual will succeed in taking his own life some day. For many families, this is not at all surprising. Perhaps they have taken the patient to an emergency room many times thinking that he has succeeded in taking his life this time. He may be someone who contemplates the idea of death all the time. He likes to read macabre fantasy or real life tragedies. He fantasizes about the afterlife or the possibility of reincarnation. He entertains the idea that he could reincarnate into a more pleasant way of life. One young woman fantasizes about returning as a cat. "Life is great for a cat. They don't have anything to worry about." Interestingly, she failed to realize that most major world religions that incorporate reincarnation as a part of the cycle of life emphasizes the working through of conflicts in each life cycle in order to move forward.

Sometimes, the family has been through this type of crisis so many times that they know that they are becoming rather callous about it and may not always be as eager to take the patient to the emergency room one more time. These families are aware that there is an accident ready to happen or a serious suicide intention by the patient that will be missed because they could no longer be as vigilant. Even the superficial cutting that goes on each day can turn into a deadly accident. Some of these activities are done in private or secrecy but most often, the family is quite aware of such acts of self-injury. Again, families and friends may rush him to the emergency room at first but after a while, they no longer do so. Here, they realize, is another tragedy at the waiting. What if a routine cutting went too far? An act of self-mutilation can turn out to be as deadly as any intentional suicide.

Paralysis

If families are not so numb to the chaos around this individual, they are usually terrified that they are going to find him dead in the near future. This is what prompts that panicked call to 911 or going to the emergency room every time he harms himself. At their wits end, most families are at a loss as to what they can better do to insuring that this patient can remain relatively safe. Sometimes, others around him would do practically "anything" to keep him safe. They feel that they would shackle themselves to him if necessary. They take turns staying up at night to keep him safe. They support him with everything they've got. They might even give in to whatever may be his whims and wishes. They are just afraid that they may not be doing enough and this can lead to grave consequences. They are well aware of the "storm" that can start at any instant if he is the least bit frustrated. They know that he needs a lot of "attention" and support and they dread the day that they "fail" at providing adequate support. At that point, everyone's greatest nightmare would come true. He could be found dead. Cause of his death could be an intentional suicide or it could be the result of a major accident stemming from another set of self-mutilation or perhaps a suicidal gesture. Accidental death is well within possibility. In this family session, we would spend time talking about the very realistic possibilities of death for this individual.

He is so extremely unpredictable and impulsive that death resulting from an accident while inflicting self-harm is not at all beyond imagination. His family members are all too familiar with this possibility but this discussion brings relief to everyone because it is a fact of life for this individual but few have been willing to verbalize it previously. It is also worth mentioning that, even on the inpatient unit in a hospital, it is not possible to guarantee absolute safety. If anyone is committed to hurting oneself or killing oneself, it is highly unlikely that even a hospital can truly keep him safe.

Of course, the one safe solution is to use seclusion and perhaps restraint while under constant observation. This would have to go on indefinitely because this individual's condition is not going to improve after a short segment of seclusion. In this session, we talk about how "locking someone in the closet and putting a camera on them" is not conducive to life either. Most everyone in his life would want to avoid this kind of scenario. But it is very easy to end up feeling that locking someone up in a padded room just might be a solution. There appears to be no empirical evidence that clinical intervention have any systematic effect on suicide completion (Maris RW 2000).

For me, if "safety plan" is meant as "coping skill" and that it is done at the right time and in the correct context, as I will discuss in the **Three Steps**, then safety plan can be immensely helpful. If "safety plan" is nothing more than a support network of people that this patient can contact at any moment of crisis, then it can perhaps be an effective method of keeping him alive in a life full of crisis but one has to understand that this may not contribute to helping him to do the work of healing and emotional growth. Here lies a great conflict. This is a conflict with many layers. This is an interpersonal conflict. This is a professional conflict. This is a moral and philosophical conflict.

We all want him to live. Family members, relatives, friends and even mental health providers can become paralyzed and run to solutions such as repeated hospitalizations and other highly restrictive options. Other measures of paralysis are such things as offering the individual with BPD unlimited access to everyone in his life. Support for him is then set up around the clock and everywhere possible. All this is done in the name of a "safety plan." Such extreme solutions constitute paralysis. One patient I worked with said that he routinely called the Crisis Line when no one within his crisis network could be tapped to fill his sense of the pain generated from internal emptiness. At times, he would even need to feign a crisis in order to access the Crisis Line.

For the most part, safety plans are good but I will explain here why some "safety plans" are created out of paralysis and in fact can promote greater dependency for this individual rather than help heal psychological pain. It has been found that short-term containment strategies and biological treatments do not provide a "fix"; therapists often find it necessary to tolerate suicidality over extended periods (Fine MA 1990, Maltsberger JT 1994). "When clinicians spend too much time worrying about suicide completion, this treatment process becomes derailed" (Paris 2002). "Coercive bondage" takes place in the therapeutic relationship when the clinician feels forced to take up extreme measures to prevent suicide completion (Hendin 1981, Rachlin 1984).

Whether on the inpatient unit or in an outpatient office, when the therapist becomes paralyzed by the patient's self-harm or suicidal risks, little attention can be paid to covering treatment issues. The therapist then busy himself or herself in setting up the best safety net possible and spends time checking to make sure that it is still working. Therapist countertransference could run rampant but there is little attention given to this problem due to the much greater concerns related to the entire ongoing crisis. This is therapist paralysis.

Not offering instant help and support seems counter intuitive in every sense of the word. But, what kind of help or support would work? What has not already been tried? When I look around in the family session at this point, I usually do not see any faces in support of the existing way of working with this individual. If my preparation of the patient for this work is done fittingly, I have now gathered around me a set of people who are completely exhausted from their work with this individual that they are able to understand what I mean by paralysis and they do not want to be paralyzed anymore. They may profess care and love for this individual but they also want a solution that will contribute to his healing and progress in treatment.

Death as a Reality

Once again, as a conclusion to this segment of the talk in the family session, I reiterate the reality of death for this individual. Hence, if we were to proceed without further paralysis, then we would all have to recognize the high possibility of death. The patient could die in the middle of treatment. It has been found that borderline patients with comorbid substance abuse and major depression were more likely to complete suicide than those without these comorbid disorders (Stone 1990). I want the patient and his family to really take this reality in and seriously consider it. The borderline patient and his family have to accept that his premature death may be inevitable rather than just a passing possibility. This is such an import message at this point that I would take a long pause and let everyone think about it for a moment. If there were any questions at all, I would entertain them at this point before proceeding.

When thus impressed with the magnitude in which this individual's acuity has caused treatment paralysis could this patient and his family to finally allow treatment to actually take place. As morbid as this discussion can be, I believe that this is the portion of the work that actually decreases the overall high risk of death for this patient. Bringing this issue to the surface does not condone the acts of self mutilation or suicide. Later in this talk, I place the act of self-mutilation and suicide in the context of acting out behavior. Once I am fairly sure that I can not ponder and proselytize about the risk of death further, I move on to the next phase of this treatment discussion.

A Caveat about Risk

A crucial clarification is warranted here in distinguishing the near constant crisis, characteristic of the borderline condition, from that of eminent danger that also arises periodically as would be expected in the borderline patient. *No therapist should ignore the plea for help from a patient feeling that life is without further options except to take his own life.* At such moments, all routine treatment considerations are off and the goal is simply to keep this patient alive. If adequate treatment discussions and preparations have already taken place, the patient, his family and the therapist should all be aware that no treatment will be rendered at such times and perhaps, treatment may be halted temporarily while everyone regroups in order to take up treatment earnestly after the initial crisis.

Predicting the risk of suicide of another human being is incredibly difficult and something therapists do poorly (Pokorny AD 1983, Goldstein RB 1991). At times, it is exceedingly difficult to predict which acts are self-mutilation and which is a prelude to an actual suicide attempt. Many factors go into suicide risk assessment. The patient's demographic should be considered. The patient's physical and emotional health plays an important role in determining his ability to cope with adversity. The stresses that he faces in life and the support that is available to him all play a critical role in determining how he copes with environmental and life event changes.

I would encourage the reader to further review the assessment of suicide risk in the literature given that this is a very important skill used in the daily work of therapy. If the risk of suicide appears quite high, paralysis in treatment can set in to hinder treatment. Outpatient treatment may not be safe or feasible at this point; inpatient hospitalization using DSA should be considered. If the decision is to keep to treatment on an outpatient basis, then a review of the great risk involved as described earlier in this chapter should take place with the patient and his family.

Summary

The foregoing discussion points to the ease in which all of us can become terribly conflicted and become paralyzed in our work with the patient who is frequently in extreme crisis. It is critical that the therapist recognizes such paralysis and works toward making therapeutic movement possible for the patient and all involved. In this process, the therapist has to be keenly aware of the risk of suicide, even though this is not possible to predict, and intervene as necessary. Treatment requires an alliance with the family in order to inform them of the rationale behind treatment and to educate them about the management plan. Involving the family and obtaining their cooperation in the treatment of chronically suicidal patients decreases the likelihood of litigation (Packman 1998). The therapist's display of confidence and care in this regard will earn him the needed therapeutic relationship for the work ahead. To prevent further paralysis and assure movement in treatment, it is imperative to have a reciprocal working relationship with an inpatient hospital setting that can initiate or carry on the treatment using DSA.

·VII·
THE CUP

"If you want to become full, let yourself be empty."
-Tao Te Ching

The Universal Cup

Still in the context of the family session, we can now move to our discussion of the understanding of the "self" within us. Thus it is, as I hope, that the "cup" is an easy metaphor for people to understand and accept the pain of emptiness within. Kohut describes the self as theoretically having a structure that has a history- a past, a present, and a future. Metaphorically, he makes the suggestion that the self is a structure that can become fragmented when "one's self-experience seem no longer coordinated or fitting together" (Wolf 1988, p.13). I find Kohut's theoretical understanding of the self very amenable to the self as viewed through the cup in DSA. Meares, similarly influenced by Kohut, wrote, "the experience of inner life goes in a kind of container, an inner space, which of course, is not real space but a virtual space like that behind a mirror, which we perceive but know is not there. This space is not merely psychic; it includes the body." "Experiences of the spatiality of self, of the body, and of the background emotional tone are all altered, in an episodic fashion, in those with disorders of self, fluctuating with the form of relationship with the social environment" (Meares 1993, p.24). As discussed here, the fluctuating content of the "cup" is symbolic of the variability of the self in relation to person, time and place.

It would be a sensible clinical assumption that, in psychotherapy, a patient may enter into treatment due to some sort of psychic pain, but most individuals require a convincing reason for making changes. A strong emphasis is placed on helping the borderline patient become acquainted with a language that helps him relate to his interior feeling world but still allowing him to take ownership of his experiences. It is my clinical experience that an illustration with a cup is a highly effective way to help everyone relate. This cup is useful as an analogy for understanding the workings of the self. It is a way of picturing how the self holds together in the best of times and how the self fragments at the worst of times. Thinking of the "level of content" in the cup allows us to gain a better sense of the transitory nature of how we might experience good moments and bad moments in life. The individual with borderline symptoms often has difficulty remembering that the sun is going to rise again the next day and that life is going to feel differently tomorrow. The cup of the borderline individual may experience wilder fluctuations, but he must also keep in mind that this variation means there are fuller periods as well as empty periods.

In this session, I ask everyone to imagine the ownership of a cup within. At this point, I draw a simple cup on the white board. By the way, in this day and age of the power point presentation, I still find it most effective to walk up to the white board and illustrate with big simple pictures in various colors.

A nice and clean projection can not make the same impact that I can make sketching figure 7.1 on the board. This metaphorical "cup" is nothing fancy and it is the same size, same shape and made of the same material whether you are king or pauper. We all have to answer to the state of the cup regardless of our station in life.

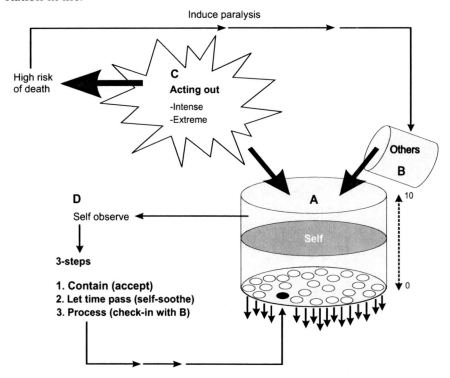

Fig 7.1 *diagrams the relationship between the "cup" and the actions that fills it as well as the actions that repairs it. Hypothetically, there are two main variables of input, B and C, into this cup. The drainage at the bottom should be thought of as a constant action.*

The cup is charged with holding the emotional "stuff" that we obtain from various activities in life. This "stuff" is not necessary good stuff or bad stuff; it is just "stuff". One might consider this "stuff" to be consistent with our general usage of the term "transference" that is taken to loosely mean the emotional exchange that takes place between two people based on their history and relationship with each other. This "stuff" helps us get through life. It sustains us in life. This is usually the love, the care, the attention, the support, the guidance, the validation, the encouragement, the approval, the dependence, and all that qualifies as exchange of emotional material. This material comes from the vital interpersonal relationships in our life. People pour this "stuff" into our cup on a daily basis; we can also call this transference. We receive their input simply by our routine daily contact with these individuals. Sometimes we seek this contact and at times we are simply thrown into contact with them by the nature of our daily life. This occurs in such a seamless fashion that we do not usually notice these very subtle exchanges. "I suggest that responses from others who fit an evolving personal reality have an effect, often quite subtle, of evoking a positive emotional tone, a state of well-being of which the individual is usually only dimly aware. An accumulation of these moments leads to a relatively enduring positive feeling about one self" (Meares 1993, p.59).

In a time in which the cup has sufficient content on a consistent basis, this stability of core source allows for this individual to feel comfortable, satisfied, confident, secure, patient, creative, playful, happy and sharing. *However, one should note that these positive attributes of feeling good are inaccessible to the individual who attempts to fill this emotional system with alternative content from acting out behavior.* In theory, temporary and rapidly fluctuating contents from inappropriate sources likely generates a semblance of "feeling good" without achieving the more stable and deeper emotional contentment. *Clinical experiences tell us that a steady state in the condition of the cup provides for a higher quality of internal experience regardless of cup content.* People generally identify the short term feeling good of excessive acting out as unsatisfactory and lacking any sense of security or confidence.

Examples of the people in box B:

- Parents

- Significant other

- Siblings

- Relatives

- Friends

- Classmates

- Teachers

- Religious mentors

- Co-workers

- Employer

- Therapist

- Inpatient staff

Figure 7.2 *is a partial list of possible relationship input to the cup. Keep in mind that this is probably a very fluid list given the interpersonal dynamics of BPD.*

My colleague who teaches DSA on our inpatient unit routinely discusses with his patients the differences in substance input into the cup. He likes to point out that clinical experiences would suggest that acting out input into the cup is like filling it with this emaciated, toxic material that lacks true substance, although, at an emotional level, this material feels satisfying. Conversely, the vicissitude of appropriate positive emotional input into the cup could be characterized as more viscous, wholesome and healthy. Clinically, patients often describe their input scenarios that closely resemble this metaphoric cup. Borderline patients often concur that it is easy to fill the cup with quick acting out input that seems "thin" and leaks out rapidly. Patients also tend to voice that more positive inputs last longer and appear to have a qualitative difference from that of acting out input. The primary purpose of using the cup in this model is to allow for easy visualization of good and bad input.

Not only do we receive the "stuff" but also give this to others. This mutual exchange is as basic and essential to relationships as water is to life. Analogous to our lungs, which go about the business of breathing without conscious efforts, the cup also operates seamlessly. For the lungs, air is only notable by its absence; at which point, the gasp for air takes precedent over the quality of air. When functioning properly, the cup goes about making sure that the good stuff that we get are stored and kept for as long as we can. Keeping the cup full is not something that most of us have to think twice; it is automatic and self-maintaining. In most instances, any repairs that are needed are done automatically to insure that the system operates fluidly and that the storage process is provided without fail. This is assuming that the self is intact, healthy.

There may be a natural self-healing tendency in someone with a strong sense of self. When examined closely, this individual probably has a natural affinity to following the rhythm of person, place and time in handling the events of life. This probably makes coping with stress easier especially in someone who maintains a fairly healthy cup. This self-maintenance is critical since the content of the cup is valuable beyond compare. When the cup is fairly full, we experience a great sense of contentment and fulfillment; we could feel at peace with ourselves and there is great calm in our world. As Kohut might suggest, this is a time when we feel highly creative and capable. In effect, we feel whole and complete. We are thus more able to deal with any difficulties or challenges in life. We have more to share with others. We are more willing to share with others. We can give to the cups of others.

Transference Filling

It is essential to include the therapist in the list of potential individuals who give input to the cup. "The therapist must become an appropriate selfobject or extension of the patient's self by providing appropriate gratification and mirroring responses in order to create a narcissistic equilibrium and to help the patient defend against painful self-esteem fluctuations, affective instability, and fragmentation of the self" (Masterson JF, Klein R, 1989 p.83). In the metaphor using the cup, it is easy to see how transference with the therapist can rapidly occur given that the patient's demand of the therapist is no different from what he required of others. For the narcissistic patient, he mostly wants the therapist and others in a mirroring transference in which everyone would listen admiringly to his transgressions. Oftentimes, the borderline or the narcissistic patient is also invested in the idealizing transference in which he feels the therapist can "magically" cure him (Masterson JF, Klein R, 1989 p.106). Thus, idealizing transference can function to allow the therapist an inroad into developing a therapeutic rapport with the patient.

It is upon the understanding of these types of transference that one can now picture the metaphor of the "filling of the cup." It is important to think of the "filling of the cup" in terms of mirroring and idealizing transference as well as the most general sense of transference. The reader may notice that I am using the terms "transference" and "filling of the cup" in an interchangeable fashion. In this work, I do consider the concept that transference is the source of the "material" that is poured into our cups. Understanding the importance of transference can help us understand the importance of the cup. *Transference plays a critical role in our relationships and the direct management of transference is at the core of our work in DSA.* Transference is a very powerful dynamic operating in our daily life; often, it leaves us in a very tangled web indeed. Such transference takes shape in many forms and under many situations; within our usage of the term, it can be a conscious or subconscious act. The reader will find that this work is about the appropriate recognition of transference, containment of transference and management of transference to promote a healthy sense of the self. In other words, healthy relationship leads to a healthy self.

In addition to the therapist, many others can act on the individual by giving input to his cup. In so doing, many people are involved in the transference dynamic with this individual. It is fruitful for the patient to be aware of his transference relationship with the number of people providing filling to his cup. "The damaged person has an almost intuitive realization that some fundamental lack in the sense of existence can be overcome in a relationship in which there is not only approval but also a sensitive responsiveness to one's most central personal experience. An idealization pervades this kind of relationship" (Meares 1993, p.170). Going beyond the immediate issue of the filling of the cup, transference can play an important role in his state of dependence or independence from his selfobjects and others. Through the work with DSA, the patient then learns of the dynamic he maintains with everyone in his life via his reliance on them for rescue input into his cup. It is important for the patient to realize the prevalence in which we all rely on each other to fill our cups; it is often useful for him to take an accounting of the staggering number of people he attempts to surround himself with in order to experience a semblance of good function. Despite corralling a staggering number of people into position to provide constant input to his cup, he inevitably feels that he is very alone and empty.

Managing the "material" input into the cup as a matter of transference brings awareness to the relationship between the self and the internal world of objects. The self has to feel secure in belonging to a network of human relationships (Jacobson 1964). A disruption in this network brings about a painful pathological experience consisting of a "predominant sense of emptiness and futility of life, chronic restlessness and boredom, and a loss of the normal capacity for experiencing and overcoming loneliness" (Kernberg 1985, p.213). Observing that the self is sustained within a network of interconnected relationships paints a picture similar to the propagation of seizure activity from a single node of irritability in the brain. For the vulnerable individual, one single breakdown of transference relationship can escalate to a seeming crash of the whole network.

Possibly, those he utilizes for input may even be the ones that he detest and dislike. This may seem improbable but real life is full of examples in which an individual appears to rely on his most problematic relationships for some sorts of emotional sustenance. Typically, this is the victim who seems unable to extricate him or herself from an apparent abuser. This is the victim of abuse who seems to gravitate toward individuals similar to the original perpetrator. In a different manner, this is the narcissistic individual who aggressively disqualifies a selfobject in his near orbit, in order to tolerate his hatred and envy for this object, yet continues to feed off this tense relationship with his sworn "enemy". In this work, extremes in relationships are said to provide a type of input into the emotional system that is experienced with equal acceptance by the cup. Through the cathexis of such an intense interpersonal interaction, he is inadvertently engaged in the transference input into his cup; this type of input consist of both interpersonal transference input as well as acting out input.

Thus, in the accurate understanding of our internal emotional system, one has to be truthful in our awareness of just how we obtain input to the cup. We must be aware of the myriad of possible input in order to avoid filling of the cup through channels of dubious quality. Most of all, one must keep in mind that we all have a choice in what types of input we allow in our cup. In this theoretical model, the ultimate condition of the cup, or the health of the self, is critical in contributing to our ability to exercise the choices each one of us has to make regarding our selection of input to the cup; it is all too easy to settle for something of lesser quality when one is constantly under distress. It is salient to keep in mind that the choices we make regarding transference input into the cup are not generally conscious decisions, that is, until such insight about our internal workings that allows us to become more mindful of the conscious choices that is at our disposal.

Transference input is often out of our grasp when one is in the throes of experiencing guilt or shame. At such times, the best of mirroring and idealizing transference may be insufficient to overcome the negative self concept. Regardless of our health of the self, at moments of guilt or shame, our fundamental propensity for cognitive distortion takes precedent and our ability to receive proper transference at a critical juncture in life is hindered. It is due to this dynamic that an individual in profound despair appears practically inconsolable.

Although the dynamics of transference will never be at the forefront of our consciousness, one can still manage to exercise control over transference input by fully understanding the issue regarding one's internal drive for input. Even though his earliest emotional hurt came from the blatant "betrayal" by a loved one, he continues to seek short term comfort from those who promises to love him with a special condition attached. "You are very special to me but you have to keep this a secret." Through his fundamental pain of disjunction, this individual suffers the anxiety of disintegration that threatens his very sense of self, an intolerable affect. Not surprisingly, he goes ahead and accepts such a transference input despite the toxic attachment involved; in emptiness, one is made to be even more acutely aware of the sense of powerlessness. A psychodynamic analogy comparing his fear of disintegration to that of a state of emptiness of the cup offers him a strategy toward making the choices of transference input.

The Role of Transitional Object as Input to the Cup

Of course, in our discussion of transference filling of the cup, one has to keep in mind a common way that is utilized to fill the cup; the use of the *transitional object*, a kind of selfobject substitute. This is a method of filling the cup that we all turn to at some point or perhaps, quite frequently. This is a reasonable way of coping and filling of the cup but is often beyond the reach of the teen or adult lacking sufficient selfobject introject.

Input from the presence of a transitional object may require one ingredient that is missing from the borderline individual's life, a connectedness with important selfobjects. One young man on the inpatient milieu turned to borrowing a teddy bear from a peer, being envious of the apparent comfort that another was able to derive from such an object. After a day of walking around with a borrowed pink teddy bear, he finally gave it back. For this patient, his problems with earlier selfobjects became evident in his difficulty in developing a workable relationship with a transitional object; thus, at times of crisis, not even a transitional object is available to provide transference filling.

Transitional objects "are special toys or playthings that act as maternal substitutes" (Cashdan 1988, p.41). Through internalization of the selfobject and the reliance on transitional objects, children are able to achieve sufficient constancy to separate from the mother by three years (Kaplan 1978, p.29). However, through childhood and into adulthood, most individuals likely continue to rely on some symbolic transitional objects. Kohut speaks of transitional objects as things that we use, even as adults, to maintain cohesion of the self (Kohut 1977). It has been thought that children can use toys with selfobject representation to play out the good self and bad self split experienced internally (Winnicott 1971, p.5). In our work, we will consider the transitional object as representing primarily the good selfobject and thus, capable of injecting positive input into the emotional system comprising the cup.

The Leaky Cup

If indeed the metaphor of the cup stands true in relating an emotional system that resides within each of us, there is almost no doubt in my mind that imperfection is sure to exist. The early developmental years are an obvious critical period for the healthy formation of the cup. As discussed earlier, numerous developmental theories suggest the notion of original anger which paves the foundation for our understanding of the imperfections of this emotional system. For most individuals, some mishap or trauma in the first few years of life may not matter greatly unless these problems translate to chronic lack of attunement with selfobjects. In addition, many individuals benefit from the resilience and adaptive ability of the young child to undergo some type of self reparative process that leaves them relatively unscathed from early developmental issues. Nature seems to allow for a window of opportunity for automatic repair prior to the latency period of development while the consequence of severe damage to the cup becomes highly palpable by the pre-teen and teen years.

Most leaks are more like trickles and it is of no concern. Genesis of the leakage is a matter of debate and scholarly deliberation. I will render a hypothesis based on object relation's theory as to the development of the holes in a following section. Regardless of the cause, the borderline individual functions as if he or she has developed a massive and constant drainage from the bottom of their cup. Effective treatment visualization of the leakage should resemble that of a showerhead; the water is draining out in a torrent. If the cup is the crucible for the self, then, this ache of emptiness has to be palpable.

A good conceptualization of the leakage will allow us further understanding of the transference filling of the cup. In this regard, we can borough from the cognitive behavioral tradition in its notion of the cognition distortion to account for the tendency toward leakage. Cognitive distortion can hinder effective transference which can result in limiting input into the cup. The self doubt and distorted perception of a situation will likely reduce transference effectiveness. Toward the bottom end, leakage might be understood through cognitive distortion such as, "My friends seem nice during our dinner but I know they would rather spend time without me." Thus, what appeared to be reasonably enjoyable time at dinner was quickly reduced to the usual sense of emptiness for the borderline patient; a leakage has taken place.

Drawing attention to the leakage of the cup, for which there is no better substitute than a big bold diagram on the board, the listener is treated to a bit of dramatic theatrics. The aim of this session is to effectively convey the seriousness of such leakage in its impact on the state of internal emotions. Illustrating the leakage with an actual demonstration by pouring water through a cup with many pinpoint holes helps to deliver a sense of tension as the container goes dry one more time. This simple demonstration in conjunction with the drawing on the board brings validation to the unstoppable emptiness the borderline patient experiences while suggesting the devastation of such an illness for the family to comprehend.

Wading into the metaphor of the cup, it is often the patient's own experiences with the capricious nature of his moods that readily draws him into this image. The ups and downs of his emotions set the stage for him to be able to easily relate to the rapid filling and emptying of the leaky cup. Quite often, patients and their family concur that while spending time with each other, the patient is prone to feeling content and even euphoric while the cessation of that activity leads to the patient feeling as if no togetherness ever took place. For the borderline patient and his family, it is their own testimony that gives credibility to the metaphor of the cup.

Life is rarely static. After misfortunes in life, we all hope for periods of improved fortune and an opportunity to regroup and heal. Perhaps we happen upon a total stranger who turns out to be our guardian angel or a kind friend or relative steps in to lend us a hand. Through such benevolent interchanges, encouragements and validations, our "cup" heals a little at a time. Most world religions do refer to similar concept as the Bodhisattva in Buddhism to attribute the random or not so random act of total selfless kindness from a stranger who comes into one's life at just the right moment to alter the course of our lives and open up new horizons for us. Through life's wild permutations, one would hope that our luck or fate can change and be prepared to seize upon the opportunity for change. I picture this to be the process in which we all learn to heal and happen upon change that allows us to grow stronger and live with a fuller cup.

The metaphor of the cup is very easy to accept and embrace because it is non-blaming and non-judgmental in nature. People often express feeling a powerful sense of disquiet on visualizing this drama with the cup. This is then followed by a sense of relief gained through having developed some insight about their own emotional world. The visualization of the cup releases them from the blaming and judging of self and others. In our society today, there are still many who feel shame and guilt regarding any ills of the mind. It is hoped that the metaphor of the cup takes the mystique out of mental illness and gives it a palpable form for repair.

Reflecting on Control, Dependence and Narcissism

In an earlier chapter, the matters pertaining to control, dependence and narcissism was discussed. In the approach to treatment that is described here, it is implied that the above issues arise out of an internal emptiness that is highly variable with or without external influence. Taking the metaphor of the cup further, we can then develop a better understanding of the psychodynamics of control, dependence and narcissism. In this understanding, control, dependence and narcissism are really not so different from our inference about BPD.

Borderline patient's frequently display struggles for control in attempts to gratify various dependency needs. His needs of others can be a direct helpless dependence on significant others or it could be a dependence based on the need to feel needed. Having discussed this earlier, I wish to remind the reader of the continuum in which the pathology of the self is viewed. Hence, when viewed on a continuum, the borderline and the narcissistic individuals have comparable clinical presentation. When these dynamics are seen through the metaphor of the cup, it is even more revealing of the similarity between these two personality entities.

Based on the analogy of the cup, it is then possible to picture the narcissistic pursuit of exquisite control could well have its origin in the painful emotions of emptiness. Ultimately, patients with issues of control and dependence tell of a sense of emptiness that is very much the same words used by borderline and narcissistic patients. The narcissistic patient may function better overall, as

Kernberg has asserted, but a deeper probe of narcissistic traits reveal the fragileness of his existence and the desperateness to temporarily restore his selfobject needs. A common sentiment amongst therapists is the challenge of helping a patient with control and dependence issues to recognize his fundamental responsibility to the self. Just as the narcissistic individual, the patient with control and dependence issues may have difficulty in capturing the essence of his behavior. Many excuses, blaming and rationalizations later, his plies for control and dependence seems, on the surface, to be a way of coping with the external world but in fact, the overwhelming pain is internal.

Without additional foresight, it is unlikely that he will develop the insight or the motivation to make changes. To understand this patient's resistance to change is to comprehend the powerful motivation of "feel good" acting out behavior based on control, dependence and narcissistic characteristics. The attempt at interpretation of such "feel good" behavior is generally a test of the limits of psychotherapy. The cup, as a metaphor for the internal emotional pain that drives the individual toward extremes of acting out, offers a approachable solution to understanding very ingrained psychologically defensive postures.

Sex, Drugs and Rock and Roll

Not everything is innocent about the cup. Look again at the cup and one would notice that it is quite *indiscriminate* in what it will accept; hypothetically, the cup will accept many types of input (Figure 7.3). This is a very important differentiation to understand about the functional dynamics of the cup; many people get into tremendous trouble in life without understanding the reason. We have already discussed the "stuff" or transference filling that is the input from important people in one's life. The cup will also accept content from some pretty surprising or perhaps not so surprising sources. Acting out behaviors as one of the primary sources of input into this emotional system is probably the most counter-intuitive concepts in this work; yet, it is central to the hypothesis of this approach. Having alluded to the fragmentation of the self, Kohut described "disintegration anxiety" as a fundamental anxiety involving the fear of inadequate selfobject response; similar to that of insufficient transference input to out cup. In this view propounded by self psychology, drug abuse, self-mutilation, sexual promiscuity, perversions and eating disorders reflect "an emergency attempt to maintain and/or restore internal cohesion and harmony to a vulnerable, unhealthy self." (Baker 1987, p.51)

Patients who perform self-mutilation provide a most intriguing glimpse into the intra-psychic world. Going beyond what authors have written about this inner space, borderline patient's reveal a great deal about his internal emotional life through describing the way in which self-mutilation seems to ease an emotional pain. These patients relate with a high degree of certainty that some types

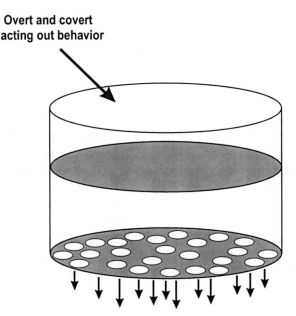

Overt and covert
acting out behavior

Figure 7.3 *The potential input into this emotional system using the product of acting out behavior can be quite counter-intuitive but must be understood as an integral component to this approach to treatment.*

of activities, labeled as acting out behavior here, can bring about a temporary quiescence of an internal disquiet. These behaviors reduce that intense sense of loneliness, emptiness and disconnectedness. This would imply that, in terms of the metaphor of the cup, this internal emotional vesicle can be pictured as potentially capable of accepting acting out input.

As far as I can judge, there appears to be an evolutionary purpose to such a multiply supported system in nature. "No complex instinct can possibly be produced through natural selection, except by the slow and gradual accumulation of numerous slight, yet profitable, variations." (Darwin 2004) Profitable or not, as the ever more complex mammalian system evolved, there became a requirement for multiple system backup or viewed differently, old useless appendages (such as the appendix) may remain to cause occasional complications. In the regular course of evolution, as the organism evolved from a strictly emotional system (think of ants) to that of a feelings system, in order to perhaps accommodate to higher intellectual functioning, the old system and the new system has to find cohabitation in the same sphere. The primitive emotional system operates on intense reactions and the more modern feelings system relies on a sense of connectedness with the selfobject world. Hence, the two types of input to the new refined emotional system are rather opposite and mutually incongruent but is possibly a witness to the process of evolution.

From the perspective of DSA, the lack of selfobject experience can contribute to a destabilization of the self which is illustrated by the decreased or lack of input into the "cup." With the pain and the hunger of an empty cup, he begins to engage in the search for quick filling to the cup. With such intense emotional pain and the inability to regulate distress, he is highly likely to turn to short-term self-soothing behavior and disregard impulse control (Tice et al. 2001). However, ordinary events in life, events that are not intense, extreme or high risk, would not serve to fill his emptiness and void. Given the severity of his emptiness, few selfobject, if any, can meet his needs. It would seem that ordinary events, activities and selfobjects are insufficient stimulus. He requires stimulus of higher arousal potential. Reading a good book, conversing with a good friend, relaxing at a nice spa, exercising, playing with your pet, doing something creative as well as a host of other activities are insufficient during a crisis of emptiness because such low arousal activities are no longer sufficient to fill the void.

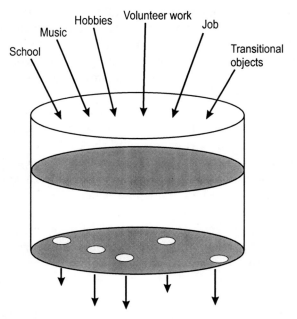

Figure 7.4 *Under more normal circumstances, filling of the cup can be achieved through lower intensity activities that reward the individual for the sense of personal accomplishment. These activities tend to be less effective in fulfilling the cup's needs at times of crisis within the apparatus.*

This patient is also unable to couple lower arousal activities with an adequate selfobject experience to make these activities meaningful from the perspective of the self. (Figure 7.4) As a result, this individual will have to reach for high intensity and high arousal activities or behaviors to find gratification and calm. Paraphrasing a patient, one stated, "If someone punched me, it would fill that void." Feeling calm or perhaps, liberating, could be the most reported end result of high arousal activities by the borderline patient. The borderline individual often reports use of such high arousal activity as drug and alcohol use. They can easily move from minor experimentation to severe drug and alcohol use due to the requirement for greater intensity. The same could be said about his use of sexual behavior as an act of high arousal. This is a patient who would frequently engage in severe acting out behavior, aggression and even antisocial acts. Perhaps, the thrills of breaking the law and the attempt to elude the authority are one of the most stimulating and high arousal activities available. Frequently, we witness the borderline patient turn to self-mutilation as a method of filling the cup. Once on this path for self arousal, the behavior can quickly escalate seemingly out of control. But, in fact, such behavior as well as any number of behaviors discussed thus far can give a false sense of control. Whether it is sex, drugs, aggression, risk taking, thrill seeking or self-mutilation, the hidden agenda is that of a sense of control in a world that is at risk of fading into nothing. I would include the contemplation and planning of suicide a potential acting out behavior. One patient commented, "In thinking about suicide, it just felt so good in my head." For this individual, fantasizing and planning a suicide can improve his feelings to the point where he would no longer feel that he has to carry through with it, at least until the buoyant feeling started to fade again.

This is not to say that this individual could not be serious about suicide. The suicide rate in the borderline population could well be higher if one takes into consideration the broader definition of those who suffers from pathology of the self. In a 20-year cohort study, patients who have engaged in deliberate self-harm was 10 times more frequent than expected for death from probable suicide (Hawton 2007). Many borderline patients dwell on the thoughts of suicide long before it became a serious determination. They may discover such contemplations are of very high arousal value and inadvertently turn to it as another route for the filling of the cup. At times, this act goes from a morbid exercise in the mind to engulfing all those around him when his contemplations are no longer private. When this occurs, this activity acquires further heightened arousal value.

I hope the reader can now picture how acting out behaviors can quickly become a vortex that draws the user into high risk behaviors even if it only provides temporary sustenance for the cup. In conclusion to this section, I want to remind the reader that there are essentially two types of acting out behaviors that is utilized in satisfying the cup. The first type is the ones that can pass for normal life activities but not done in accordance with the socially accepted expectation for person or place or time. The second type is acting out behaviors that are clearly not socially acceptable. Both types of behaviors are done for the purpose of filing the cup.

When Anger Makes Us Feel Good

What anger is doing in the background of our everyday life is one of the least understood aspects of our psyche. Even as anger is about to consume us and destroy our world, we still are unlikely to attribute our trouble to anger. Sometimes, anger actually makes us "feel good." Take the example of the teen girl with an extensive history of assaultive behavior who declares one morning in the inpatient milieu that she is having a much better day. Since arrival in the milieu, she has been a picture of depression and talked about feeling an intense sense of inner tension. On this day, however, she says that there has been some "drama" in the milieu that has troubled her. She is contemplating whether or not she should confront the person who is spreading some rumors about her. On exploration, it seemed that "feeling pissed" and ruminating on this issue actually allowed her to experience a sense of vitality that she normally does not get to enjoy. In her world, the intensity of such cognitive deliberation helps to fill her emptiness; a bout of physical altercation would be even better.

Acting Out Behavior is Intense, Extreme and High Risk

The characteristics of the more negative input into the cup can be summed up as activities that are intense, extreme and high risk. Some of these activities are not always inappropriate or even generally considered as negative behaviors. For some normal activities in life, doing it at the wrong time, wrong place or with the wrong person can make it an inappropriate acting out behavior. Some normal daily activities can become acting out behavior when it is used or indulged excessively. An example of this is excessive food intake or overly restrictive dieting. Occupational work can be taken to the level of workaholism and it then becomes acting out behavior. The common denominators to activities that are considered to be acting out behaviors meet criteria of being intense, extreme and/or high risk.

To make an indelible impression on my audience at this juncture, I would announce that the cup will accept "sex, drugs and rock and roll!" Not that rock and roll is necessary a bad thing; it just rolls off the tongue nicely and most people will remember this better than a stale list of unpleasant acting out behaviors. When does a normal life activity become an inappropriate way of feeding an indiscriminate cup? If sex is such a "normal" part of life, how do we know if it is used to fill the painfully empty cup or a normal life activity? Work is a normal part of life; but when does work becomes acting out activity that is used to fill emptiness? However, to understand the impact of these activities or events on the individual with BPD, we must keep in mind the manner in which these activities are used.

Food consumption is another very normal part of everyday life. However, some people eat excessively, beyond the need for nutrition and satiation. Some individuals restrict food intake beyond the bounds of what is considered a healthy diet. Where is the point in which one would consider these behaviors to be conscious or unconscious acting out? Acting out behavior are activities that contributes to the indiscriminate filling of the cup. Use of alcohol is seen all around us in everyday life. Its use and its role in society have cultural characteristics as well as genetic predisposition. However, any observer of alcohol use in any given culture would be left wondering about the precarious manner in which alcohol is used by some. Is it addiction? Or is it acting out behavior that has deeper psychological roots? Most casual observer might say the same of chemical dependency. It appears that beyond experimentation by some individuals, there are those who do it seemingly out of desperate need to escape from some terrible reality. One might comment that this individual is "self medicating" an emptiness.

Street substance use can then be seen as acting out behavior beyond the "I just like it" rational. It is easy to see how activities such as alcohol and drug use can become acting out behavior. What about activities such as sex, food and work? Where do we draw the line as to when these activities become acting out behavior? The rule of thumb that I use to gauge the difference between what is normal life activity and what constitute acting are covered under the terms: *intense, high risk, and extreme.* In other words, most acting out behaviors meet criteria of being intense, high risk, inappropriate or extreme in one or combination of the previous. Additionally, use of the concept of person, place and time can help make the distinction between what is normal everyday behavior and what constitute acting out behavior.

Not all intense and extreme activities are necessarily acting out behaviors. Most importantly, an activity is acting out if the individual can identify a feeling of great unease and emptiness prior to the search for high arousal activities. A notable sense of emptiness that regularly precedes the intense feelings of boredom differentiates this from the more plebian complaints of feeling momentarily bored. The difficulty in recognizing emptiness confounds the identification of acting out behaviors, which then results in the delay of doing good treatment for many borderline patients.

The Rollercoaster Life

Now that we have discussed what constitute inappropriate feeding of the cup, I will address the more blatant types of acting out behavior used by the borderline patient as temporary filling of the cup. Severe acting out behavior can generally be seen as actions that bring about heightened arousal. Frequently, borderline patients talk about a profound sense of "boredom" that clearly goes beyond the general usage of the term. It appears that the usual activities of everyday life can seem dull and uninteresting. He seems unable to appropriately entertain himself because the routine activities of daily life are never quite sufficient to keep his interest. He also seems unwilling or unable to utilize his own creativity or imagination to hold his interest in an activity. As a result, he could be seen searching far and wide for some excitement that can inject a dose of aliveness into his life. He presents as endlessly restless while rejecting any reasonable suggestions for activities he could do.

For any one activity to maintain the fresh intensity of a new and novel experience is very difficult. Predictably, many extreme and even high risk behaviors or activities lose its luster as soon as it is repeated a few times. Very often, the second attempt is already not quite as intriguing or intense as the first. This is all because physiological tolerance as well as emotional tolerance is the bane of human experiences. Therefore, the next rollercoaster ride always has to be faster, higher and with a new twist; the rollercoaster aficionado has to keep looking for the next big ride. The extreme sportsman has to keep looking for the next big wave or higher mountain.

Seeking of thrills can just be the pure pursuit of an extreme challenge but it is bound to disappoint if it is done for the purpose of filling an emotional void within. As emphasized in the previous section, the presence of a baseline sense of emptiness is a prerequisite to ferreting out the role of the extreme activity. Akin to the search for the next thrill ride on a rollercoaster, the borderline patient will steadfastly escalate his or her acting out behavior in order to overcome the natural development of tolerance to the initial emotional and physiological intensity. Many time, patients have related that superficially scratching oneself on the body no longer hold any meaningful experience because it is not an intense, extreme, or high risk behavior anymore. They may have to cut deeper, more widely or perhaps, do it in front of an audience or have others do the cutting on their body.

The ups and downs of the rollercoaster life have its consequences. With the escalation of extreme behaviors come the criticism and condemnation by others. Many such activities grind against the grain of our own moral and ethical judgments. The loss of self control evokes a drop of self-esteem. Hospitalization, incarceration, expulsion from school, loss of job, being grounded by parents, all can worsen one's feelings of shame and guilt. The ultimate consequence of the rollercoaster life is death when one tests the limit of an extreme way of living. There is a risk of pushing the rollercoaster to its limits and there are multiple risks in filling the cup with high risk activities.

Overt versus Covert Acting Out

In teaching our patients about acting out behaviors, it is far easier for most people to grasp the concept of overt or "hard" acting out. These are the various aggressive types of behaviors and the substance use as well as many other obviously high risk activities. Covert, or "soft" acting out is altogether a very interesting class of acting out behavior that is most interesting to discuss and most challenging to confront of our patients. The need to experience super control is covert acting out. The drive to fulfill a dependency need with significant others and the narcissistic penchant to lash out at others are all soft and possibly subtle acting out behaviors.

Covert acting out behavior is much more evident when viewed through the concept of *intense, extreme and high risk* behaviors. However covert or soft the acting out, the behavior is often of high risk, intense or extreme in nature. Someone who is unwilling or unable to come in touch with his internal feelings might find that he is physically unable to get out of bed all of a sudden. An extremely angry individual feeling powerless to change his circumstances in life finds that he is mute one morning. Although these symptoms can indicate affective disorders or conversion disorder but the differential diagnosis should also include the consideration of covert acting out. In our discussion, covert acting out can include those activities that are beyond our conscious awareness, as long as they suggest intense, extreme and high risk behaviors.

Consider the young man who woke up one morning with an inability to speak. He could not make one sound and no medical etiology could be found. Whether an unexplainable numbness of a limb or a mysterious muteness, these can be examples of covert acting out in that each symptom brings with it the experiences of emotional intensity. In DSA understanding, these symptoms garner intense interpersonal transference and therefore, filling of the cup. Hence, the experiences of covert acting out is joined by transference to create a rather powerful source of input to a desperately empty cup.

The patient should be aware that excessiveness or overdoing of any activity could potentially be deemed "acting out." Extreme nationalism, overt religious fervor, feverish political activism, ruthless work ethics, habitual gambling and excessive Internet immersion are just a few of the possible examples of acting out. This is not to suggest that any hard working person is subject to being labeled with pathology of the self. One has to keep in mind that the presence of a powerful pain of emptiness is one of the prerequisites to this disorder and the subsequent manners of coping might be inappropriate in the context of this emptiness. An executive working tirelessly to save his company from bankruptcy is not necessarily doing this to stave off the pain of the emptiness of the cup but simply facing a reality of life.

Covert acting out can also involves activities in which we are quite purposeful. Purposeful does not necessarily mean consciousness, selfish or intentionally hurtful of others, but rather, one has the expectation that one will feel better through this behavior. Sleeping too much and eating too much or too little are commonly encountered behaviors of soft acting out. Excessive shopping spree, gossip, ideological extreme and sexual addictions are just a few examples of covert acting out. Unconstructive criticism of others in reaction to perceived personal threat or competition is emblematic of narcissistic acting out. The perpetrator of such acting out does anticipate a sense of importance, confidence or satisfaction derived from the attack of others. Narcissistic rages are examples of acting out behaviors. Most, if not all forms of overt and covert acting out are rooted in defense mechanisms of splitting, denial projective identification, omnipotence and primitive idealization (Kernberg 1985, p.229). These are just some of the common examples of covert acting out.

Person, Place and Time

There is an appropriate person, place and time for all activities in life. It is my opinion that anything in life that is done outside of these parameter could potentially become a problem through the seeking of intense, extreme or high risk activities. As human beings, we naturally fall into the habitual pattern of structuring our life according to the precept of person, place and time. There is a particular time for meals. There is a particular time for work and school. There is a particular time for play. There is an appropriate time for a young girl to try on makeup. There is an appropriate time for the eager young boy to get behind the steering wheel of the family car. There is perhaps an appropriate time for a person to experience the first taste of alcohol. There is an appropriate time to explore the excitement of a first date and there is of course an appropriate time to experience sex.

Around the middle school years of development in which Erikson termed identity versus role diffusion, a child faces nascent ego identity and group identity. Confronted with the preoccupation for appearance, hero worship as well as ideology, the young individual most often finds himself or herself in the throes of following the pack. Not yet in the phase of individualism or independence, the pre-teen or teen seeking acceptance through sameness will have great difficulty awaiting the appropriate opportunity to experience life according to person, place and time. If this is the first time the child hears about the need to delay gratification until the appropriate time, with the appropriate person and do so at an appropriate place, he will surely find himself in conflict with the authority figure asking this of him.

When this understanding is instilled in a child from an early age, then this concept of the person, place and time becomes a very natural part of everyday living. A child who grows up understanding this concept will be able to easily accept the need to wait and be patient with so many of the things in life that he wants to explore. Picture a child who is willing to wait until she is older to try makeup. This is also likely to be a young child who will be more willing to wait and not be tempted to keep up with the most cutting edge of adult fashion. You see, this will be the older teen who is excited about trying out makeup for the first time. The message to the child is that when it is the right time to try makeup, "mom and dad will buy you a really nice set and you shall learn to do it well."

Along this line, when he or she becomes a teen, he is more likely to tolerate the admonition to refrain from experimentation with drugs and alcohol. He will understand that, when it is time for his first taste of alcohol, his mother and father will introduce him to this cultural aspect of life. This same concept can be applied to times when the young child is pushing hard to experience life ahead of the appropriate time. "When it is time, I will help you with it."- is the reply from his or her parent. Once a child understands this concept, he understands that when he is told that he could not have something or allowed to do something, he is aware that he has a chance to do it in accordance to appropriate person, place and time. With this understanding, it is much easier for him to allow time to pass before it is his chance to do all those things he could not do as a child. When it is time to do these activities, he then could do it as a more independent and mature person. When these ordinary events in life are done in accordance to the precept of person, place and time, then one is more likely to feel rewarded and fulfilled. When, finally, it is his time to try the activity, he is more likely to feel a sense of accomplishment and satisfaction and he can use this positive feeling to fill his cup.

Often, many ordinary events in life are done out of the context of person, place and time. An ordinary event in life can become a problem when it is not done at the right time, when it is not done at the right place or when it is not done with the right person. This is the teen who experiments with alcohol early in life by stealing a drink from the parent's alcohol cabinet. This is the teen exposed to sex at an early age due to abuse. He or she can then become a teen who is acting out sexually in discord with person, place and time. Most often, these young people express a sense of shame and guilt with such acting out behavior and realize in full, how short lived the gratification. If insightful, this individual might even identify a profound sense of boredom or even "emptiness" as driving force to the acting out behavior.

When these ordinary activities are used at a time when we experience profound emptiness within, suddenly, these ordinary activities are no longer quite so ordinary or innocent anymore. For the young person, sexual activity is not appropriate for many reasons including cultural and developmental. For young people and adults alike, sexual activity driven by a sense of desperate loneliness and emptiness can be highly harmful emotionally. Under these circumstances, people have described their indiscrete sexual activity as unrewarding and perhaps guilt inducing.

Moreover, such indiscrete experiences, whether forced upon this individual as in the case of abuse or self driven, will likely deprive this individual of the proper developmental growth. Thus, many victims of sexual trauma at an early age presents as if they have suffered from a degree of developmental arrest. This is why the damage of trauma can run so deep; it leaves an indelible mark in the psyche of the individual and freezes the development of the self. The teen who starts experimenting with alcohol at an early life with equally young peers miss out on the support and validation of this activity from significant figures in his life. The anorexic patient who makes a control issue out of the daily routine of food intake is deprived of the celebration of family at the food table experienced across all cultures. These are just some of the examples of how person, place and time plays an important role not only so that the individual is appropriately patient with life but this is important in the proper development of the self as well.

If a developmental pathway frequently eschews the context of person, place and time, the healthy development of the self would come into risk. Activities pursued outside of this triad tend to suggest high arousal activities that are intense, extreme and high risk. These activities may not be the genesis of the pathology of the self, but the maintenance and perpetuation of these activities works against the healing of the self. Eventually, these activities could evolve into sources of covert acting out.

Attention Seeking versus Self Soothing

Having discussed the severe acting out behavior, we now turn to behaviors that are more difficult to categorize and place. Attention is something we all need regardless of our age or station in life; but the excessive seeking of attention could be an indication of some degree of emotional pathology. Often one hears the patient's family, relatives and friends complain that the borderline patient is very "needy" of attention. In our study, I will use the term, seeking rescue, to describe an action that is more consistent with filling of the cup. Often, he asks the same question repeatedly. Often, he needs repeated assurances. Often, he complains excessively of being mistreated by the others and seeks reassurance and rescue from his victim role. Sometimes he presents as helpless and vulnerable and seeks constant safeguard. Often, he presents as sad and unhappy and blames it on others; he places responsibility on others to help him retrieve a better mood. Often, he becomes highly talkative and demand full and absolute attention from others around him. Often, unable to wait his turn and continually interrupts others to express his point of view but he is usually unable to find his thoughts. Often, he talks about feeling bored and works hard to convince someone to entertain him or to take him someplace to do something interesting or exciting. Frequently, he acts out in minor and annoying manners on a fairly constant basis to get the attention of those around him.

Most commonly, this type of behavior is referred to as "attention seeking" behavior which is attached with much negative connotations. This is generally viewed as highly willful and manipulative behavior to wrestle attention from those who may not be willing to participate. Whether we call it attention seeking or rescue seeking, it can quickly generate tremendous transference based negative feelings from others. Transference is defined as those perceptions of, and response to, a person in the here and now that more appropriately reflect past feelings about, or response to, important people earlier in one's life, especially parents or siblings. "Attention seeking" behavior can easily provoke transference with the patient's family and friends. Of course, through projective identification, attention seeking could also garner care taking behaviors from others.

These same types of behavior can just as easily provoke countertransference issues with mental health providers. When combined with negative projective identification, these dynamics can quickly breakdown any working relationship the therapist may have with this patient. A provider can come to feel highly resentful and angry about feeling intruded upon and manipulated. This is a natural reaction that likely arises from our own learning and upbringing. After all, these attention seeking types of behaviors are precisely the ones that our teachers and parents have admonished us about. In the case in which one is able to keep check of our countertransference issues, one may still experience any behavior one considers "attention seeking" to be of poor etiquette or born of poor upbringing. Whether one experiences the negative reaction to the patient's attention seeking behavior as part of our own countertransference or inappropriate behavior on the part of the patient, the outcome is conceivably that of pure loathing.

Within the DSA model of treatment, "attention seeking" behavior is viewed in the light of one's desperate need to fill the cup; this constitute an antithesis of the popular perspective on attention seeking behavior. In DSA, filling of the cup is experienced as self soothing for the individual; we all experience it and we all use it. Since we understand self soothing as a matter of our fundamental wellbeing, it is natural that the filling of the cup should also be fundamental to daily function. By understanding that self soothing is as critical as breathing, one can then make sense of the desperate need to fill the cup when it is running empty.

Given that acting out behavior or its lesser version, the rescue seeking behavior, can be easy alternatives to filling the cup, it is not difficult to comprehend how this type of behavior can be a matter of survival for the individual with BPD. This view of acting out behavior and attention seeking as self soothing behavior motivated by the need to fill the cup can help us better deal with countertransference issues and our loathing of such behavior. There is less of negative connotation and less sense of manipulation with this perspective. Henceforth, it would be easier for the therapist or the inpatient staff to address attention seeking behavior in a more productive and treatment focused manner.

One particular inpatient scenario reminded me of the importance of recognizing the difference between attention seeking behavior and self-soothing behavior. A female teen patient with severe pathology of the self who is often teetering between reality and psychosis suddenly decided that she desperately needed to get the attention of a particular male peer. As she ran down the hall and started to flirt with this peer, staff attempted to intervene and reminded them of appropriate boundary expectation on the unit. This intervention quickly melted down to the point in which the female patient had to be physically contained for her safety as well as that of the others. The boy was mildly amused by the girl's approach and the staff was just doing his job to maintain appropriate interpersonal boundary but the situation deteriorated badly.

The question here is whether or not the staff could have intervened in a more effective manner in order to avoid such an escalation by the patient. Because this patient behaves in a constantly provocative fashion to engage the attention of others, she leaves most people feeling that she simply loves attention and enjoys being in the spotlight. This behavior does not garner much empathy or compassion from most people. In fact, this behavior often draws competition from some of her peers who could not stand to watch her get all the attention. Unit staff have an equally hard time maintaining neutrality in the face of such behavior and in the case of this particular incidence, they may have been more harsh and confrontational than need be. Instead, if one were to view her reckless attempt to get the attention of this boy who was practically a stranger to her, in spite of the strong prohibition of such mingling on the unit, as a desperate bid to fill the practically empty cup, one may be able to be more compassionate in one's approach toward this patient. A more productive intervention would be to assist her in recognizing the emptiness in her cup at that very moment and help her to identify this as a possible treatment opportunity. If she has sufficient understanding and investment in treatment at that point in time, she may be very willing to reconsider her action and take an alternate route that is more productive. Interestingly, many such interpersonally dependent patients are willing to put this agenda on hold once they truly comprehend this dynamic through DSA.

Just as frequently, the unit staff or therapist observe with concern that several patients who are normally quite needy of attention are suddenly rather content to leave staff alone and appeared to be rather distant. In querying the patient about the state of his feelings, he answered repeatedly, "I am just fine. There is nothing wrong." This commonly encountered scenario on an inpatient unit is fraught with complex treatment issues. Realizing that the decreased demand on staff is a temporary respite from the needy frenzy that may characterize this patient's daily life on the unit, the staff does anticipate trouble for this patient within a short time. In addition, as staff look around the milieu, he or she is likely to see that, perhaps, one or few of the other patients seems rather quiescent as well. On one hand, things appear on the surface to be quiet and calm, why disturb such peace? Now, to an experienced staff, this could raise serious concern about the treatment milieu.

In a treatment program that is not based on DSA, this quiescence on the unit could be interpreted as an indication that this patient or a group of patients are generally coping well, utilizing the skills taught in treatment to tolerate distress or possibly, this calm is the result of recent insight development in individual or family therapy. Not to down play the role that psychotherapeutic insight development can bring about in the course of treatment, however, one has to keep in mind that such breakthrough in treatment is difficult to achieve and infrequent even in the course of intensive and long term therapy work. From a DSA perspective, this decreased engagement of the patient is worthy of concern for several reasons. Firstly, these patients may simply be resisting treatment and therefore, not engaged with the program. Secondly, even though this patient is not engaged in working with staff on treatment issues and not seeking much of staff attention; it is conceivable that he is able to somehow satisfy his internal emotional needs through some other avenue. Thirdly, as I have endeavored to emphasize, one must be aware of the continuous leakiness of the cup.

In the DSA manner of consideration for treatment, the therapist has to take into account the constant sense of the emptiness that this patient has to contend with in his every moment of wakefulness. From this consideration, one would then anticipate that he will try to fulfill his needs through another mode of self-soothing if this is not achieved through seeking rescue with staff. As it turns out, staff investigated and found that several patients have formed an alliance of sort to meet each others needs. On observation, staff reported of poor physical and emotional boundary involving undercurrent covert behavior. The intense focus on each other and establishing the "us against them" mentality toward staff only fueled the propensity for splitting in a milieu generally prone to such dynamics. In so doing, these individuals are demonstrating their usual mode of function in daily life to cope in a fashion that is minimally functional; ineffective and inappropriate self soothing took precedence over treatment focus, this codependent style of coping will sooner or later break down to another episode of the crisis of the self. It is important to note that this manner of self soothing is not consonant to the 3-steps to be described in the next chapter. In further review, the treatment team decided that this dynamic is not conducive to engagement in treatment of any modality and certainly not treatment according to the concept of DSA.

In helping to bring his focus back to treatment, for a patient who is versed in the DSA model, the team only needed to articulate the importance of being mindful of the state of the cup. This was exactly how the team confronted a group of patients by reviewing the dynamics of such codependent, rescue seeking behavior as being wholly for the purpose of obtaining input from group B in diagram 7.1. Why is this behavior inappropriate? The heavy reliance of input from B can be inappropriate in the context of the patient's sole dependence on this input while neglecting the leakage at the base of the cup. Most often, it takes just such a brief reminder for individuals to further understand the significance of their action in relation to the cup and make immediate correction to become more invested in treatment.

Aren't Friends Supposed to Help?

"What do you have against friends?" Borderline patients have frequently been puzzled by the seemingly incomprehensible prohibition against friends when trying to understand this work. Many have felt flabbergasted at the apparent suggestion that relationship input from a friend can somehow be inappropriate. The notion that friends are supposed to be helpful goes back to the dawn of man in which alliances and allegiance were critical to survival.

"Let us state, he said, that a friend is one who is both thought to be helpful and also is; one who is thought to be, but is not helpful, is thought to be a friend, but is not" (Grube 1974). Friends are supposed to be helpful; this response pertaining to the definition of friendship arose in a dialogue between Plato and Socrates.

One of the most outstanding technologies today is the advent of the popular availability of communication method using the Internet and the cell phone. As a result, a significant majority of teens and adults are never without this mode of indirect companionship. Beyond chatting in the hallway or the cafeteria, sometimes even text messaging in the classroom, the young person could also continues to talk on the phone and message deep into the night. In this constant connectedness, it has been found that co-rumination contributes to increases of depression and anxiety, especially in teen girls (Rose 2007). Co-rumination is defined as "excessively discussing personal problems within a dyadic relationship", consisting of mutual encouragement of problem talk, rehashing problems, speculating about problems and dwelling on negative affect (Rose 2002). Related literatures hint at the connection between depression and emotional problems with that of over involvement in others' problems as well as excessive reassurance seeking (Joiner 1992, Prinstein 2005, Gore 1993).

Viewed from a DSA perspective, friendship serves three fundamental functions. Firstly, in the interpersonal orbit, friends provide a consistent and predictable source of relationship filling. This type of filling of the cup mostly arises out of spontaneous or otherwise unscripted daily interactions. (A further discussion of this issue in regards to daily interactions with treatment staff takes place in chapter 3.) Secondly, Socrates suggested that the essence of friendship is the willingness to be helpful. Even today, the notion of friends helping friends is precisely the expectation held by individuals, societies and geopolitical systems. As a result, friends often do come to our rescue when one is in emotional crisis or in an emergency state. Finally, in respect to BPD, friends are often called upon to provide the relationship filling in the ongoing emotional emptiness of the borderline or narcissistic individual.

It is this potential misuse of friendship that is the treatment concern in DSA. Although co-rumination may bring youth into closer friendship, authors in the 2007 study suggest the concern that "youth in friendships characterized by co-rumination may go undetected by adults, thus leaving them vulnerable to the development of emotional adjustment problems." The borderline individual has to come to sharp awareness of the counter productive nature of this demand in a friendship in his longer term health of the self. In the context of treatment using DSA, friendship filling of the cup outside of routine interchange and specific crisis intervention is considered to be interpersonal rescue; this is distinguished from normal interaction through the recognition of the emptiness within. Sitting in group therapy session, a teen lifeguard capitalizing on his experiences to comment about his tendency to become enmeshed with others by expounding that, "I am rescuing in an ocean of emotions."

A Developmental Perspective on the Cup

It is helpful to have a hypothetical understanding of how this "cup" forms as part of the psychological makeup of a person and relate it to classical developmental understanding. From the writings of Jean Piaget, Margaret Mahler, Sigmund Freud and Erik Erikson, we understand the ages of zero to five to be very critical developmental years. Although this cup is imaginary, I like to think of it as an organ like any organ such as the lungs, heart, liver, kidneys and brain; each organ matures in its developmental course and has its stated function in the body. In our discussion, the cup symbolizes the fluidity and stability of the self. It is then useful to have a developmental picture of how such a psychic structure might develop in an individual over time. The manner in which I portray this developmental process is perhaps simplistic, but I do think that it is sufficient to serve the purpose of our discussion.

The Developing Cup

Picture, if you can, an amorphous material flowing amongst the primordial ooze that comes together to form the cells of a fetus in the uterus. This liquid material gradually gels over time to form a rudimentary vesicle of sort. It is initially a very incomplete structure that barely suggests the forms of a container. This is how one could imagine the "cup" of an infant. It is not yet a truly useful structure. It is full of leaks. It really does not serve much of a purpose. So, what does this pre-cup do for the infant? This is precisely the point here. For the infant, we can speculate that he or she lives from moment to moment without any real sense of history or the future. The infant is content and perhaps "happy" when his mother is there to feed him and comfort him, a reliance on mirroring and idealizing transference. At that moment, he can take in his mother by vision, by hearing, by smelling and by tactile senses.

If one were to consider this state of existence for the infant further, one can begin to get a glimpse of the terrifying state of existence an infant can face when he is all alone. The human infant is not able to fend for itself in any way or manner. He is one of the most vulnerable creatures on the planet. He is completely dependent on his mother or his caretaker. He is endowed with very little instinctual ability to function or survive in life but he does have the inherent ability to recognize his consistent caretaker. He is able to show joy when this mother figure is around and he panics when his mother is away. Of course, we all know that his mother is not really gone. His mother may have just stepped out of the room to get him another bottle. When the infant sees his mother leave the room, he has no idea if she is ever coming back into his life. He does not know if she is coming back to feed him and comfort him. He does not know if he will ever again enjoy the love and comfort that he relished when she is present. In essence, the infant has to learn to *accept* this fear and *contain* his urge to act out. These rudimentary coping skills will then form the basis of the 3-steps to be further discussed in a later chapter.

In the discussion of projective identification in Chapter 3, idealizing and mirroring transference were described as important elements that help support the early infant self. The combination of the idealizing and mirroring transference together with the attention the mother lavishes on the infant, this is sufficient to allow the infant to form the illusion of a cup that sustains him through infancy. The infant lacks the capacity to store any of the good "stuff" that he gets from his environment; he is not able to store the sense of comfort, love and safety that he is able to enjoy when his mother is present. He is truly living in the moment. It seems to be the classic saying about "out of sight being out of mind." Anyone who spends enough time around infants could readily identify with the vulnerability of the infant at this stage of life.

Infant Learning to Cope

We don't know precisely how the infant would feel at a time of unease but his sobering cry may give us an idea of just how distressed and upset he feels. Does the infant just have to accept this state of existence? Does the infant need to go through this traumatic experience repeatedly? Conceivably, the mirroring and idealizing transference may not be enough to assure constant stable sense of self at this stage in life. It probably does not make developmental sense if the infant goes through this convulsion between calm and high anxiety on an ongoing basis. From an evolutionary and developmental standpoint, one would expect that some type of coping has to take place until such a time that the infant is old enough to take in the reality of how life around him operates.

The fact is that, in reality, we do see the infant coping elegantly with those empty moments when his mother is not present. We see the infant making attachments to such inanimate objects as a toy, teddy bear, blanket or the pacifier. These items appear to be used by the infant to soothe himself temporarily. How long can the infant soothe himself in this fashion? He may not soothe himself for long; soon, he is going to require the return of his mother or caretaker to feel secure and satisfied. The objects that he picks up to cuddle or to suck on are only for short term coping. These are transitional objects; these items allow him to *let time pass* while awaiting his mother's return.

At this juncture in the family session, I would talk about the continuing coalescence of this amorphous material in the primordial ooze that is the beginning of life. I would get everyone to picture how this material is starting to form a shape that can now be recognized as that of a container of sort. As the infant continues to mature, this material is also maturing and forming a "cup" that is more of a container and therefore able to start to function in its purpose to hold the "stuff" of life that the child is receiving from the people and the world around him. This container is perhaps not perfect at this stage and still can allow much of its contents to leak out. However, it is holding in far more of its content than it was before. We can observe the progress of the formation of the cup by watching the infant mature into a toddler and the toddler mature into a young child. At each stage, we can witness the greater emotional stability and self-confidence of this young person to explore, wander away from his mother and play independently.

Internalization of Maternal Figure

As the child develops the ability to tolerate the absence of his mother and starting to be in touch with his own feelings, this newfound independence and sense of the self is reflected in the development of the internal cup. In the language of developmental psychology, this process of maturity is termed the internalization of the selfobject. Due to the lack of integrative capacity of the early ego, this early cup is still functioning in a limited fashion and maintains the self in a separated good and bad split as well as maintaining the object in a similar split (Kernberg 1985, p. 25). In our use of the cup as an analogy for understanding the degree of security in this process of maturity, the young child begins to possess the ability to hold this maternal figure within his being.

However, the early rudimentary cup can swing from being very full when there is immediate input to being quite empty when instant input is not available. In the DSA perspective, when the cup is full, the self and object can be experienced as good and when the cup is empty, the self and object can be experienced as bad. The integrative capacity is improved as development progresses and the cup becomes a more mature vesicle for holding its content. If, however, frustration and anger pervades his existence, which leads to fear, anxiety and guilt in analytical terms, splitting and projective identification can result. This is not conducive to the healthy development of the self and in the language of DSA, translates to the porous base formation in the cup.

Given a normal trajectory in development, the child matures and become more capable of holding the transference relationship that he receives from his mother, he is now able to keep a part of his mother with him even though his mother may not be physically with him. This is a very critical part of a child's development. For the practical purpose of discussion and understanding this complex developmental issue, we are going to say that the child "holds his mother in his mind and in his heart" by placing this "stuff" that represents his mother in the internal cup. We will use this very important concept of the internalization of the maternal figure to help us understand how this very critical developmental phase can give us clues as to how best to help the individual with BPD.

First Sign of Independence

Having a maternal figure ever present is likely unnecessary as well as, perhaps, problematic for the young child. Margaret Mahler talked about the Rapprochement subphase and Erik Erikson talked about the Autonomy vs. Shame and Doubt to emphasize the importance of independent function by the toddler. There have been suggestions that less than perfect parental attentiveness is still quite adequate because it means the child has to sort out how to cope on his own. The temporary absence of the maternal figure allows the infant and toddler to acquire experience of relating to the transitional object as well as experience the consistent return of the mother. Some children with a highly available maternal figure early in life may actually delay the utilization of the transitional object until pre-school probably as a result of the need to cope with greater independence required at this age. If development for this child progresses as expected, one would find a child who is now more secure when his mother is absent. Secure development encourages the child to experience greater ease to explore his surroundings away from his mother.

The healthy development of the infant and the young child requires that he exercises the essence of the 3-steps on a daily basis. Waiting for his mother to return with another bottle, going to sleep without parent's help, coping with a moment of loneliness and learning to play by oneself are all daily examples of the child's use of the 3-steps. In the context of the 3-steps, he now becomes more secure in the trust that his mother will return. As he becomes more familiar with his own feelings of fear and uncertainty and copes with these feelings successfully, he can now better take on greater exploration of the world around him.

Based on infant developmental hypothesis, I would like to share with my reader an intriguing clinical example that may serve as a synopsis of our discussion here. A certain young girl of nine entered the hospital milieu following repeated failed foster placement. Instantly, she went about demonstrating her capacity for violence when she did not get her way. Through biting, spitting, hitting and kicking, she demanded absolute attention from her staff. As if engaged in sibling rivalry, she jealously guarded her time with staff but seemed never feeling secure or happy about her existence. For this young child, no amount of traditional therapeutic intervention and teaching mattered at times of outburst.

To test our object relations understanding of child development, the treatment team decided upon a rather unusual approach. This nine year old actually comes across as an infant/toddler by her behavioral presentation. Her sense of insecurity speaks loudly of a lack of object constancy. The team then provided her with a one to one relationship with a "mother" and placed her in a "nursery." We were under pressure to complete our work in two weeks and thus, divided the treatment into three phases to fit into this span of time. For nearly a week, she was in an exclusive relationship with her "mother" and the staff was instructed to start to set up scenarios based on the 3-steps as soon as the third day. Fortunately, she was able to "bond" fairly quickly and adjusted to the engineered separation from staff with minimal difficulties. Once staff is able to successfully extricate for brief periods of time and reliably return to her without overtly frustrating her, she seemed much more comfortable to operate on her own. Subsequently, she was able to reenter the general milieu and interact with others with greater ease. Has she attained object constancy? It is highly doubtful that such progress could be made in the extremely short amount of time but further study is needed in better understanding the dynamics of this work.

True Self, False Self and Dissociation

Maintaining a healthy core self, the cup, is reciprocally dependent on the appropriate balance of the true and false self. These three entities are so closely connected that one can not exist without the others. Yet, we want to view the mechanism of emptiness in a separate state from that of the workings of the true and false self. It is also useful to examine the true self and false self on a continuum. On this spectrum, whether it is weighted more toward the true self or the false self, one must keep in mind the notion that at any one time, both aspects of the self are present. With these principles in mind, one can now study the intricate manner in which the internal emotional world operates.

An important aspect of healthy development of the cup relates to the opportunity for the young child to be able to experience a true sense of the self. This is when a child gets to feel that he is respected as an individual, his feelings count and his thoughts and ideas are valued. He should learn to trust that his feelings are all his and does not belong to another person. When he falls, the degree of excruciating pain that he feels on his knees are for him to determine and this pain does not belong to anyone else and therefore, he will cry if he wants to or perhaps, he will not cry at all.

If on the other hand, after falling, an adult comes around and appeared so extremely distressed at his wounded knees that this adult's visible distress caused him to falter about how he should really feel about his own knees, then he is likely to feel quite frustrated about whether to cry or to choke back the tears. If instead, after skinning his knees, the adult approaches him with consternation and demanded that he keep a brave face and not make a fuss. This too can be rather confusing to him about what is an acceptable feeling to have at a time like this. Such are the examples in which the child is left feeling unsure of the ownership of his feelings and the acceptability of his feelings; either way, he is deprived of an opportunity to be in touch with his true self.

True self or authentic self often refers to our ability to access our real feelings and the comfort to express ourselves without influence from others or in response to our own projections. Projective identification is the scour of humanity and comparable in magnitude to the worse of disease epidemic while allowed to sneak by as a minor player on the stage of suffering. False self is the lackey of projection. I believe that it is often far easier for the false self to take center stage given that our social world is often too hostile for true self to be counted. True self represents the respect others offer us and foster within us. Most importantly, authenticity of the self can only happen when the cup is in healthy condition and reasonably filled.

Much like Jung's four archetypal figures of ego and shadow, representing the good and bad split in all of us, the persona and soul-image, representing the face we wear for society and the projected dream, myths and fantasies, one might view our emotional system as composed of opposites vying for attention as well (Hyde 2005). In this view of the emotional system, there is a reciprocal influence between the conscious and unconscious components of our psyche. In such a system, the cup is considered a conscious component and it co-exists with two subconscious entities, the false self and the true self. This is a very dynamic system whereby conscious and unconscious parts of the self interface with the external world through the cup.

This hypothesis makes the assumption that the true self and the false self exist simultaneously while one may be more dominant at any given time depending on the state of the cup. (Figure 7.5) Thus, early anger and frustration promotes the presence of the false self; this is a person who is anxious, jealous, envious, spiteful, sad, insecure, overly confident, artificially happy, obsessive and/or full of rage. He is unauthentic in trying to be everything to everyone which usually ends sadly in his failure to please anyone, including himself. When frustration looms, he is likely to retreat further from true self, surrendering to the false self in which the opportunity to be authentic is lost to his anger and resentment; thus is the damage to the cup of the core self.

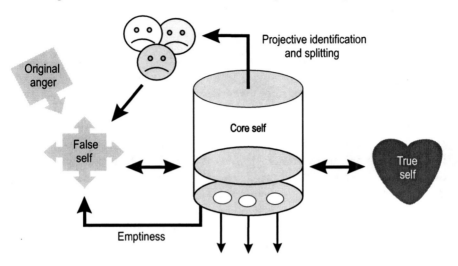

Figure 7.5 *Original anger promotes the formation of the false self which in turn damages the core self. False self, attempting to be everything for everyone has arrows pointing in all directions. True self, false self and the core self exist in oscillation with each other. Beyond the early damage by original anger, sedimentation of original anger in the cup tends to bring about projective identification, a threatening dynamic that maintains the prominence of the false self. As the false self is inflated, the true self becomes anemic and contributes to a lesser share of the core self.*

Looking to the clinical descriptions shared with us by our patients, it is clear that conscious and unconscious components of the psyche are all acting in concert to function as a whole. To this conclusion we must deduce that beyond the early impact of anger and frustration on the false self that there must be a current manner of reinforcing the false self as well. We can now further appreciate the immense power of the projective identification and splitting defense mechanisms. (Please review projective identification and splitting in chapter 9) As the cup, representing the conscious self, becomes drained, sedimentation of original anger is now dispersed toward those standing nearby in the form of projective identification. Now, others may take on an appearance of threatening stance that makes it difficult to differentiate the reality from that of projection; thus, the false self is further activated.

Furthermore, the concurrent psychological pain of emptiness at this juncture also contributes immensely to promoting the use of the false self. One must keep in mind that the core self is primarily concerned with survival. Thus, the false self serves as a type of survival function when the self is in fragmentation. In this mode, one can enter into a host of personalities such as strong, vulnerable, fragile, angry, comical, serious, uncaring, concerned, ingratiating, belittling, involved or aloof. In extreme cases, use of the false self in conjunction with severe regression may involve dissociation. On the principle that such an unconscious strategy has the purpose of regaining the function of the self, one might view the false self as attempting to engage others, or perhaps, the selfobject, in transference input.

Through this brand of understanding, it is important to remember that the activation of the false self may have the primary purpose of surviving the destitute of emptiness. Through acting out behaviors as well as rescue seeking, the borderline individual may achieve a level of emotional fulfillment. But we have every reason to believe that this satisfaction is not only short lived but of questionable quality. Therefore, while in this state of pathological filling, this patient is unable to experience the authentic self. He has learned long ago that the true self is insufficient in garnering input to the cup. This is not surprising since it takes the forfeiture of true self in order for this patient to access intense pathological input. We may further infer that acting out inputs are conducive to inducing scenes of shame and activation of doubt, which further fuels the prominent use of the false self.

These remarks highlight the insidious nature of emptiness and the influence this has upon the formation of the false self. With respect to this view, true self becomes a state that is more difficult and complex to reach. Authenticity of the self could not be reached simply by will or cognition; it could only be accomplished through an adequate repair of the cup over a period of time. Many patients do indeed retrospectively recognize the overt presence of the false self but are unable to truly make changes through simple coaching. Even on the chance of appropriate selfobject input, as long as the self is suffering significant developmental injury and "leaking", the rapidity of the loss of content does not allow for the stable construction of the true self. Emptiness must be overcome through the gradual repair of this constant drainage.

Summary

As I have emphasized throughout this work, the metaphor of the cup is simply a way to visualize and understand the developmental potential of an individual as well as the behavioral aspect of the borderline patient. The behavior of the borderline patient is intricately linked to an unstable internal state attributed to the inability to sustain the fruits of the selfobject experience. This instability accounts for the unpredictable mood and brevity of positive interpersonal experiences as well as the tendency to incorporate severe acting out behavior in daily life. The cup is an analogy for the emotional dynamic at play in each person and the "filling of the cup" is a metaphor for the psychological drive and motivation behind many of our behaviors.

I would maintain the notion that the lack of emotional regulation, the leakiness of the cup, tends to be a steady state once established in the early years of life. However, it is plausible that further damage can be sustained by the cup in severe trauma or frustration prior to completion of developmental maturity. Without repair, the cup remains in an unsteady state of dysregulation although, on observation, the individual's behavior in addressing this disrepair could appear to worsen as he seeks inappropriate filling and continuing the access of the false self. As an adult, severe invalidation, lack of attunement or chronic use of insidious feeding of the cup results in the fortification of split self and object representation. Through ongoing invalidation from the selfobject, he remains hesitant, insecure, frequently fragmented and out of touch with his true self. It is in this abnormal developmental state of the leaky cup that this individual will have to traverse the vicissitude of daily life.

·VIII·
The Three Steps

"In Chinese, the word for crisis is wei ji, composed of the characters wei, which means danger, and ji, which means opportunity."

-Jan Wong

Self-observation

The foregoing discussions have led us to addressing the daily work of therapy. Up to this point, I have engaged the patient and the family in the opening discussions to pave the way for starting treatment. We have weighed the high risk of death whether treatment is rendered or not. Then we got to understand some developmental theories and how this relates to our understanding of the treatment issues using the metaphor of the cup. Following the intensive preparatory work with the patient and his family, I am now ready to start the core aspects of treatment by emphasizing self-observation and reflection.

Presently we will talk about the work involved in making repairs to that leaky cup. In this approach to the treatment of BPD, the developmental discussion of the cup and the 3-steps are implemented in a complete introductory package. My clinical experience informs me of the benefit to complete the overview discussion of this work in one extended session of about sixty to ninety minutes. Although busy with information, the audience of this session should arrive at a general impression of this work. If without a complete understanding of the work ahead, he should at least derive a sense of the importance of engaging with this therapy.

Having alluded to the presence of the aversive inner tension that resides within, it is essential that the borderline patient comes to accept self-observation as a matter of working in treatment. Indeed, the overture to the 3-steps begins with self observation. Much of this work focuses on understanding the internal emotional world as the foundation of embracing treatment while self-observation is the key to starting in therapy.

A Balance in the Work Relationship

Treatment is at its best when the therapist and the patient strike a nice balance in taking the responsibility for the joint work that they are doing. Most therapists would agree that psychotherapy is all about the power of healing through this treatment *relationship*. If one partner in this work oversteps this delicate balance, then the dynamics of this treatment relationship shifts and the therapy is less likely to be as productive. The goal of the initial acute intervention should be that of independent function without acting out. For the individual with BPD, he can be highly dependent on others, while at the same time, highly dependent on acting out as well.

Through this work, he should become more insightful of the interdependent nature of his pathology. In this work, I strongly promote a degree of patient independence through the encouragement of self-observation and the 3 steps; this will require the therapist take a strong support and guidance position without having to coach the patient excessively. The artful balance of this position is critical to the productive outcome of treatment for the patient. One of the principle emphases in DSA is that of encouraging the healthier independent function in the context of interactions with significant selfobjects.

A Review on Emptiness

To begin the work with the 3 steps, I first ask my patient to work on identifying the sensation or the feelings of emptiness within. This is likely an inner tension that is at the baseline of his daily existence and he is generally highly familiar with this feeling. Therefore, when asked to make note of the existence of this feeling, he should have no trouble doing this part of the assignment. However, the introduction to this treatment can be challenging for the borderline patient because of his propensity to subconsciously turn to various distractions and rescues from the internal pain. Most likely, his instinct is to act out, even before the full onslaught of the familiar pain within.

Often, the patient would describe feeling "stressed" and would in the next instant turn to engage significant others in an intense interaction or conflict. When "stressed", he may turn to the use of drugs and alcohol. When "stressed", he may turn to self-mutilation. A frequently encountered problem when patients are asked to identify the emptiness within is that he has been coping with it by ignoring it for so long that he is not used to stopping and looking closely at these feeling states. What is even more challenging is that he has now rationalized why he has such apparently poor coping; he often blames others. His avoidance of feelings may lead him to comment that these feelings are of no consequence. "If you have a feeling you don't like to feel, would you stand there or would you find the first thing that takes this feeling away?" At times, he may say, "If it feels good, why stop?" About his self-mutilation, "I just like doing it." When he turns to peers or "friends" to seek escape from his pain, he proclaims, "They understand and they make me feel good." See case 9.1 for illustration. To achieve good movement in therapy, he needs to begin with a good conception and acceptance of the emptiness within.

The work of self-observation is for the patient to take note of any feeling state or the lack of, into account. One individual suggested, "It's not like it is empty. It is full of something negative." For these individuals, the state of emptiness is experienced as an intense sense of hollowness that parallels awareness. For others, this is a feeling state that is incredibly difficult to comprehend and describe. As opposed to a sense of feeling happy, angry, embarrassed, envious, jealous and the more "common" set of "feelings", the individual with BPD is most often battling with a sense of feeling numb and empty most times. In contrast to the heaviness and immobility of classic depression that barely lifts as the hours of a day passes, the borderline patient can have moments or even extended periods of feeling without great emotional burden when "all the stars align", as one individual once accounted. Of course he is capable of feeling happy and angry as well as a host of other feelings but notably, the sense of feeling empty is the predominant driving force behind the bulk of his pain of daily existence. At this point in treatment, I want him to identify this emptiness and this tremendous pain within. I want him to understand that I will not be frightened off if he was to bring this pain out into the open.

Therapist Acceptance of the Patient's Emptiness

The therapist must be aware of the patient's projective identification as well as his own countertransferential issues. In the context of therapy, the projection of this internal emotion most often is done subconsciously. It is conjectured that even the infant is capable of discerning the subtle changes in the mother following the infant's projected distress. "The normal infant needs to be able to sense that her mother is struggling to tolerate her projected distress without major disruption of her maternal function. The mother will be unable to avoid giving the infant slight indications of the way she is affected by her infant, and it is these indications which allow the infant to see that the projected aspects of herself can indeed be tolerated" (Carpy 1989, p. 293).

I want him to feel comfortable that I am interested in his internal pain state even though I may not have a similar experiential background to understand precisely what he is going through. He may be skeptical that anyone is capable of understanding his suffering but the therapist, a professional, is in the best position to validate his pain. The showing of compassion by the therapist then leads to a gradual development of empathy toward the patient's position. I want him to understand that this is not a discussion to challenge his feelings but an effort to work toward validation of his internal pain. He should feel comforted that he does not have to justify or prove to the world that he has such unbearable pain within. This is an opportunity for the patient, in the context of the therapy, to perceive that the therapist is affected by the patient's projected communication and then to witness the struggle by the therapist to tolerate the negative affect and ultimately to contain it without acting out (Pick 1985).

With adequate coverage of this issue in the family session, he is hopefully comfortable that the significant people in his life are accepting of him and his condition. With sufficient trust and validation, he can now safely identify his sense of emptiness within. In so doing, I now want him to identify this feeling state as often as he can. We are in fact going quite the opposite to the avoidance of such pain but instead, to be very much in touch and embrace the existence of this state. This should be quite foreign to anything that he has experienced in the past. He no longer has to hide his pain and operate in secret. If he wants to, he could be given a work sheet that allows him to document the frequency in a day in which he can stop and take note of the existence of such sense of emptiness.

Recognizing the Subtleties of Dependence

Once he is willing and able to identify the sense of "emptiness" within, he has a very important choice to make regarding a commitment to the work of healing. This is a highly critical juncture in treatment. He has to understand that identifying and embracing his feelings is notable but the challenge lies ahead. The goal of this phase of the treatment discussion as well as the upcoming days and months in treatment is to help him to truly recognize the subtleties of his acting out behaviors and the extent to which such behaviors are often ignored. In this session and in subsequent sessions, his resistance to treatment will have to be confronted aggressively. Treatment will also have to include a clear set of understanding and expectations to prevent any confusion about what constitute healthy interpersonal interaction.

The therapist has to remind him that his ongoing method of coping with this pain of emptiness has been to act out in some fashion. In terms of the cup illustration (fig. 7.1), he could reach reflexively toward input B (people) and input C (acting out) as he has done in the past for the temporary satisfaction of filling a desperately empty cup. Even though the mostly positive input from people is seen as reasonable coping, it has to be recognized as a method of temporary coping. In his denial, he may reason that his level of interpersonal interaction is nothing unusual or pretend that it is all done in normal social interaction and not for the purpose of emotional rescue. If the patient still maintains the belief that his interpersonal interactions are well within healthy limits, the other participants in the family session may disagree. This is why it is so crucial that family or significant others should be involved in this treatment session to make certain that everyone comprehends the importance of doing this treatment as prescribed. Of course, the people that he accesses most often, because his cup is practically always empty, are prone to chronically feel burned out and exhausted from emotionally supporting him. As a result, people may start to drop out of this set and he has fewer and fewer individuals who are going to be there for him at a time of need.

A suicidal teen who was repeatedly confronted regarding his lack of focus in treatment was in fact enamored with a female peer. At the conclusion of a DSA feelings exercise in which each individual is asked to refrain from interacting with others for only a few minutes to focus on his or her own feelings of the moment. In so doing, he later reported of experiencing the familiar aversive emotional sensation during the initial phase of this exercise. His therapist commented, "I saw that the two of you spent some time together seemingly really enjoying your time together. Were you feeling good just before group session started?" His answer was "yes." Therapist then added, "Now, only a few minutes later, you are reporting of the same empty feelings that you always get." This patient's eye lit up with an alertness that was not observed previously and he indicated a sense of surprised recognition of a basic frustration in daily life. The point of this interchange was to help the patient realize that no amount of gratifying interpersonal input will remove or replace the pain of emptiness.

In some rare cases, there are instances in which the people in his life may insist that they can provide unlimited and unfailing support for him. They encourage his dependence on them with a stoic sense of self sacrifice. There may be family members or a significant other who is willing to provide whatever support that may be demanded of them. Some people may consider this to be the best reflection of their commitment to this individual. They may even say to this individual that what is offered is "unconditional love." Arguing squarely from the court of common sense, one might prudently point out that such "love" is neither feasible nor sustainable. Besides, the borderline patient may already be aware that such "gifts" often comes with strings attached and the acceptance of such a gift is to keep the true self hidden. "Unconditional" can often lead to "unlimited" and in DSA, unlimited input into the cup is neither desirable nor welcomed. Instead, in DSA, through the use of the 3-steps, it is reliability, predictability and sincerity that hold the most value for those who want to help him heal a very injured cup. Furthermore, through the 3-steps, the borderline patient comes to realize that he can still be loved even if he functioned independently.

Generally, most people are interested in making progress in life. Most people do want to be healthier and happier in life. All of his previous ways of coping with his pain of living has to do with bringing about a false sense of feeling better in life. Therefore, when faced with the prospect of continuing to cope as usual and continue to deal with a leaky cup or try something different and perhaps discover a better sense of fulfillment in life, most are likely to opt for the later.

Working Together in Object Relations

With respect to treatment, once the individual with BPD indicates his readiness to start this portion of the work, he has already accepted a number of important and fundamental underpinning to this approach to treatment. The understanding and acceptance of this approach to treatment requires a profound paradigm shift for the patient and the therapist. The traditional notion of overcoming an impasse through the careful exploration in psychotherapy is not the expectation in the acute intervention. What matters most at this stage of treatment is the patient's acceptance of a model of disease or disorder that fairly accurately conveys his internal state of emotions. In this case, the model of the empty cup in our diagram is used as a representation of such a state. It takes a certain degree of faith in the therapist for the patient to accept such a model of disease. This portion of the work with the 3-steps continues to require that the patient accept this model of disease that I have proposed thus far.

A strong cognitive acceptance of this model of disease is important because the result of this work is not going to be readily experienced. This reality is more so in the work with DSA than perhaps other modalities of work given the interpersonal balance between the patient and others. DSA is an emphasis on the trust that is negotiated with the selfobject without overt reliance on the object through the use of the 3-steps. Even if he accept the earlier discussion of how the cup is a receptacle of the "stuff" of life, he is now faced with quite a challenge to picture how all of this work is going to translate into improving his being. I have found that *my own conviction about the effectiveness of this work has a dramatic impact on the patients that I have worked with.*

In many ways, the work of any kind of psychotherapy relies greatly on the therapeutic relationship and the respect of the therapist as a professional. Of course, the work of therapy is much more effective if the patient is experiencing such "pain" that he is willingly seeking help. Given sufficient therapeutic alliance and adequate preparatory work to help the patient understand the model of disease with the cup, we are hopefully ready to move on to the final discussion with the patient and his family about how the repair of the leakage in the cup will take place. Most likely, we are still in the marathon session with the family present when I discuss this final section in treatment. I have found that this treatment approach is best presented as a whole in one session if possible.

Pre-3-Steps: Introspection

The initial foray into the work of the 3-steps is not easy. Prior to this point in the work, the emotion of emptiness has already been identified and its existence has been accepted. This section refers to the pervasiveness of this emotion. For most, identifying a sense of emptiness at times of conflict and crisis is all too familiar but taking note of this feeling at other times can be rather challenging.

This is despite the acknowledgement of his pervasive emptiness. His ability to monitor this internal state is a keystone to success in this treatment.

In the thralls of rage, it is not difficult for the patient to realize the presence of intense emotions. However, the ability to observe feelings at any given moment and to relate this to the pervasive emptiness is important to his treatment and must be practiced with skill. "I feel great. Nothing is bothering me." These are, in practice, very worrisome statements to the discerning clinician working with borderline patients. It should be quite apparent that such moments of feeling well is not to last and that the inevitable storm of emptiness will soon take center stage.

Despite the various benefits in the practice of the 3-steps, this work is less meaningful without the concurrent mindful observation of the pervasive presence of emptiness. For some individuals, their suffering is a very private business. They become even more isolated in their depression and rarely do they act out in any easily detectable external fashion. Even though they may act out covertly through extreme isolation and seclusion, without a profound insight about emptiness, they are not able to truly take on the work of healing. Hence, the proactive analysis of one's internal feeling state is a highly critical step. Therefore, the preamble to the practice of the 3-steps involves a self-observation and reflection that is highly relevant.

Through clinical experiences, many instructors of DSA have developed their own methods of assisting their patients to come in touch with their internal emotional distress. Through written assignments, group sharing, mindful focus, meditative exercises and individual coaching, patients can rapidly gain the confidence to engage emptiness. In so doing, the therapist has to be sensitive to the patient's underlying ability to tolerate the palpable emotional pain that can be evoked through the pre-3-steps. It is advisable for the patient to partake in these exercises in small segments in order that he is not overwhelmed. In-depth exploration of past traumatic events should be held as separate sessions from that of experiencing emptiness.

Many patients report that the exercise to bring to awareness of the internal emptiness is much harder than explorations of past traumatic events. It is quite possible that the continuous engagement of defense mechanisms tend to strip away the immediate rawness and pain of trauma. Furthermore, emptiness is hidden or covered up through incessant focus on the filling of the void within. For the novice patient, these exercises to familiarize oneself with the pervasive emptiness can be both enlightening and rewarding. He is enlightened in the realization of the insidious nature of emptiness and he is rewarded in his beginning effort to master the control over this emotion. Therefore, the self-observation of the pre-3-steps is an indispensable part of this approach to healing.

Upon the observation of that feeling of emptiness within, the patient can now proceed to the implementation of the 3-steps. The steps are to contain, let time pass, and process in this order. I would emphasize that these steps have to be completed in this order for apparent reasons that I will explain later. Another important rule to follow is that the first two steps have to be completed by the patient alone. The final rule in working the three steps is that the third step is highly critical to the healing process and should never be skipped if healing is to take place; the first two steps only accounts for best coping. When the 3-steps are viewed as engagement cycle and accomplishment cycle that finishes with a joint celebration, the purposes of the steps become more apparent.

Step One – (To Contain/Accept)

Now let us turn to the patient's choice of actions following his awareness of the aversive tension within. Turning to interpersonal rescue or acting out behaviors is not conducive to his long term wellbeing. In choosing the work of healing, he is to exercise the containment of any urge to act out. Not acting out means to refrain from the contemplation of death, self-mutilation, substance use or any number of self destructive behaviors as well as covert thoughts of extreme ideas or concepts. If the patient is suitably secure in his understanding of the pain of emotional emptiness, he will now show some interest in finding a way to heal and discover a better way to cope with emptiness.

The adherence to refrain from any overt or covert acting out behaviors is arduous. In this step, it is required of the patient to delay any instant gratification. He will not feel a reduction of emptiness or internal tension except for the small amount of fulfillment in doing step two and three. The strenuous pain of the emptiness is still hovering over him or stirring within. To contain his urge to act out in his usual manner is not natural or instinctual to him. Hospitalization may be an appropriate consideration for the borderline patient who is very emotionally unstable or actively under the influence of drugs or alcohol. If necessary, the inpatient setting can offer him a degree of external containment that is beyond him at this time. Even though his choices for self destructive behaviors may be restricted in the inpatient setting, it is unlikely to contain all of his acting out behaviors.

In DSA, he is discouraged from approaching other for comfort or soothing at the first sign of emptiness. In his world of profound sense of loneliness, he is actually asked to refrain from attempting to seek some sort of joining with another individual as is likely his habit. To contain means that he should not reach reflexively at just anyone to save and rescue him from that moment. In the past, he may try to engage others by any means possible at a time of emotional crisis. In so doing, he has come to rely overly much on what others can do to soothe him at a time of crisis. He may have grown so dependent on them that he feels completely at their mercy for the attention and soothing that he needed from them. In 1958, Winnicott proposed that a child's "capacity to be alone" is preceded developmentally by his attempt to act as if alone in the presence of the selfobject. The child then achieves more advanced functioning through the use of transitional objects if the selfobject does not take on the role of the transitional object. Subsequently, if the selfobject allows the child some independent function, the child can then adopt the use of the transitional object to achieve a sense of ownership of his psychic life.

As has been discussed in an earlier section regarding co-dependence, he may have been an unwilling or perhaps, willing victim of a relationship that requires him to neglect his true self in order to avoid the expression of his real sense of anger and frustration. It is likely that he has some undercurrent resentment for his unwitting dependence on others or perhaps, he has a great degree of anger for their seeming lack of response to his needs. Either way, there may already be a great deal of the love/hate relationship between him and just about everyone in his world. In turn, others often feel ineffective in helping him. They may feel that they have given him as much as they could; they feel drained and exhausted. They too are human and in terms of DSA, they too need to work on filling their own cups.

In actuality, life is such that when he is in need of someone, there may not be anyone around. What about his therapist? Isn't his therapist supposed to be available for just such a time? Well, it depends on one's perspective on psychotherapy and how a therapist should function in the context of treatment. In DSA, the therapist does not hold the unique role of being the sole proprietor to the work of helping the patient heal. The therapist is seen as a professional who will guide the individual with BPD in his treatment and encourages him to be mindful of the concepts in treatment. In DSA, the therapist is not viewed as a coach, who is generally someone highly directive and advise giving, but rather as someone who fulfills the selfobject role and eventually helps the patient to internalize the whole object, consisting of both the good and the bad parts of the object. Internalizing the whole object is the same end goal of being able to hold the object within, as if within the cup, for long periods of time without the constant input of the selfobject.

In DSA, the borderline patient is discouraged from accessing his therapist prior to the completion of the firs two steps. When the patient accesses his therapist before the completion of the first two steps, he should be aware that this is a choice to fill the cup for the short term and is not a part of the work of healing. Contacting the therapist prematurely with the request to review and clarify treatment steps is a rare occurrence and mostly unnecessary since there are only three simple steps to follow in this protocol. Therefore, it has to be very clear to him that reaching out to feel good through acting out and prematurely reaching out to access others are not effective methods of coping at times of emotional pain. *However, an absolute crisis is a time to put treatment aside in order that others may step in.* In DSA, premature involvement of others without mindfulness of the 3 steps is viewed as a treatment conundrum regardless of whether the treatment involved is DSA or other modalities. Once he is able to see the limits to the few options that he has, the pre-requisite to contain would seem far more achievable.

To contain one's instinct to seek rescue or to turn to acting out behavior is an exercise in facing the realities of the internal pain. In some modalities of treatment, the patient can at times arrive at the perception that, "I have to fake it until I make it." He may be given to the feeling that once he is indoctrinated to a type of work, he has no excuse to feel poorly unless he is somehow resistant to treatment. Human intelligence and cognitive ability are at times valued above all else in certain models of therapy. When his intellect fails him, he has little recourse and once again, feels the sting of shame. This can contribute to the frustration that many therapists and families face in their work with a borderline patient after many years of work. However, the whole of DSA is based on the premise of helping the patient accept the pain of emptiness while making a concerted effort to partner with the patient in recognizing the depth of this emotion. Promoting a greater sense of connectivity, the borderline patient works on establishing an awareness of his internal emptiness through introspect in preparation for another moment of mirroring and idealizing transference with a selfobject in the context of the 3-steps.

The therapist should also be reminded of the importance of respecting the 3 steps in one's therapeutic interactions with the patient. All too often, the therapist, through the patient's projective identification and the therapist's own countertransference, reacts in accordance to the patient's projected distress and attempt to offer a solution prematurely. In this case, the therapist fails to offer the emotional containment in balance against the patient's chaotic turmoil. The patient needs to be made aware of the therapist sensing and regulating his own as well as the patient's affective state. "The essential step in creating a holding environment in which an affect-communicating reconnection can be forged is the therapist's ability, initially at a nonverbal level, to detect, recognize, monitor, and auto-regulate the countertransferential stressful alterations in her bodily state that are evoked by the patient's transferential communication" (Alhanati 2002, p.37). Premature intervention or interpretation can represent a therapeutic misattunement. A better way as Sands (1997) states, "…if I allow myself to be taken over by (the patient's) experience, successfully contain it (and wait until later to interpret it), she becomes calmer and more organized, and her need to communicate through me decreases in intensity."

To Vent is Just to be Angry

All too often, the common misconception that venting can rid us of anger is played out with the advice to buy a punching bag, to hit a pillow or the prescription to scream in an organized therapy group. "The idea of getting rid of our anger by giving vent to it has some dramatic appeal and in a way might even sound like fun, but the problem is that this method simply does not work" (Cutler 1998, p.254). In describing a scene in therapy in which a child was using puppets to sling vitriol at one another, his therapist commented in his writing that, "As fascinating and alive as the play was, I reminded myself that simply venting feelings does little to help a child understand or manage them" (Bromfield 1992, p.99). In DSA, anger and hatred has another face; it is the reflection of one's emptiness within. An emotional disconnection acts like the fragmentation of a mirror in recall of a more distant time when an important selfobject failed us. "However, extreme maternal failure to adapt impinges on the baby like repeated loud noise. The embryonic self is, for these moments, obliterated" (Meares 1993, p.115).

Feeling a sense of rejection by an important other can lead to the sudden emptying of an already leaky cup which could then be experienced as anger, envy, jealousy, guilt, shame, hatred and so on. Whether the anger is the direct result of the emptiness within or the evocation of original anger (discussed in a later chapter) through which projective identification is manifested, the external expression is that of aggression and the internal dynamic is that of an attempt to seek emotional balance. Externalizing anger through acting out aggressively is experienced as temporarily effective in making up for the low level in the cup. For the individual with pathology of the self, anger is experienced frequently as would be predicted by his sense of emptiness. This type of anger is not to be confused with the sudden flash of anger expressed by an individual faced with an extraordinary circumstance. Many subject matters, such as crime, war, terrorism and other inexplicable brutality, induce anger and hatred in contexts beyond ordinary frustration. Anger in the setting of these types of atrocity is not the target behavior for which DSA is to serve, but step-one, the effort to contain, can nevertheless be valuable in accomplishing the virtues of *patience* and *tolerance*, the teachings of His Holiness the Dalai Lama (Cutler 1998).

Achieving Containment

For the indoctrinated patient, the work of containment can be a much more sophisticated affair. Whether through his own mindfulness or simple coaching from a selfobject, he is able to connect his acting out urges to the internal state of the cup through constant introspection. He needs to avoid any potential use of covert acting out as discussed earlier. The more advanced patient should also be made aware of the existence of splitting and projective identification. True containment can not be achieved in the presence of rampant splitting and projective identification. An awareness of such defense mechanisms should point to the intrinsic pain of emptiness and trigger the need to exercise containment.

Insight regarding the use of classic analytical defense mechanisms allows the borderline patient to achieve a higher level of success in his treatment work. Defense mechanisms are often steeped in intense feelings about another that ties us to anger and hatred. In so doing, we are inadvertently exercising a type of acting out that defeat one's attempts to contain all acts of inappropriate filling. Appropriate containment is an individual matter. Absolute containment may not be achievable especially in the case of individuals lacking in psychological readiness for this level of insight. A fair degree of containment from the most severe of acting out behaviors would suffice for a patient just entering into treatment. The maturation in therapy consist of the transformation toward better awareness of all potential acting out.

On occasion, the therapist may encounter a patient who has surrendered all hope of feeling better and insist that "I feel empty but I am fine." This patient will go on to maintain that he or she has no reason to contain any acting out urges because "I mostly don't act out." To such an individual, the work of the 3-steps can seem meaningless and the resistance to treatment can be great. The insistence that he has no need to contain is often misguided because this individual is likely engaged in various covert acting out through entertainment of extreme ideas or disposed to intense sense of self loathing. The intensity of such cognition in combination with emptiness will undeniably result in covert acting out. And thus, this is clearly an individual with a need to contain the emotional pain of emptiness in order to further treatment.

Step Two – (To Let Time Pass/Self-soothe)

Once containment has been achieved, he has a chance to do the work of healing. The second step is to *let time pass*. This is a very interesting step for several reasons. This is the step in which I picture the coming together of many different disciplines in therapy. In this step, I tell my patient that he is free to exercise this portion as he pleases as long as he does not seek help prematurely from others or to act out. Depending on his creativity, there is actually a great deal of latitude in this step. He could utilize any number of relaxation techniques. He could use the multitude of cognitive behavioral methods of coping. He could work, play, relax, meditate, sleep or exercise, as long as these activities are done with moderation and within reason.

It has been suggested mainly through self psychology that one also has the option of utilizing an inanimate object to help bring about cohesion of the self. This is akin to experiencing the remnant of transitional object such as the infant pacifier. Certain familiar items can be infused with selfobject introject that represents the symbolic good mother. Whether turning to one's favorite music, clutching to a cherished figurine or sitting amongst a special collection of books, these things we seek at times of uncertainty. At moments of fragmentation of the self, these symbolic items can offer us some comfort and refuge from the pain of emptiness.

A crucial rule of thumb at this juncture being that the first two steps have to be completed by the patient without any assistance from others. Any help from another individual at this step could be considered as his attempt to seek rescue and soothing at a time of emotional dysregulation; to fill his cup when it is draining empty. The insipient involvement of the therapist would be highly counterproductive at this moment. Whether for the purpose of feedback, guidance, problem solving or expression of support, his therapist must refrain from the professional urge to instantly engage him. For the patient, the impetus of the second step is to gain a sense of accomplishment and self preservation.

For most therapists, practicality makes it prudent that one's patients should make appointments ahead of time so that the therapist can better manage his work hours in an organized and collected fashion. It is the rare instance when a therapist would allow his patients to call whenever he or she is in need of consultation and make this the routine as opposed to the exception; it would indeed make even more hard work of the challenging life of a therapist. In most cases, we urge our patients to make appointments. This is a request that would already set some therapeutic expectations in motion. Because the appointment time is set sometime in the near future, the implicit understanding is that the patient is expected to somehow manage the best he could until the designated appointment time and date. At the appropriate appointment time and at the designated location which would be the therapist's office and with the therapist in person, would then the issues and problems of the recent past be reviewed and discussed.

This is in keeping with the concept of the person, place and time that I have mentioned in an earlier section. To conform to the concept of the person, place and time, means the same as asking the patient to handle the 3-steps on his own while waiting for the time of the appointment. In this respect, the first two steps in this work is nothing new at all. The crucial difference is regarding the treatment of the moment of crisis by the therapist. The individual with BPD would be expected to have frequent crisis moments and his tendency to be highly dependent on his therapist to support him through these crises is characteristic of the clinical dilemma that faces the therapist. Some therapist may advocate a style of treatment that is to provide full support of the patient through the current crisis. Consistent with this type of philosophy of treatment, a non-DSA therapist may encourage the patient to make contact when he begins to experience the urge to act out in response to an upset in life or if he is insightful, the pain of emptiness. In a similar vein, some therapists are willing to provide the patient powerful medications to sedate and calm the patient "through the crisis".

The complication in these methods of intervention is obvious. This is a patient who is expected to have frequent and severe crisis. This would translate into very frequent contacts with the therapist outside of the designated person, place and time. At best, the therapist can play the role of a coach and assist the patient through the crisis and hope that the patient can learn some skills through this interaction that could be generalized to a future crisis moment. Most likely, the result of such intervention would only contribute to the greater dependence of the patient toward the therapist and in the case of medication usage, contribute to the over reliance on medication at time of crisis and perhaps, leads to addiction.

In DSA, the approach to treatment is distinctive in that, at the onset of the crisis of emptiness, the therapist would not necessarily intervene. At the most, the therapist cues the patient to be mindful of the treatment protocol and the interaction should be kept to a minimum. In noticing that a particular patient is starting to behave in an agitated fashion, the therapist or the staff may comment, "It appears that you are experiencing a difficult time. It is important that you begin to think about the 3-steps of treatment. I'll be back to check on you." The therapist may choose to be more specific in order to assure the patient of the therapist's return by stating, "I will be back in ten minutes." Please note that the amount of elapsed time stated is judgment on the part of the therapist in accordance to how much time he or she believes the patient can tolerate distress at this point in treatment.

A very concerned parent posed the question of how best to handle the frantic phone-calls from her daughter on the inpatient unit reporting of yet another crisis in her day. It has been very difficult for the parent to resist the urge to hang up the phone and rush right in to help her daughter resolve the eminent crisis. Having been introduced to the treatment protocol, the mother wondered about how she could best handle these calls. When this borderline patient calls her mother, the dynamic and dilemma is no different from her crisis contact with her therapist outside of the designated session time. Being a distance away by phone, it is difficult for the parent or the therapist to accurately asses the situation. Therefore, it is advisable that her mother should receive the call with compassion and make available the attunement and validation that befit the stated crisis of the daughter. However, it is imperative that the daughter understands that this phone-call is not consistent with the treatment as discussed and agreed upon. If this patient neglects to utilize her treatment skills at this moment or utilize a coping that is inconsistent with the work discussed previously, a review of the treatment skills would be warranted. In this work, a distinction is made between interpersonal filling of an internal void and the proper therapeutic work of the repair of the self, *no blame is placed even if the patient reverts to acting out or interpersonal rescue.*

Encouraging the patient to tolerate a degree of distress is in compliance with the earlier discussion and understanding that death or severe injury is a likely risk for this patient but repeated protective measures by others would not mitigate the risk; in fact, it could worsen the risk and become an obstacle to treatment. Risk of death is an undeniable reality of life for the individual with BPD. It is imperative that the patient and his family are clear in their understanding of this risk. Therefore, at the next moment of crisis, when his cup is approaching empty and he is reacting to this in his usual fashion by reaching toward acting out behavior, the therapist's response to encourage the patient in the use of the 3-steps would not be a surprise to the patient and his family. Moreover, a similar approach by his friends and family would be clinically constructive and highly therapeutic in this work.

Quite often, the patient will continue to test the limits within the context of treatment and could refuse to try the work discussed. Given that this is the phase of treatment most consistent with basic behavioral management technique for the modification of an undesirable behavior, it is expected that the patient should challenge and test the limits of containment. Generally, one would expect such a testing of limits to last up to several weeks even if the management technique was applied consistently. The borderline patient continues to act out and may even comment that he is not interested in getting better. At this point, the therapist will have to be consistent and persistent with the message of the initial discussion about the 3 steps.

Of course, this is not to say that this patient is to be left completely to his own making. Feeling abandoned is absolutely not the purpose of this exercise. As a matter of fact, it is imperative that the therapist is there for the patient when he has successfully *self managed* to get through the first two steps of containing and letting time pass. Invariably, there will be a moment when the patient will somehow manage to complete the first two steps by purpose or by chance and it will be up to the vigilant therapist to take note of this and step up to complete the third step with the patient.

Going back to our earlier discussion about the developmental growth of the infant, the important issue in the infant and maternal dyad is not for the mother to be forever and constantly available but it is more important for the mother to be consistent in returning after a brief retreat. Just prior to and during the rapprochement subphase, Margaret Mahler shares that, "it begins to dawn on the junior toddler that the world is not his oyster; that he must cope with it more or less "on his own," very often as a relatively helpless, small, and separate individual, unable to command relief or assistance merely by feeling the need for them or even by giving voice to that need. (1974, p.100)" I believe that it is this powerful dynamic of experiencing the return of the maternal figure that is most germane to healthy development in the first few years of life. The basis of DSA is to help the individual with BPD re-experience this very important aspect of development.

The keen reader may already be wondering as to how much time should pass for each round of the three steps. What I will describe about this could appear arbitrary but it is I believe quite the opposite. There is no formula to calculate the precise amount of time that is appropriate but I think that it is also not necessarily complex. This is where one's familiarity and understanding of the individual patient would pay off. Being aware of his tolerance of his emotional pain and the rapidity in which he would resort to acting out behavior would be important in creating a behavioral program that is effective and encouraging to him. Like any behavioral management program, which this portion of the method resembles, it is imperative that he is asked to make goals that can be achievable. It is especially important that the initial "buy in" period to this work is attainable. To achieve this compliance to the program, I may only ask him to contain and then let only a short time pass before he progresses to the process portion of the work. To stress this point, I sometimes suggest that even one minute of letting time pass might be sufficient in the beginning of this work.

A well regarded therapist from our inpatient program is known for taking her patients through a meditative exercise to help the individual arrive at some comfort at facing his or her disquiet of emptiness within. In this work, the patient is asked to sit quietly by self in a non-distracting environment to focus on experiencing the pain of the emptiness within. This patient is prepared for this exercise with an understanding of the cup and the 3-steps. In this context, he works to feel the emotional pain but maintain containment without instantly easing that pain with accessing others or acting out. This meditative process can be very brief for beginning patients. On completion of the first two steps, the patient meets with his therapist to check in about the experience. Many patients express an enjoyment of this simple exercise for the ease in which they can experience success as well as conveying to the patient the very real threat of the emptiness that looms beneath the façade of daily drama.

Let Pass A Reasonable Amount of Time

One may question how the elapse of a small amount of time would be helpful. However, what is really important is the principle of the idea that he is going to help himself even for just one minute. *Steps one and two are differentiated from otherwise idle passing of time by the purposeful attempt to address the pain of emptiness.* Earlier, I made the statement that there is no better time to start the work toward greater independence than right at this very moment. I hold strong conviction about this statement. In so doing, I am also communicating to my patient that I do believe that he is eventually capable of happiness in conjunction with greater independence. I often urge the patient to be really honest about what is a tolerable amount of time for self-soothing at that juncture in treatment.

With sufficient treatment connection with the therapist and with adequate motivation for improvement, most patients are able to understand the push for greater honesty on his part in determining the length of time that he should tolerate for step two. The amount of time to let pass should be proportionate to his current function in treatment. His therapist needs to take into consideration his most recent episodes of overt and covert acting out behaviors and weigh these acts against his ability to tolerate the pain of emptiness that drives these events. As he becomes more successful at one length of time in step two, the subsequent amount of time would then be lengthened. In this fashion, he is asked to contain and let time pass for longer and longer period before the requisite processing with a selfobject. However, overly lengthy periods for the purpose of self-soothing are also not productive, especially in the beginning of treatment. One must keep in mind that the purpose of the 3-steps is also to create yet another opportunity to connect with a selfobject.

Three Levels of Self-soothing Activities

Several important learning and developmental growth occurs while working with the activities of self-soothing. He gains confidence regarding the types of activities that are appropriate and are effective in allowing time to pass. The prerequisite to contain and let time pass often forces the patient to confront the issue of how to entertain self in an appropriate fashion for the first time. Most of his pursuits are for fast and intense payoff that could quickly fill his cup. Activities such as drawing, reading, writing, gardening, simple games, walking the dog and playing music may never have been a part of his distressed existence. He has not cultivated many of the mundane activities that bring enjoyment and satisfaction to others. Spending time by himself to just relax and do little is perhaps completely alien to him.

Effective coping at times of distress requires some proactive consideration and preparation. Fundamentally, there are three levels of activities for self-soothing. The most basic level of activities for self-soothing consists of simple actions or activities that one can engage in without any special material or equipment. Refocusing one's attention (appreciation of the texture on a rock), simple relaxation exercises (deep breathing), prayer, positive self statements, thinking of positive experiences, imagery and counting are examples of activities that requires no tools and one can do almost anywhere. The next level of activities may require some ready access to simple items or tools to accomplish. Some of these activities may also require some basic skills to be of use. Jump rope, shoot basketball, reading, writing, coloring, listening to music, walking, walk dog, wash car are some examples of level two activities. Taking an approach from self psychology, one might consider using a special transitional object such as a special tool to perform a task of some sort. The final level of activities involves investment and commitment. These items include acquiring skills in a sport, joining a sport team, taking up a special hobby, painting a picture, playing a musical instrument, work a job and school. Although these activities may not be readily accessible to the borderline patient at first but he should be encouraged to master some skills that will eventually provide him with greater rewards. Some pre-planned activities such as camping, shopping and vacationing can also be useful. Of particular relevance to the second step is the use of various cognitive behavioral skills (i.e. dialectical behavior therapy).

A special comment should be made about the use of journaling as a skill to self soothe. This allows him to document his feelings at that very instant in time so that he can have an accurate account of his experience to relate to his therapist later. This act of documenting his feelings also helps him to understand that he is not alone in weathering this moment and that he will be sharing this internal experience with a selfobject subsequently. The patient should be cautioned against use of extreme writing in which he indulges in the entertainment of morbid or gory images and ideas in the name of journaling; such acts are better labeled as covert acting out.

Focus on the Senses

Kaufman, in his writing about the psychology of shame discussed the refocusing of attention as a tool for releasing shame. This is accomplished by "becoming immersed in external sensory experience, particularly visual and physical" (Kaufman 1989, p. 183). It is literary the act of stopping to "smell the roses" that can assist us in our efforts to gain momentary cohesion. This technique holds close resemblance to Kohut's discussion of the use of transitional objects in bringing about the cohesion of the self. The mindfulness of the classic Japanese tea ceremony is the quintessential example of the focused awareness to bring about a total cohesion of the self (Kakuzo 1956).

Shame, likely a proponent of the false self, has an existence that may fluctuate greatly through our consciousness and evoked by a sense of emptiness. Tolerating the affect of shame and emptiness require a powerful commitment to acceptance of this most difficult of feelings and will test the best laid plan to let time pass. I find that *refocusing attention* is a highly effective technique to assist the patient in getting through intolerable moments of self consciousness. It is also a method that is simple enough for most to find achievable. "Turning the attention outward effectively interrupts shame spirals, thereby allowing individuals previously held prisoner by shame to enjoy various solitary or relational activities, from public speaking, dancing and sports, to sexual pairing" (Kaufman 1989, p. 183). In refocusing on a spot in a painting on the wall, one young woman expressed a sense of relief after engaging the feelings of emptiness in an introspective exercise. Overcoming the moment of shame and emptiness allows for cohesion of the self in that instant in time and improves our daily function.

Creativity and Play

Beyond the simpler and more basic activities that one could utilize to allow time to pass, there is the more important role of letting time pass through the use of creative activities and symbolic play. Sigmund Freud once commented, "In some things the great Leonardo (Da Vinci) stayed all his life a little bit infantile; you can say, that all great men have to stay a bit child like. He was still playing when he was an adult and became of that to some contemporaries he was weird and inapprehensible." Erikson points out, "Play, then, is a function of the ego, an attempt to synchronize the bodily and the social processes with the self" (1950, p.211). Play and creative activities may be more available to individuals who have access to a healthier self. However, creativity and play are the area that the borderline patient moves into as he achieves greater consistency in the self. At a certain level of basic functioning of the self, the activities of *letting time pass* can contribute to the psychological healing of developmental hurt.

Heinz Kohut suggested the term *transference of creativity* to describe one's dependence on others or sometimes, an object that represents the selfobject experience that strengthens the self sufficiently to allow the individual to realize his creative potential and productivity (Kohut 1976). The central hypothesis in self psychology states that beyond the inborn tendency to organize experience, the self also requires the presence of others, technically designated as *objects*, to help evoke the emergence and maintenance of the self. This is termed *selfobject experience* and abbreviated as *selfobjects* (Wolf 1988). There are perhaps many example in history of famous individuals who have relied on special trusted others to insure optimal functioning of the self. On the use of a transitional object, keeping his favorite book of poems on his desk, a gift from a revered grandfather, provides one author the needed selfobject experience to be confident and productive in his work. Kohut and Wolf give some examples of such exclusive relationships (Kohut 1984, Wolf 1988, p.29).

When the cup is empty, he is neither creative nor fulfilled. In the treatment utilizing DSA, one is advised against the direct and complete reliance on selfobjects to fulfill an internal emotional need. However, the use of a symbolic selfobject such as that of a favorite and meaningful inanimate object can be highly helpful in the stage of self soothing and letting time pass. This is highly reminiscent of the infant using the teddy bear to self soothe while awaiting mother's return.

At yet a more sophisticated level of functioning, Meares (1993, p.175-181) described the close relationship between play and the selfobject experience. In his view, the therapist should not become an impediment to the patient's growth by focusing on the factual and the interpretation while straying from the feelings, wishes and imaginings that underlies the patient's words. Individuals suffering from developmental disruption live in a zone in which experiences come, overwhelmingly, from the outside world. "Consequently, the story they tell deals with events, troubles, and difficulties rather than imaginings. In terms of the metaphor of the play space, they live in the real playroom." Frequently, the disruption and disjunction of zero to five years of age has the greatest impact in causing a child to turn so outwardly in his coping that he forgoes the opportunities to truly experience and be validated for his inner life. It is likely that the coping mechanism of developmental hurt are many, but whether turning inwardly or focused outwardly, compartmentalize the self or merge with powerful others, the end result is often the neglect of the true self.

The drive to play can be manifested in the desire to do something that one can call one's own. In the transitional object, the child exercises a kind of magical thinking that links the aspects of the mother to an object such as a doll or a blanket. Additionally, his inner experience is projected upon this object like a metaphoric screen. Thus, an object such as a doll has the function of representing the internal world of the child, but it also signifies the existence of the mother. "The awareness of the mother penetrates into the intimacy of every wish and thought." It is through this experience of the other as selfobject that is necessary for play to begin and to be maintained (Meares 1993, p.39). The use of the transitional object assist the young child to cope while mother is away; likewise, an older child, teen and adult would similarly require the use of a transitional object to optimize his daily function. For the adult, his use of the transitional object may be more artful and perhaps, subconscious. A writer may intentionally rely on his favorite fountain pen while, habitually, a ballplayer finds his special handkerchief indispensable during a game. Is this superstition or object relations?

Whether through the use of a transitional object that conjures up the secure feelings connected to our selfobject, or the enjoyment of play that links us by memory to a time of positive transference, both transitional object and play could have similar functions. Play space can be a transitional space; it can be a bridge to our developmental beginning. From the manner in which the early developmental years were described by the pioneers in psychology, this stage of childhood can be quite a terrifying time. In normal development, it appears that the human infant has evolved to cope with all of the uncertainties in a most elegant fashion; he found play and the transitional object. Regarding "child's play", a child needs to adjust to a difficult situation by learning to manipulate new objects, toys and to conclude by receiving recognition, interest and pride from his mother (Erikson 1950, p.218). In abnormal development, disruptions serve to interfere with healthy play and proper use of transitional objects. In theory, such disruptions lead to developmental pathology. Therapy has to help restore the loss of the true self and step two introduces the borderline patient to the use of play and transitional objects as bridges to the developmental beginning.

What is most notable about someone at the cusp of being able to play is a change in their demeanor from their usual external focus of attention to that of a more ethereal internal focus. One particular patient with a dependent relationship with others through enmeshment and overt acting out, gradually came to enjoy talking about his special love of the food and arts of a particular culture. In his conversations on this subject, he appears to enter into a zone of his very own and relished these moments seemingly without the need of any other. These are often the times in therapy in which a patient produces something of his own creation and presents it seemingly without expecting approval but simply to share his enjoyment. If the individual has generally in the past focused on the short term gratification to fulfill an internal emotional need, as he began to engage in play, he seems to exhibit a greater sense of the future and broader tolerance of time, especially time spent by self. If he appears to be more preoccupied internally, this is done without actual isolation from others. Metaphorically, instead of staring into the eyes of another with an intense demand for connection and attention, he would rather show you what he sees through the telescope of his minds eye.

True play has to be cultivated. As was suggested by Meares, play has to occupy a specialized zone that conjures up imagery and imagining within. This conception of play can involve such activities as meditation, work, chores, exercise, sports, hobbies, writing, painting, playing music, etc. In essence, play =work and work=play. If this can be achieved, an individual's functioning in life is said to be optimally effective and well balanced.

At a theoretical level, the activity of play set in the general context of the natural "3-steps" way of living may be instrumental in helping the young child overcome some of the instinctual terrors of childhood. The classical notion of the death instinct and castration anxiety has to be resolved effectively within a designated period of time for the child to progress into the next phase of development. Neutralizing the castration anxiety may require more than the child's alignment with one or the other parental figure. However, one way or another, most children appear to deal with this phase of development without further ado. In observation, the activities of a young child appear to be focused on learning of language and to partake in play in a multifaceted and multilayered fashion. Communication and play then allows for the child to experience mirroring and idealizing transference optimally. In so doing, the play of a child has the additional purpose of helping him to address the inexplicable anxieties of development. Perhaps, in a proficiently orchestrated performance, the transitional object, toys, mirroring and idealizing transference and play all come together in a concerto with the child at center stage as object relations become strengthened.

Learning to Fill One's Own Cup

A most rewarding goal of the second step is for the individual to learn to fill his own cup. For many individuals suffering from the disruption of the self, the greatest challenge can be the inability to use routine daily activities, leisure activities, work, creativity and play to fulfill the emotional requirement within. All too commonly, the borderline individual scoffs at the simpler things in life as ineffective. The borderline patient has difficulty utilizing these activities because most average life activities lack the necessary intensity to be of meaningful filling for the pervasive emptiness. As he abandons these "normal" activities in life, he will have to rely increasingly on behaviors of questionable credibility to satisfy the emotional hunger.

Accompanying the repair of the cup is the improved economy of function of the emotional system. Whereas previously, in a leaky system, he is highly dependent on some specialized input that can be a further detriment to his overall function; in a better repaired state, he is able to make use of more types of acceptable input that ultimately helps to meet the needs of the system more efficiently and consistently. Short term and long term projects of various sorts as illustrated in fig. 7.3 are example of healthy input enjoyed through constructive daily activities.

The natural tendency for many is to stop at the second step with an activity for self soothing. "I felt better already so I didn't do the third step." It must, however, be made clear that the pursuit of these activities alone is insufficient in the work of repair without coupling this moment to the third step. Without the third step, the borderline patient will soon become disenchanted with these activities and come to confirm, once again, that such low intensity activities are not worth the effort. A lack of completion of the third step is a lack of mirroring and idealizing transference and devoid of developmental healing.

Step Three – (To Process/Check-in)

Assuming the patient is successful at attending to the first two steps, he is presumably safe and in reasonably good emotional shape but not necessarily feeling better, to attend the therapy appointment at the designated place and time. This should be a very rewarding moment for this patient. Each time he successfully attends a session with his therapist is an achievement independent of what they might address during that session. He should be made very aware of this unique credit in therapy. In keeping with the basic tenet of DSA, the process step is more about the arrival of the whole rather than the detail of the individual step. *It is fundamentally about unconditional positive regard,*

trust, confirmation, connection, validation and empathy. "The essence of the psychoanalytic cure resides in a patient's newly acquired ability to identify and seek out appropriate selfobjects…as they present themselves in his realistic surroundings and to be sustained by them." (Kohut 1984, p.77) It is through the completion of the third step that this treatment parallels the selfobject development of the infant. Naturally, this step should best be carried out with someone with a certain degree of familiarity to one's experiences in life, an authentic selfobject.

The final step of "process" is analogous to that of the joyful reunion of the mother and child after a brief period of separation. It is precisely because of this reason that this is a step that should never be left out or overlooked. At times, a patient may relate feeling that once he has implemented the first two steps, he feels rather calmed and gathered that he in fact no longer feels the need to process or check-in with anyone. The purpose of this treatment is not about achieving independence through isolation. He should not become isolated or feel abandoned and ignored. Therefore, the third step is a very integral part of the three steps concept in this treatment.

This step is as important as the maternal figure's return for the infant. After all, the purpose of the infants coping by containment and letting time pass (such as the use of the pacifier or blanket) is to ultimately be able to celebrate the return of the mother. If the mother was experienced as inconsistent in her return to care for the infant, then the world of the infant could easily collapse. This type of anxiety would certainly interfere with the appropriate and healthy development of his cup/self. In the early infancy, his mother may need to return more often given that he does not have a well formed internal object sense of his mother (lack of a true cup to hold his mother within) at that early stage in life. As he got older, the toddler can tolerate the absence of his mother for longer periods of time.

In the case of the individual with BPD, it is prudent that he or she sees the connectivity with others as an integral part of treatment and relate with consistency rather than do it on whim or when absolutely necessary. For many individuals with BPD, their tendency is either feast or famine in their approach to interpersonal interactions. This patient's manner of approaching others may often be based on the vicissitude of his past experiences. Perhaps the exposure to physical and sexual abuse contributes to his reluctance to trust authority figures. Often, the victims of abuse come to feel that he or she was somehow deserving of the maltreatment and come to experience a great deal of guilt and shame; this individual may not approach other selfobjects with the trust and openness to heal earlier hurt. He may keep away from others altogether and become as inconspicuous as possible. The patient who has come to feel that his self worth is completely based on the attention and recognition lavished on him by the selfobject will feel compelled to force his way into the consciousness of others to seek the affirmation of his existence. As a result, he tends to overindulge in his accessing of selfobjects. Both of the aforementioned scenarios involve individuals who are highly needy of others while one accesses excessively and the other retreats with distrust.

The desire to be totally and completely understood rests at the center of human existence. This indeed becomes the unspoken fantasy of infants and young children as relates to idealizing and mirroring transference. Upon encountering excessive misattunement in early life, the frustrated child continues to seek the unattainable emotional alliance in selfobjects. A need for merger is not necessarily the same as a desire for "love". It may not be love that a patient seeks from his therapist but rather, a feeling of absolute understanding. Many patients express feeling that, try as they might, little can be accomplished in conveying their innermost emotions for those who profess to care. Possibly relating to the frustrations of misattunement, this patient may continue to seek complicity in his hopeless dream of exclusive comprehension or runs away from further trying. Effective and appropriate connectivity is the goal in the third step.

Therefore, in hospital treatment, he is encouraged to have contact with his therapist on a consistent basis. His therapist will need to maintain consistent involvement with regularly placed appointments. Much like the regularly scheduled outpatient appointments, it is productive to have a routine and structure that is conducive to building trust and to meet the patient's needs in this treatment. Such structured appointments help to maximize the patient's chance of success in this treatment by providing an ongoing opportunity to complete the 3-steps regardless of the specifics of daily life. Often, even without mindfulness of treatment, a patient will inadvertently complete a round of the 3-steps as part of his daily life. In this case, the therapist should take this opportunity to praise the patient for utilizing his coping skills and give him credit for a round of the 3-steps. (See case 8.1)

For the beginner, carrying out the 3-steps can feel like a very artificial process. This is to be expected and the patient should not feel discouraged. He or she should be encouraged to exercise the 3-steps in a scripted manner even if it feels unintuitive. He is to do this work even if he does not feel particularly empty or in distress. Even though he will have fuller periods in his cup, he has to be reminded of the constant leakage and this supports the need to consistently be mindful of repair. Through repetition, the steps will become a natural part of his daily interactions.

On the inpatient unit, the structured appointments take place through the daily rounds. On a good day, his cup could be relatively full, but the structured rounds take place routinely and this assures the patient additional opportunities to complete his 3-steps. Other than his contacts with unit staff members, his psychiatrist and in the case of our facility, his program therapist will each visit him once a day; this is another very predictable opportunity to complete the 3-steps. Additionally, there are also chances to check-in during special groups designed to do so in a group setting. It is critical that his therapist make clear to him that it is within the context of the 3-steps that they now have an opportunity to meet. "In reviewing the chart and hearing reports from staff, since my last visit, you have managed to contain any acting out urges and utilized your skills to let time pass. In so doing, you have avoided self injury that would require emergency room visit or containment otherwise. You have attended most treatment activities and refrained from using staff to maintain your sense of wellbeing or rescue you. As a result, I am able to meet with you as is our routine and this constitutes a completion of a cycle of the 3-steps."

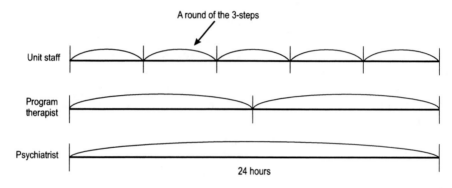

Fig. 8.1 *This illustration shows the various frequency of interface between providers and patient. In fig. 8.3, a macro level of interaction is shown.*

The additional significance of processing with a selfobject is an opportunity for the patient to gain a type of unconditional validation. If the experience of emptiness can be equated with shame, then, through imagery, the patient can "take inside" his therapist and by this new identification which provides healing for the self and overturns maladaptive old scenes of shame (Kaufman 1989, p.210). Often, I teach the inpatient staff to "just listen". This is not a time to correct, redirect or even to give advice. Listening should be done with an attitude of compassion and better yet, with empathy as well. In the daily work of treatment, it is sufficient to just listen to the patient reporting of his implementation of the three steps with the best concentrated listening I could offer at that moment and end with an appreciative smile and a comment of encouragement. It seems, in most instances, a sincere listener is all that the patient needs.

Mears viewed the therapeutic task as one in which "the therapist must, together with the patient, metaphorically gaze toward the play space." He spoke of the empathic stance of the therapist in bringing about a state of play, if left without the tampering from the therapist, allows the patient to own the experience. "It is the therapist's task to somehow liberate this activity, the movement of which resemble those of the dream. In those with disorder of self, its first manifestations are brief and largely hidden in the linear language of adaption" (Meares 1993, p.185). The patient moves gradually toward a liberated sense of play through cycles of therapeutic relatedness in which he starts with an idealizing transference of the therapeutic relationship and end with a sense of disjunction with the inevitable empathic failure of the therapist. With each round of this cycle, the patient recovers from the disappointment of a selfobject experience to gain the permission to be free to play and to briefly own an experience that was, at the same time, valued by another (Meares 1993, p.177).

As I have maintained throughout this work, the 3-steps should hopefully not just be viewed as glorified time out. In fact, the 3-steps are not time out, with the usual connotation for punishment. When appropriately implemented, the 3-steps should provide the structured and disciplined interaction between two people that enhances the self and object relations as well as contributes to developmental healing gained through the therapeutic play space. The specific ideas about what activities or imaginings that constitute the individual patient's true play, like that of the play of a three year old child, can not be prescribed but should come from the patient.

This then takes us to the contemplation of the many forms of the 3-steps that takes shape in practice. In the inpatient hospital setting, I tend to encourage the literal use of the 3-steps as a way for staff and patients to experience each other in a structured and developmentally appropriate fashion. This has obvious benefits such as milieu management, interpersonal boundary, relationship building and trust. The resolution of transference, disjunction and corrective emotional experience occur in the context of doing this work.

In the outpatient arena and for the patient involved in longer term psychotherapy, there is the opportunity for some patient's to begin to graduate toward a more advanced way of experiencing the 3-steps. Assuming the patient is able to partake in this work for a consistent period of time, his therapist is able to demonstrate attunement and attentiveness in a trusting fashion within this setting. Hence this patient has a chance to work through his anger and frustration in accordance with object relations basis. Heralding the success of another week of independent function, the patient informs his therapist that he looked inwardly for any hint of aversive tension and applied the 3-steps frequently. As the patient is able to increasingly achieve the introjection of the selfobject, he should become increasingly more comfortable at his own ability to let time pass. In particular to this method of work, the patient then enjoys greater meaning and value of the 3-steps as he applies this work over time; clinically, there is reason to believe that most patients find it easier and more desirable to engage in the 3-steps as his therapeutic relationship strengthens.

Depending on the sophistication of the patient at this juncture in treatment, the therapist can move the patient toward a more symbolic understanding of the steps rather than staying concretely on the particular of each individual step. The patient then has the option to discuss his coping in a more general sense rather than with details of individual episodes. Furthermore, this patient may not see his therapist so frequently and the discussion of each individual episode of the 3-steps would be too cumbersome on meeting. Instead, the patient and his therapist now engage in a session in which the 3-steps are the general spirit of the work.

An astute young woman once made the remarkable comment that she should not spend too much time processing with her staff during the third step. She then confessed that she has at times lingered in this step in order to gain added transference input to further fill the cup. She felt that, in so doing, it could then motivate her to seek more frequent input in such a fashion and jeopardize her treatment. She realized that a balance is required in exercising this work; overt focus on the third step is likely to compromise the true purpose of this interaction.

Having completed a few intensive weeks of inpatient DSA, one young woman seeking treatment for the injury to the self began to express doubts about the sustainability of her progress. She explained that even though she feels quite comfortable with her current staff, she is apprehensive about her ability to work with others outside of this facility. To this most important question, I gave her this answer, "Through your sincere effort to work in this treatment, I feel that you have been able to incorporate many of the core staff into your inner emotional world; this will allowed you to lateralize your sense of security to working with many of the interim staff as well. In effect, I feel that you have taken in the hospital as a whole to become a part of your internal emotional world; this represents a feeling of security about important others in your life." Hence, with this newfound confidence, she should hopefully be able to lateralize this trust toward working with many more people in her life. This ability to generalize an internal sense of trust is the essence of forming object constancy.

The most important achievement in therapy should not be that of simply developing a supportive network around the patient. The therapist who is prone to engage in complex academic discussions with portentous psychological jargon with a colleague will often resort to providing simple supportive measures for his or her patient without striving to help the patient achieve long term selfobject introject. The unfortunate result of this manner of work is the patient who will appear stable only when his therapist is available. Doing a type of non-DSA work, one patient's comment was, "I had to be so fake. I could not be myself," feeling that she had to "pretend to not have bad feelings or bad thoughts." In DSA, the therapist strives to help the patient gain a sense of connectedness through the natural course of disjunction and then corrective emotional experience in a trusting setting, an approach that seemed easily embraced by many patients.

Even though the patient may experience a sense of disjunction with others in the initial phase of doing the 3-steps, gradually, feelings of disjunction give way to secure independent function. Through this process, he can now better tolerate his frustrations of pervasive emptiness and come to achieve a better presence of the selfobject within. It seems that introjection of the selfobject is most effectively performed through the cycles of disjunction and unification in the context of trust and attunement. This is the essence of object relations work. Through self psychology we learn that the selfobject can help us get through the most challenging of times and through object relations theory, we learn that object constancy comes from learning to trust the most important people in our lives.

On Completion of the 3-steps

Once a round of the 3-steps are completed or credited to the patient, a symbolic repair occurs; a small imaginary leakage is plugged at the bottom of the cup. The borderline patient should be aware that his cup is full of enumerable tiny leakage and each round of the 3-steps would only plug one hole. As is the belief in most types of therapy work, progress made is progress kept. Each hole that is repaired is a leakage that is seen as permanently plugged. A patient may do his treatment haltingly but he should be made to understand that this treatment work is cumulative. Furthermore, this repair work can be performed as often as he desires, resulting in more profound and rapid improvement if the 3-steps are undertaken frequently.

The patient is rewarded in mainly three ways when he completes the 3-steps. Firstly, he benefits from the act of self soothing. Secondly, he has the satisfaction of having made a repair to the cup. Thirdly, he has just received an interpersonal input into his cup by engaging a selfobject in the third step to check in. This repair and input is gained through obtaining a bit of trust, validation and self confidence in the play space offered though the therapeutic context of the 3-steps. Although he has had to accept the pain of emptiness while pursuing the completion of the 3-steps, he can now experience a bit of relief by enjoying the input derived from mirroring and idealizing transference. By engaging his selfobjects in the context of treatment, these others are going to be more welcoming of his interactions with them now and in the future.

The patient's experience of the 3-steps can vary greatly because this is an interaction based on the involvement of two people. On the aggregate, the patient's sincerity in the completion of the 3-steps is going to be easily apparent to the therapist or the selfobject. If he attempts to get by without actual completion of the 3-steps, the therapist can confront this by commenting that routine contact and touch base will take place but he should be aware that these are not true 3-steps. It may not be productive for the therapist to be critical about the patient's failure to complete the steps given that this only furthers his sense of shame. However, once the patient begins to show some completion of the steps in a quality fashion, it is imperative that the therapist help the patient distinguish between honest approaches from that of false attempts.

Even the most astute patient may lapse into thinking that each round of the 3-steps should bring about instant reward of feeling emotionally improved. Despite the self soothing measures and the interpersonal transference input by the selfobject, the very emotionally empty patient may not experience noticeable change in his sense of wellbeing at that instant. This lack of instant satisfaction in contrast with the immediate reward of various acting out behaviors can often seem like a gulf in the mind of the patient as he ponders which choice to take in future crisis. It is fruitful for the patient undertaking this work to fully understand that the purpose of the 3-steps is not necessarily to bring about an instant cessation of pain but focus on the ultimate importance of repair. Reflecting on the core purpose of this treatment, the highest level of priority is the development of trust and the introjection of the selfobject. Thus, temporary cohesion of the self as achieved through interaction with the selfobject takes place within the mechanism for developmental repair to the cup.

Living the 3-steps Life

Because the 3-steps truly mimic the healthy and natural coping process that most people gravitate to in their daily life, it is fascinating to see what patients do with the steps once they understood the basic concepts. Frequently, I encounter variations on the 3-steps that, at first, may not resemble the 3-steps in proper sequence but on further examination, the steps are all there and more. One common example is to utilize a shorter second step of letting time pass, due possibly to the patient's inability to tolerate a longer period of time and connect two rounds of the 3-steps together to address one particular moment of difficulty. This means that there is one act of containment and two rounds of letting time pass and two rounds of processing. (Fig 8.2)

Indeed, the tapestry of life is full of many wonderful permutations on the 3-steps. Despite the natural occurrences of the 3-steps in all of our daily lives, for the borderline patient in treatment, it is important to be particularly scripted about the implementation of the 3-steps. How this could be accomplished in the inpatient setting or the home environment is particularly cogent in the successful application of the steps. With careful observation, the therapist or the staff can easily spot positive behaviors consistent with the steps. Taking advantage of the natural occurrence of the 3-steps in daily life, it is highly engaging to point out and give credit for the steps.

One's natural tendency to provide transference input is often contingent on the state of our mirroring and idealizing transference as well as perceived projective identification for both the self and the selfobject. In a reciprocal fashion, transference input between any two individuals operate in much the same manner with an emphasis on mirroring and idealizing transference as well as projective identification. As a result, what comes to pass between a staff and a patient in an inpatient milieu requires a certain sense of mutual gratification for both parties to experience adequate meetings of each other's needs.

It can be argued that many of life's highly structured activities have built in qualities that allow one to strengthen and pursue a healthier sense of the self. Such activities are usually characterized by the inherent structure and the presence of consistent selfobject or selfobjects. The selfobjects often play the role of a highly regarded, respected and perhaps, feared individual with authority. These selfobjects perform the task of protector, coach, spiritual guide, teacher, commander or boss. Our lives with these individuals expand on our original object relationship with our parents.

Stories abound in the popular press of individuals lost in their own misguided search for meaning and sense of the self, comes to discover a particular sense of belonging and connectedness in some sort of disciplined activity. In the presence of an appropriate selfobject, many individuals find solace and calm in the context of these relationships. When examined, these relationships all operate with the same common denominator; the requirement to contain and let time pass is commonly expected in exchange for the reliable presence of the selfobject. One memorable story from the Seattle Times in 2006 told of a troubled teenage boy who discovered his true self in the jungle temple of Cambodia. Probably angered and shocked at the unwitting transition from suburban United States to a minimalist Buddhist temple life style, he found that the monks were not in the habit of catering to his every interpersonal whim. Additionally, in the jungle, there was a lack of the usual acting out outlets familiar to him. Within this structured setting, he learned to cope with the harshness of life and discovered an inner calm likely related to a newfound sense of connected with others.

In the foregoing case, his family might well ask as to why his calm could not be achieved in his usual environment back home? I am partial to the understanding that effective 3-steps has to be experienced in a non-distracting environment in order to allow for effective mirroring and idealizing transference and selfobject introject to take place. No doubt it is not feasible for many of us to experience selfobject relatedness in the peace and quiet of a jungle temple but such extremes can be avoided if each of us maintains mindfulness of the importance of the 3-steps in daily life.

Thus, it is not uncommon to hear of successful stories of change that took place within a highly structured environment with the attributes of the 3-steps.

The presence of the developmentally needed object relations experiences seems built into many of life's activities. Sadly, many such opportunities do not fulfill a developmental need due to man's general lack of insight regarding proper selfobject role. From the head of a household to the leader of a society, the greatest purpose of such authorities in life is often unrealized. The CEO of a company, the governor of a state, the president of a nation are all individuals who have the obligation to fulfill the role of the selfobject to call upon the lost and the suffering to seek proper actions in life. Without an insight about living in the 3-steps, life and productivity can neither be efficient nor stable.

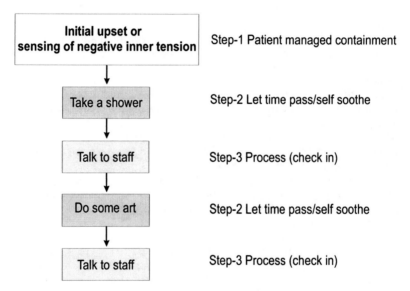

Fig. 8.2 *In this diagram, we can see how this one patient combined two rounds of the 3-steps to help shorten the amount of time in step-2 while effectively meeting treatment protocol.*

Toward a Cohesive Approach to Treatment

Case 8.1: Doris is a 14 year old ward of the state. She meets people with a big bright beautiful smile while appearing rather shy and aloof, as if questioning why anyone should pay her any attention. For someone who came into the hospital after repeated attempts to cut and kill herself, one will instantly notice her eyes as very alive and full of life. Next, one is taken aback by the multitude of keloid scars on her arms from self-mutilation. These scar tissues have grown and roiled on top of repeated cuts with barely any appearance of original skin. In between old scars, there are new wounds of varying freshness. Thus she presented on the inpatient unit under court order.

The first five years of her life was full of strife. Her mother was a drug addict and a prostitute. The mother took all of the children and moved frequently without informing any relatives of her whereabouts. Thus, the severity of the children's suffering was never clear to anyone at first. In this fashion, the dawn of this patient's early life was spent with people who were negligent of her care and abused her in unspeakable manners. Finally, she was found wandering a school playground with a soiled diaper at age five and Child Protective Service was notified.

Although in the care of the state, the years to follow were no less traumatic in some sense. She moved frequently from foster homes and group homes due to her constant conflict with others. Despite her demands for attention, she was unable to establish trusting and lasting relationship with others to satisfy her needs. She wanted her needs met instantly and was prone to severe aggressive outbursts when frustrated. On top of the stealing, lying, running away and destruction of property, the development of self-mutilation was beyond what these foster families were able to tolerate.

Impressively, the state, represented by her guardian and a host of social workers, managed to keep her out of the inpatient psychiatric setting until now. In past efforts, they cobbled together various crisis intervention plans ranging from extra aid for the foster families to special group homes. When problems arise, they would exert extra effort and attention to distract her and buy time in hopes of weathering the crisis. Such efforts would of course include a visit to her therapist's office but little could be gained given the lack of an effective systematic approach to treatment. If in need of greater intervention, Doris would find herself at yet another doctor's appointment trying to explain, in her limited ability to communicate, her difficulties. Explaining her behaviors generally turns out to be a highly shaming procedure given that she could never quite understand her own actions. Inevitably, she leaves such visits with yet another change in medications and the accompanying side effects.

Under the pretense of seeking stabilization, the most recent of her group home snuck her into the psychiatric inpatient setting and then promptly announced that they will not be taking her back. One can only chuckle about the desperateness of such a measure but it speaks volumes about the frustration that her outpatient providers were facing. On arrival, she slept for some time having been given hefty doses of antipsychotic and benzodiazepine medications at an emergency department due to her combative behavior. She was then placed on involuntary treatment hold and transported via ambulance.

Upon awakening from her medication induced fog, she shook off her lethargy and took a look around and decided to yell. Every demand and verbal exchange was delivered in top decibels with the likely intent to annoy. Her treatment team pondered the psychodynamic significance of this behavior in view of her interpersonal relationship and past history of abandonment and disappointments. In observing her from a distance, it is obvious that she is completely dysregulated emotionally. She seems randomly high and low emotionally in the most incomprehensible fashions but on closer examination, a vicissitude of daily life can upset her intensely. Minor interpersonal slights or disappointments, any sense of guilt and shame, people approaching, people leaving, are all events that brings great emotional disturbance to her.

With the gradual adjustment to the milieu and some minor titration of her medications, she reached a more quiescent state in the hospital. She has experienced just about every medication in every psychotropic class available and none were ever beneficial in the longer term. Of course, this initial calm is typical of many patients and shortly thereafter, she began to escalate fiercely once again. In the milieu, treatment as usual did not offer her much comfort or satisfaction. When CBT skills were added, she found it intriguing only as far as the added attention she could gain by pleasing her staff through superficial compliance periodically. At other times, she goes about her usual manner of acting out in abandon. All staff personnel came to feel a great sense of impotence in their daily work with her, feeling that the time they spend in processing, exploring, and connecting with this patient appears to just contribute to temporary calm only to be followed by worsening symptoms and behavior on the part of the patient. Staff's comment was, "Some days she may seem highly invested in the treatment but it seems that she may just be trying to seek my approval and attention."

The foregoing remark by the staff set off a search for another approach to this very challenging clinical case. This unit has been moving toward the increasing use of the DSA. Staff members are now more informed of this work and expressed readiness in trying this new approach to working with a patient that has essentially defeated every therapeutic idea thus far. Staff also did not want to maintain the status quo by means of heavy medication use or physical containment to keep her safe until she was discharged to another facility. Everyone on the treatment team held the sentiment that DSA could be her best chance for treatment at this juncture.

The introduction of DSA was met with initial trepidation by Doris. This treatment team has experienced reactions ranging from a bit of skepticism to outright scoff in this regard; this patient's response was not a surprise. Initially, Doris acted as if she would have nothing to do with it, but on further inquiry a few days later, she revealed that she did not quite take in all that was discussed with her in the first introductory session. With a review of the key features validating her powerful sense of emptiness and understanding the origin of the leakage of her cup brought her to greater insight about her internal pain and additional motivation to accept treatment. She even expressed great excitement about the work and said that she has never encountered any approach in treatment that made more sense than this model. Her enthusiasm at this phase of treatment would be short lived.

At this juncture, all staff members were determined to not allow Doris to just use DSA as another fresh topic in treatment to garner additional attention without a semblance of investment in the work. Everyone carefully followed the easy directions set out by the 3-steps and Doris was given frequent reviews to better understand the nature and dynamics of the cup. Her understanding of the dynamics of the cup is critical to her development of true insight about the purpose of treatment, an area of weakness in the work of many such patients. The foregoing remarks about her leaky cup did not automatically engage her attention toward repair; in general, most individuals do not make the instant connection between what they learn about the cup and the vicissitude of one's mood throughout the day.

In the first place, much of this work requires constant learning from one another. Doris learns from the staff as to the identification of feelings within and the alternative rewards available through skillful therapeutic work. Staff members learned of her ability to tolerate the internal pain of emptiness and how best to cue her to use treatment coping skills. All who worked with her had to maintain the strictest of boundary according to the 3-steps. Each round of processing in the 3-steps was an opportunity to reinforce her understanding of the functions of the cup. Every effort was made to gently confront her pathological use of interpersonal interactions to support a very fragile self while providing the needed input to her cup when in the context of the third step. On those inevitable moments when she turns to severe acting out measures to appease the jagged pain within, staff would need to maintain compassion without upstaging treatment; the handling of this impasse in treatment is critical to the overall success of this work. The treatment provider has to communicate compassion and support for this patient while firmly conveying the meaninglessness of interpersonal interactions following an act of self-harm or aggression.

For the therapist, the greatest difficulty in implementing this work comes from the rather counter-intuitive principle of engaging the patient only in the third step. Many unit staff and therapists find it difficult to disengage from the patient at the moment in which the patient starts to provoke an engagement through acting out. (Overt acting out feeds the cup and the covert acting out of engaging staff in a negative or non-productive manner also feed the cup.) Often, staff takes action preemptively to avert patient self harm or harming others. (Keep in mind that the high risk of death has already been discussed with the patient and her outside community case management team.) Premature engagement with the patient will only result in the powerful secondary gain of such acting out, not reacting to such provocation is truly a monumental struggle of the will between the patient and her staff. For therapeutic execution, staff are taught to *monitor from a watchful distance*. Treatment team members will require a great deal of processing and support amongst each other to carry on appropriate therapeutic engagement.

For a period of time, Doris was in a state of denial and avoidance about treatment. She appeared to be aware of her internal emotional pain and seemed very conversant of the treatment work but lacked true motivation in doing her work. Often, she cites her overall good behavior as evidence that she is doing well and no longer needed to do treatment. Of course, these periods are always followed by quick negative turn of events. Even though she has not been mindful of the 3-steps, she has periods of containing her impulse to overtly act out. At such times, it is useful for staff to review her effort in treatment and confront her about the lack of true repair work in her therapy. Doris has to understand that this type of session is certainly outside of the context of the 3-steps and does not contribute to the repair of her cup.

Doris, "I have been on good behavior for many days."

Staff, "Yes, you have managed to be safe and stayed out of trouble with others."

Doris, "I don't think I need to be in treatment anymore."

Staff, "Do you feel that you have been mindful of the cup and used the 3-steps?"

Doris, "Not really."

Staff, "I am glad that you have been on milieu level 3 for this many days. It shows that you have made an effort to better cope with difficult times. You do have to keep in mind that obtaining level 3, without mindfulness of the 3-steps, does not contribute to true repair of your cup."

Doris, "Why do I have to do anything else?"

Staff, "You are aware that, when you are feeling good, you will be getting along better with others and not acting out; but, how long do the good feelings last?"

Doris, "Usually not long. I wish my moods don't have to swing so much."

Therapist, "Let me ask you one question. Does your cup continue to leak even on a good day?"

Doris, "I guess it does."

Therapist, "Does it then make sense that feeling good won't last long?"

Doris, "Yes."

Therapist, "When you do pay attention to the cup, you will then be better aware of the need to do the 3-steps."

On a particularly angry day, she yelled and screamed at every staff, anything and everything was not to her liking. She finally stomped off to her room. A kind staff offered her some ideas to let time pass but she dismissed him unceremoniously. Monitoring from a distance, she appeared to be safe and sat listening to music. Staff carefully gauged the amount of elapsed time before approaching her once again. Upon checking-in, she became tearful and confessed to feeling fearful that her anger may engulf her and drive all others away, which she has already done with most family. Staff took this opportunity to help her understand the projected anger that is perhaps sourced from the deep emptiness that hides original anger. (Please refer to discussion of projective identification in chapter 9) "So, you mean that when I feel angry and irritable for no reason I can think of, it is because my cup has gone dry and the mud at the bottom of my cup can now be seen and smelled. As it overflows and splatters on people, it makes them angry at me and the dirt and smell makes them look ugly and mean to me." Yes, a scene highly reminiscent of the robin attacking its own reflection in the window.

Within the course of a relatively brief hospitalization, Doris came to settle comfortably into this treatment milieu and displayed a stability that was quite scarce in her previous history. She now exudes a confidence and independence that could only come from someone with sufficient trust for the consistency and availability of others; yet, she now maintains good boundaries with all of her staff through improved independent function. She can now better enjoy her own company and takes pride in her work and creativity while spending time alone; she seems to have discovered a whole new world of activities that she abhorred previously. Interpersonally, she appeared far less reactive of disappointments. When upset, she seems to have little use of dramatic displays of affect and instead, appeared quite satisfied at the chance to process with staff following a round of self initiated 3-steps.

Discussion:
How to appropriately meet the borderline patient's intense need for input into the cup is a perpetual challenge in any environment. Despite the intensive multi-systems approach the state took to manage a very challenging young person, much of the effort probably just prolonged the inevitable frustrations that she experienced. Some individuals behave as if they require input in a never ending stream; this is not possible and can not be appropriate. Often, the therapeutic work offered to the borderline patient actually engage the patient in intense interpersonal exchange that does not work to promote actual developmental growth. In certain circumstances, the intense exploratory work of therapy does not contribute to greater insight development but instead, encourages greater dependence on others for the unease of internal affect.

In other instances, the patient can cleverly engage the therapist in a game of pursuit that leads to increasing departure from good therapeutic conceptualization. Often, these conversations stem from the borderline patient's need to relive the extremes of a behavior through the retelling of an intense story to anyone willing to listen. With each repetition, a new iteration of the story is formed with greater details and images. It is as if the original story loses a certain degree of intensity and new versions are established in order to satisfy the hunger for acting out. Thus, even the telling of a story becomes an act of covert acting out; not because she is lying or creating a story, the hunger of the empty cup can only be satiated by something of intense substance at that very moment. Unwittingly, the therapist can enter into a realm of therapy that is unilaterally under the manipulation of the patient and partake in the replaying of the patient's ineffective coping methods. This can occur despite the therapist's best intentions to help the patient through transference interpretation. One should not be surprised at the need for caution even on the fundamental therapeutic task of listening.

Linehan advocates a biosocial theory of personality functioning that describes dysfunction of the emotion regulation system as resulting from biological irregularities combined with transactions with dysfunctional environments over time (Linehan 1993, p.42). Many of Doris's wild mood swings and the dramatic manner in which she experiences world about her can be understood through this type of biosocial theory of dysregulation. However, until more scientific knowledge is available to describe the inner biological workings of the emotional life, one is left with a certain aspect of dissatisfaction in resting on this view of dysregulation alone.

Elsewhere, it has been suggested that interpersonal theory and object-relations theory are fundamentally based in a dualism of drive versus relationship. "Either personality is conceived as organized and structured around innately unfolding drives or it is viewed as organized and structured around interpersonal relationships." "Neither relationships nor drives are primary; affect is primary. Tomkins conceives of affect as the *primary innate biological motivating mechanism*. It is affect that gives texture to experience, urgency to drives, satisfaction to relationships, and motivating power to purposes envisioned in the future" (Kaufman 1989, p.61). Here, if I may take the liberty to draw a mild connection, the discussions of Tomkins and Kaufman have a similarity to the analogy of the cup in this work. In our work, the innate drive system and affect system represented by the cup are also seen as intimately related and reciprocally affect each other.

The metaphor of the cup as described in DSA is indeed an affect based system of input and output. From this position is derived the theoretical understanding of classical defense mechanisms as well as the conditions of borderline personality disorder and narcissism. The direct effort to correlate the net gain and loss of content in an emotional reservoir to that of the use of classical defense mechanisms and character pathology makes for a model of treatment that is inviting as well as hopeful. Patients can be encouraged to work toward a reduction of acting out behavior from the onset of treatment and a ready system for positive affect (transference) replacement via the 3-steps is poised to leap into action as soon as the patient allows rudimentary engagement.

It is the nature and dynamics of this cup that ultimately appeals to the self preserving instinct of the organism to then seek tenable healing. In this work, the patient is discouraged from direct physical venting of feelings prior to self containment and self soothing. Guilt and shame are not awaiting high levels of expression, exploration and interpretation for resolution. The patient begins to work on self confidence immediately through the simple and achievable technique of interacting with selfobjects through the 3-steps. This simple method is practical and can be easily mastered by individuals of all levels of intellectual functioning regardless of whether the source of his emotional dysregulation is biological or social. Thus, an unwavering goal to achieve developmental repair makes the focus of this work easy to maintain.

Doing the 3-steps Amidst Daily Interactions

In using DSA, a frequent dilemma for those working with the borderline patient is that of knowing how to hold a common interpersonal interaction with the patient without feeling as if one is intruding on the moments when the patient should be directed to doing the 3-steps. One staff accounts, "I am in the milieu for a whole shift and I am around this patient all the time. I don't always know when to direct the patient to the 3-steps or perhaps, I tend to cue the patient to the 3-steps too often due to my own concerns about keeping him to treatment." Addressing such awkward moment is important because any hesitancy about the appropriateness of the interaction at hand will cause the selfobject/staff to appear distant, un-empathic and unsure in the interchange. Consequently, many therapy providers and parents abandon the therapeutic work in a flash of confusion about whether one is overly engaged in common daily interchange and when to cue the patient to do the 3-steps.

In the inpatient milieu, as in the family kitchen, there is the likelihood of having a number of people around and available for conversation or interactions at all time. The accessibility of this number of people should not be a detriment to encouraging the patient to be mindful of treatment. The usual greeting, communication, validation of feelings, and extension of support for the patient should not be eschewed. In most ordinary interactions, when the patient is not exhibiting disproportionate use of the interpersonal filling of the cup, it is unnecessary for the therapist or the selfobject to reject the patient's general social overture. The inpatient staff needs not be overly concerned that his interaction with a patient is too lengthy; it is far more important to focus on the quality of the moment.

It is effective to allow the natural rhythm of daily life to take its course. In so doing, the ebb and flow of individuals in this traffic of daily activities and routines will bring about natural coming together as well as separations from each other. With each separation, the borderline patient will again experience a certain degree of loss and emotional dysregulation. It is precisely this moment that he should be encouraged to not fight this separation but instead, to accept it through the implementation of the 3-steps.

Moreover, the distinction between what is a treatment conversation based on the 3-steps and that of a conversation otherwise consist of the specific awareness of the tension of emptiness. Beyond dealing with external stress, the borderline patient should purposefully focus on using the 3-steps for confronting the tension within. Thus, a clear distinction is made to delineate treatment from non-treatment conversation. The greater the distinction that a patient can make in this regard will allow him to conduct his treatment with less confusion and greater treatment efficacy.

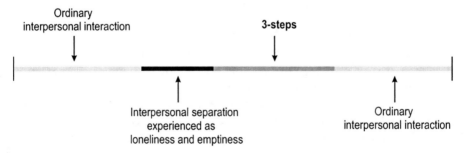

Fig 8.3 *This diagram represents a small segment of the individual's day. Each colored section can be of various time lengths. The patient has to recognize the feelings of loneliness and emptiness that follows each segment of separation; this is the cue to exercising the 3-steps.*

"I Will be Back."

Once the staff directs the individual to commence a round of the 3-steps, it is critical that he or she signal the intention to return to the patient. In the regular course of events, the 3-steps should never be viewed as a command or as a punishment. All too often, the misuse of the 3-steps is apparent when it is used to coerce the patient toward spending extra time on his own. About this issue, a major differentiation has to be made between what is encouraging the patient to self soothe in the context of the 3-steps as opposed to a way for the staff to extricate himself from an interaction with the patient. Without predictably checking back with the patient, it is simply conventional milieu management with questionable therapeutic value. The reaction commonly experienced by the patient at being told to "go contain" often involves feeling resentful and rejected.

If staff and patient separation is required, a simple statement by staff such as, "I need to take care of something" would suffice. However, the effective staff could take this opportunity to set the patient up for another round of the 3-steps by suggesting that, "I am going to be busy for a little while but if you get through your next group keeping the 3-steps in mind, I will check-in with you in about an hour." The treatment provider and even the parents of the borderline patient must always keep in mind the revolving nature of the 3-steps in daily life on the inpatient milieu or the family environment. Thus, every separation is just another opportunity to reconnect and validate.

Generally, the staff should not pause in the middle of an ongoing interaction to suddenly direct the patient to do the steps; this abruptness is likely to be experienced as a dismissal. Cueing the patient toward the 3-steps should best be done in the context of a lull in interactions.

Staff, "I feel as if you are seeking care taking and rescue from me."

Patient, "No I am not. Why do you say that?"

Staff, "Well, you seem anxious, uneasy, restless and agitated, yet you have been unable to tell me what upsets you. We have been talking a long time and I am not able to soothe you. This could be a very good time to practice the 3-steps."

Patient, "I think you are right."

Staff, "Let's plan to meet back again to process in about fifteen minutes."

In the course of doing treatment, the patient will gradually develop a greater interpersonal connectedness with his staff or therapist. As a selfobject to the patient, the therapist takes on increasing significance in this patient's world through mirroring and idealizing transference. Hence, the transference input of the therapist into the cup is sure to play an important role in their routine interactions with each other. As meaningful as this relationship is, allowing the patient to seek unlimited amount of interactions while the patient is found to be covertly acting out is clearly not therapeutically productive. This situation is ripe for therapeutic processing and not a time to fire the patient from treatment.

One may question the compassion of the 3-steps especially at a time when the patient appears to be emotionally labile and vulnerable. The totality of the DSA discussion should give the reader a powerful sense of the futility of incessantly providing emotional support without encouraging the patient to face some of his familiar inner tension. Hence, the patient must be confronted about acting out behaviors or ineffective interpersonal skills; this should be done through the context of the 3-steps. A patient who is versed in this work should only require a brief cue that his behaviors are not appropriate to the work of the 3-steps and that staff will not be available for intense interpersonal interaction at this time. Alternatively, the patient should be informed at the next opportunity to meet in the 3-steps that a previous opportunity to meet was deferred due to the patient's lack of appropriate demonstration of the work. If the patient has an adequate understanding of this work, having to forgo an opportunity to convene will be experienced as a very temporary frustration out of his own exercise of non-treatment choice; the next chance to meet is literally around the corner.

This very approach can be utilized by the outpatient therapist in that the stated understanding for the treatment contract is the following: the therapist will be available at the designated time and place for the session if the patient follows through with maintaining the safety and effective use of the treatment work. If the patient is unable to uphold this agreement, the consequences of his actions may mean that he is unable to attend the session. For example, if the patient suffered injury as a result of his acting out behaviors and had to be hospitalized, he may not be able to keep his usual appointment. When thus impressed with the importance of opting for the 3-steps, he is then aware that his staff "will be back."

Exploratory Work in the Third Step

Essentially, the therapist or others who participate in the process step have only got to listen and validate the patient's experience. However, this is a valuable moment in the course of therapy to address the here and now in the daily life of this patient. It is also a moment in therapy to further explore his historical patterns of interpersonal interactions. It may even be an opportunity to make a therapeutic interpretation. The third step can be a valuable opportunity to engage the patient in further therapeutic exploration if he is ready.

Often, his crisis of emptiness is triggered by his reaction to a perceived external conflict; this is a chance for his therapist to point out his usual patterns of response. He is likely to react to such events without careful consideration or discrimination; practically all events are experienced with similar intensity. The fragmentation of his self can occur at the slightest provocation. Given his inability to maintain cohesion of the self (appropriate and adequate filling of the cup), he is highly vulnerable to minor conflicts and perceived slights. Upon this upset, it is likely that he will quickly cut off any input from the offender into his cup and in return, the others will also cease offering their input. When this spigot of input from the other is turned off, his continuously leaky cup will surely run low more quickly. The third step is an opportunity to help him understand the dynamic in which such difficulties can occur and help him anticipate similar problems in the near future. The diagram in figure 7.1 can be an easy tool to illustrate how his interpersonal dynamics affect the cup.

In therapy, there may be selective moments in "processing" that can be utilized to further explore the patient's history, to review his strategy in coping and most commonly, analyze his interpersonal dilemma. On the other hand I do not feel that in the context of acute stabilization that there is much room for traditional exploratory or transference based psychotherapy. The fragile borderline patient may not be able to partake in such work. The initial goal of any psychotherapeutic work is to develop trust, attunement, validation, and acknowledgement. Given that DSA is a model of treatment that points to the importance for all individuals to work toward the repair of our own cup, any work that adds to trust, attunement, validation, confirmation and acknowledgement is productive work, even without initial psychotherapeutic exploration. Therefore, the cup and the 3-steps is therapeutic healing that can be highly effective without involving intense exploratory work.

The psychotherapeutic topics that can be extrapolated from the work of the 3-steps can be highly productive for the patient if he is ready for further exploration. Depending on the individual therapist's preference, issues such as abandonment, trust, validation, abuse and dependence are just a few of the common topics that are stimulated by the work of the 3-steps. Quite often, patients complain that the therapist or the staff seems not to care in the context of the 3-steps. Despite their awareness of the treatment model, patients find themselves struggling with the change in boundary for interpersonal interactions. Belying this belief, the therapist's diligent commitment to this model of work will bring about the patient experiencing the connection he wishes. Through this process of therapy, the patient has a highly efficient method of addressing transference issues related to his selfobjects.

Event Analysis using DSA

The metaphor of filling a cup is a practical way to analyze recent events and to dissect it in hopes of helping the patient gain some insight into cause and effect. The popular methods of taking the patient through a chain of events to review the cause and reaction often falls short of convincing the patient that he has anything to do with the chain of problems. Improving upon this method of assessment of an event is to combine such an analysis with DSA. The patient is guided toward understanding the impact of external events on his internal emotional life and the contribution of inner tension toward that of external conflicts. The goal is to help the borderline patient become more aware of his own responsibility in the feelings and problems he encounters. Once again, this has the purpose of strengthening his commitment to treatment.

Before engaging the patient in processing, it is important for the therapist to keep in mind the limitation in the borderline patient's ability to recall certain episodes accurately due to his tendency to activate defensive splitting in an experience. When an individual resorts to splitting the self and the object into compartments of good and bad, he will then be blinded to the truth and reality of the events at hand. In the defense mechanism of splitting, which can be closely coupled to his projection of anger, the patient's view of the other becomes all bad and tainted with his subconscious negative projections. This is another reason that simple analysis of a chain of events is not sufficient to help bring insight to the patient.

Teaching the borderline patient the proper skills to examine an event has to start from the fundamentals. The patient can be asked to take an event such as when he was looking in the mirror while brushing his teeth and think about all of the possible thoughts that could have entered into his mind during those few minutes. For example, when he looked at the tooth brush, he could have observed that there was a speck of food left on it from the previous brushing and felt repulsed momentarily. As he looked in the mirror, he was reminded of the acne developing on his nose and felt a sudden sense of resentment and a tinge of guilt for not following the skin care instructions by his dermatologist. Once he shook himself free of the guilt, he proceeded to put toothpaste on the brush; he then experienced a moment of anger because his wife bought the wrong kind of toothpaste when he explicitly asked for a specific type. As his mind percolated on this mood, he began to think about how the people in his life are just not paying much attention to what he tells them. He then wondered as to just how important he is in the life of everyone around him. In the next moment, his attention was drawn back to his mouth by the familiar twinge of a sensitive tooth resulting from the wrong toothpaste.

Such therapeutic exercises are helpful in bringing to awareness one's internal mental and emotional life in mundane daily activities. The mind is continuously active indeed. However, if the examination of an event ends with a list of external causative factors, then one can easily come to the conclusion that the problems reside in the others. A person may state, "These are the people and things that make me angry and sad." Even if one were to come to the conclusion that external events caused one to experience a particular feeling state, it is still too easy to come to conclude that the others are responsible for such tension.

If indeed the individual is aware that he may have over reacted to the chain of external events, he may not have the skills to recognize the reason for his excessive emotional response. The key here is to understand why he "over reacted." Therefore, the DSA therapist will help the patient look inwardly at the state of his cup before any exploration of the external events. Without this self realization, it is like the attempt to control and battle Mother Nature without first looking at human impact on the environment. Once the patient is aware of his own internal emotional state, he is more able to make sense of his reactions to the chain of events that has occurred.

In tracking the chain of events in the above example of a fellow brushing his teeth, the DSA therapist starts with a referral to the diagram of the cup. Following the patient's scene by scene description of images and thoughts, he is now aware of what made him feel upset as he headed to work this morning. Although he is now aware of what feelings he possessed at that time, he still has no insight about his own involvement in these feelings. His therapist will then ask him to dissect his feelings further and look to see if he can be in touch with any sense of the pain of emptiness within. If he is familiar with this baseline state, it will be rather easy for him to access this information quickly. His therapist could then refer to the diagram and review the dynamics of the cup.

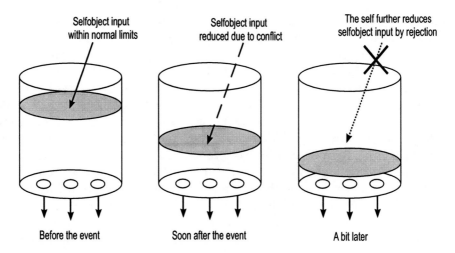

Figure 8.4 *In a state of conflict, the self could reject input from the selfobject as well as experience a reduction of output from the selfobject.*

More than just the analysis of external events, the realization of the existence of an internal emotional life is important in the work of DSA. Awareness of the state of his cup, recognizing that it was perhaps quite empty at the time of a specific event, allows him to be more accepting of his own responsibility in the end result. With experience, the patient will understand that chain analysis using DSA will allow him and his therapist to examine the issue from both sides. He will have a chance to review how the actions of another impacted his "cup" and the consequence of this exchange; thus, every problem is viewed through the internal perspective as well as the external happening. (Fig. 8.4) For a more advanced patient, a discussion of technicalities of splitting will further help him better analyze the situation. The step by step learning process that introduces the patient to DSA allows him to readily accept his internal emotional life as having a role in his external conflicts. In summary, when the borderline patient is aware and accepting of the existence of the emptiness and able to view this condition through the analogy of the cup, he is much more capable of benefiting from the sequential exploration of an event.

Disruption-Restoration Cycle

The life of a therapist is harsh, very harsh. At times, most of us have probably wondered if someone is playing a cruel joke on these bunches of poor, hapless psychotherapists. Patients often have high and untenable expectations on the therapist's unfailing ability to make him feel better. The psychiatric professional is viewed as a confident, self-assured, knowledgeable, selfless, empathic, strong, validating and reliable individual. One patient comments, "He is worth five of us." Another patient standing nearby comments, "No, he is worth five hundred of us." From such satirical comments one glimpse the deep potential conflict facing the patient seeking help from someone he perceives as authoritative. Of the astonishing complexity in therapy, it is not surprising that the patient can face certain disappointment whether he holds positive or negative transference with the therapist.

On occasion, when we get lucky, patients actually tell us that a therapeutic intervention made them feel better, but very soon, the wall comes tumbling down. The therapist is sure to disappoint. From the lofty position that the patient may place the therapist, empathic disruption can easily occur. Through such a disruption, past childhood trauma is resonated in the therapeutic setting but with a few differences. Now the patient is older and with age, comes with more maturity and resilience. Additionally, the therapeutic relationship is hopefully based on developing trust and memories of previous disruptions are repaired on the basis of trust. But, most importantly, the therapist's non-judgmental and accepting stance in treatment provides a most empathic and compassionate environment which is conducive to the restoration of the self. "The self thus emerges from the disruption-restoration incrementally strengthened by having integrated into the organization of its self-experience the contents and affects of the disruption-restoration experience" (Wolf 1988, p.104).

Theoretically, the disruption-restoration cycle is a very natural and healthy aspect of any interpersonal interaction. Thus, through each cycle of going from an idealizing transference, in which the patient seek merging with a strong and good selfobject, to the use of the defensive strategy of splitting to fend off the disappointment with the therapist, the patient comes to realize a more healthy stance with one selfobject. In DSA terminology, the 3-steps constitute just such a vehicle for the disruption-restoration cycle. The therapist's imperfection can be a disruption that awaits restoration in a purposefully prepared therapeutic environment that attempts to maximize such reparative cycles.

Furthermore, DSA prescribes an easily repeatable interpersonal interaction that can be implemented with all selfobject as opposed to limiting this selfobject experience to just the therapist. On the premise that interpersonal conflicts will occur, the patient is sure to experience disruption and disappointment. "What everyone learns early in life is to avoid, as far as possible, actual or symbolic experiences that reinstate painful affects aroused by memories (as well as misconstructions) of earlier experiences. If this means avoiding intimacy in interpersonal relationships or restricting them in other ways, that is the price that will have to be paid." Thus are the usual functions of the defensive operations to shield a person from painful affects (Strupp, 1984, p.32). In the current work, the therapist assist the patient in identifying reasonable selfobjects in his daily life and through preparatory family therapy sessions to set up opportunities for the 3-steps in the context of the disruption-restoration cycle of interpersonal interactions.

The 3-steps are to be exercised with individuals with whom one has issues or upset; for the borderline patient, this could easily be everyone in his world at one time or another. This is very much the essence of repair work through the use of this treatment technique. On feeling quite invalidated when her mother failed to acknowledge her loneliness, one young woman left her house in search of easier companionship. In the throes of her anger, she engaged in some high risk behaviors that only invoked greater shame and guilt. In analyzing such events with her therapist at the following session, she was able to recognize the hurt she felt in the cup and accepted the emptiness within. They then set up the opportunity for her to exercise the 3-steps with her mother on a regular basis which would also include times of perceived disruption in their relationship. It is generally difficult to connect with one another when one is upset, but she found that upon the completion of the first two steps, she can more easily approach her mother and discuss her feelings. Ideally, the primary motivation for her exercise of a different manner of coping was her desire to obtain healing in her internal emotional space.

Recap of Person, Place and Time

Therapy is always about interpersonal interaction. Interpersonal interaction is the most fundamental feature of human behavior and human society. It includes both verbal and non-verbal interactions as well as negative and positive interaction. It can even be said that an attempt to avoid interaction is really an interaction nevertheless. This is precisely why it is important to subscribe to some structure in order to best benefit from repeated interactions. Here, we are not so concerned about chance encounters or one time run-ins. The most frequently recurring interactions are those that we maintain with immediate and extended family. Within these orbits, there are certain individuals who play an especially important selfobject role. Beyond these orbits, there will also be some special people who do partake in unique selfobject experiences with us. Through sufficient compassion, empathy and eventually, transference, the therapist and treatment team can become important selfobject experiences for the borderline patient. How best to maximize this selfobject experience is at the core of our work.

Mirroring Transference with the Selfobject

Transferences of various types are important to the functioning of the individual with severe pathology of the self. In the very young child as well as individuals with an inability to hold the substance of the result of transference, the mirroring transference plays an important role to fulfill the needs of the self. The young child makes demands of his parents to provide the sort of unconditional admiration that bestow upon him the necessary cohesion to function in life and learning. When this child looks into the faces of his parents and sees this recognition and admiration, he is able to feel himself as a valuable and lovable person. (See figure 3.1) It is through idealizing transference, the need to merge with an idealized selfobject, and mirroring transference that binds us to important figures in our lives. We learn to rely on such object figures early in life and continue to depend on them for our internal emotional requirements as adults. The appropriate presence of selfobjects consistently in the context of person, place and time assures the healthy development of the self.

An Appropriate Place to Process

In negotiating any interpersonal interaction, it is always best to pay attention to the physical place of such encounters. This is just common sense but is often dictated by cultural elements. Certain conversations are more suitable to the therapy office and other discussions may be more appropriate to the dinner table. Some places and environments are more conducive to individual attention while other settings are designed for group activities.

For example, in the inpatient hospital setting, recreational therapy hour is usually a group activity time and it is generally not possible for staff to offer much in terms of individual attention. This happens to be one of the most frustrating times for many teens in the program given the fast action and potential for interpersonal conflict. Once an individual becomes upset, he has to be able to self soothe for a period of time, often encouraged as taking a personal time out, before a more private location is available for processing. If an individual suddenly felt the encroaching sense of wretched loneliness in the middle of a grocery aisle, finding appropriate selfobject or others in sharing and validating this moment is likely unrealistic.

Some may argue that in a world where cellular phones allow people to be in constant touch with each other could mean that loneliness will never be felt again regardless of your location. Firstly, it is exceedingly difficult to garner adequate attention in a random call to others every single time. Secondly, the quality of interpersonal connection is questionable over the phone. The phone may be a great tool for transmitting and communicating information but is can not compare to person to person contact for quality reciprocal interpersonal interaction. Recently, someone jested about never having to feel alone anywhere by mentioning that many luxury automobiles today offer a type of telephone/satellite monitoring and assistance; for an extra monthly charge, perhaps, the access to a human voice can be had while making the lonely drive to and from work. In a world in which consumer excess is only secondary to the aggregate demand for greater electronic flash and entertainment, there is sure to be a market for some type of constant companion regardless of location. Can this be a good thing? Well, hopefully, most people do not have a strong need to have constant contact with just anyone. For the borderline patient, the pursuit of constant connection with others can be significant in terms of the pathology of the self and therefore, even if such services were available, care should be taken regarding the appropriateness of such assistance.

Just as getting his empty cup filled instantly is discouraged in this work, his wife should not drop whatever she has been doing to cater to his demand to complete the 3-steps with him. Both the borderline patient and his wife have to respect the fundamentals of person, place and time. Even if he could call her on the phone, it is probably best to wait until she comes home. In the case of the patient in the milieu, he has to wait until there is a place of privacy for him to check-in with the staff regarding the 3-steps.

Finding the Time to be Together

Here, I am speaking of time as a negotiable entity. Of course, time is in a constant flow that never stops. Short of time travel, we can not manipulate time forward or backwards. Because time is highly precious and irreplaceable, most people know that they have to treat it like treasure. If so, one would dole out time as if it is money. If time is so valuable, each one of us would have to determine how we could best balance the use of our time. How much time to spend alone in pursuit of things to do in solitary and how much time to share with and include others, are just some of the issues of time.

For the borderline individual, when his cup is empty and he is feeling emotionally unwell, the essence of time may not play a critical role in daily life; remember that he is mostly in a crisis survival mode. For him, time may appear to stand still, as life seems one long dragged out painful episode, or time may speed by in a blur of barely memorable events. Either way, he may not value time like individuals with a healthier self. Here lies a high potential for tremendous conflict between the borderline patient and others around him. As we have discussed thus far, the borderline is often in need of a great amount of time investment from others. As we have also established, he is unable to maintain the positive benefit of his interaction with others and requires repeated, if not constant input. Given his enormous needs, there are few people who are so inclined to continuously give of themselves, essentially to give a great deal of their time. Often, people find themselves in a struggle to find a balance between how best to satisfy the borderline individual's needs and how best to preserve their own sense of value to their time. In this struggle, any perceived hesitancy in sharing of time can be interpreted by the borderline patient as monumental misattunement and disconnect. For him, the beleaguered content of the cup can only feel far worse at such a moment. If this is disappointment related to an important selfobject, the consequent anguish for the borderline patient can be quite profound.

Scarcely any interpersonal interactions occur outside of the proceedings of person, place and time. When we pay some attention and respect to the tempo of the person, place and time, life generally goes smoothly and productively. When efforts are made to go against this framework, the resulting experiences can be highly noticeable and unpleasant for everyone involved. The concept of the 3-steps helps to remind us that life is indeed based much on person, place and time by giving structure to our interaction with each other. For the borderline patient, the 3-steps has to be internalized, without it, he can not overcome the frustrations of daily life.

Identifying Problem Interactions

Here, I shall make a necessary comparison of routine daily interactions to that of the specialized interactions in the context of the 3-steps. I would like to emphasize here that even though the 3-steps have been characterized here as a natural part of every day life, few actually think in terms of the 3-steps in daily living. In reality, it is not necessary for most people with fairly healthy self and selfobject experiences to constantly think of the 3-steps in every interaction; for most, the 3-steps just occurs naturally out of their normal rhythm of life. For these individuals, the frustrations of daily life do not necessarily cause a fragmentation of the self. For them, even though a temporary loss of total cohesion of the self can occur with a faulty selfobject experience, the cup never completely runs dry. Because of the generally healthier internal emotional states, theses individuals would have learned early in life that they can easily manage self control in time of minor interpersonal crisis and are probably quite capable of "getting through it". In addition, most of these individuals probably have a ready set of support that they can reliably turn to at times of difficulties. Since they are not likely to be abusive of their relationships or turn to excessive use of psychological defense mechanisms such as splitting, projection and denial, he is sure to have a greater cadre of support players in times of need. For these individuals, they do not have to consciously think of the 3-steps in daily life, they just simply live the 3-steps in daily life. With far fewer leakages, it is much easier to simply refill the system and carry on with good functioning.

Against this normal backdrop of average daily life, the borderline patient has an intense affinity for interpersonal "filling". In DSA, this interpersonal affinity is viewed as both normal and abnormal, depending on the timing of its use. Some school of thought would suggest that women are more affectively connected and have greater intimacy and social support needs than men. It has been suggested that the emphasis and greater value placed on independence in Western culture invalidates a very fundamental feminine characteristic. "Indeed, it appears that there is a "poorness of fit" between women's interpersonal style and Western socialization and cultural values for adult behavior" (Linehan 1993, p.55). However, in our work here, the emphasis is on an emotionally reparative process rather than that of strictly meeting one's supportive needs. Consequently, interpersonal effectiveness in DSA is based on the proper allocation of interpersonal resource or support through heedful usage of person, place and time.

At first glance, the interactions of a young man on the inpatient unit seem quite the usual with talking, chit-chatting and laughing. As the staff moves away, he seemed quite reluctant to terminate the interaction despite a lull in the conversation and attempted to resume speaking; politely, the staff felt compelled to step back into the conversation and paid further attention. After several rounds of this dance, his listener finally makes a more dramatic move away. He then escalated by stating how depressed he has been feeling and related of a welling up of an urge to self-mutilate. In other instances of this sort, he has raised a wide range of concerns from his anxiety that he may now be suffering from cancer to reports of visual and auditory hallucinations. In each of these encounters, the attributes of normal interpersonal interaction can quickly breakdown to a frantic plea for sustained attention on the part of the borderline patient and a sense of disquiet at best but perhaps, anger and frustration on the part of the staff. In overview, it is the tipping of balance from reciprocal interpersonal interaction toward that of unidirectional flow that hints at the sudden change in the dynamics with a borderline patient.

The astute DSA clinician will carefully evaluate the manner in which the patient carries out the 3-steps. Many individuals will utilize the 3-steps in an isolated fashion without sufficient consideration for the broader purpose of the need to do this work. In alluding to the 3-steps, one young woman gives the appearance of doing the steps yet she never seems to improve clinically. Thus, upon returning to the acute inpatient setting from a residential treatment facility, the team probed into the cause of such impasse. This patient was asked, "When do you think of using the 3-steps?" She answered, "Well, I use it when I feel sad or mad." The keen reader of this material will instantly recognize that her answer is mostly incorrect in the optimal use of this work. The reason that it is partially faulty is due to the notion of the treatment of emptiness versus the management of anger.

Foremost, the 3-steps are for the purpose of bringing together a corrective emotional experience with the selfobject introject. These steps can certainly be useful in the management of anger and other emotions but this type of use eschews the primary benefit of this treatment experience. In referring to feelings such as sadness and anger, most people imply an experience that is brought on by the actions of others; this is a focus that detracts from the important focus on the aversive tension of emptiness. Therefore, this patient's answer gives us a clue as to her lack of true clinical improvement. It appeared that she uses the 3-steps to calm herself once she faces rejection from her attempts to seek extensive emotional rescue.

Theoretically, I do maintain the belief that the 3-steps under most circumstances, if done properly, can be healthy and healing for most people. However, for the borderline patient, these steps should best be performed in the context of the awareness of the emptiness within. Within the structure of the 3-steps, many issues of an individual's daily functions can be addressed but it is the working of the 3-steps with a mindfulness of the emptiness that holds the greatest healing for the individual seeking emotional stability and actualization of the true self. This point is not difficult to understand in the context of DSA; ownership of our hurt is priority number one in the attainment of motivation for this healing work.

Hence, one can now see that, in daily life, what constitute as normal interpersonal interaction may actually be an activity that can be quite toxic to the borderline patient. What he simply sees as a "feel good" thing to do may only prolong his suffering. What everyone may assume to be the best and only thing that they can do to be of help to this individual may only contribute to his disorder. What appears to be an innocent conversation or interaction can turn out to be nothing more than a temporary fill for a very empty cup. As a result of the patient's projective identification or the staff's own countertransference, the staff will generally experience a strong sense of foreboding that can warn him or her of the potential problems in this interaction. For inpatient staff and outpatient therapist's alike, confronting this transition from normal daily interaction to that of a unidirectional flow of "stuff" or input toward the patient is always a challenging dilemma for even very experienced staff. As always, the recognition of a problem is the beginning of resolution. DSA is designed to help in the recognition of problematic interpersonal dynamics.

Following the identification of another problem interpersonal moment with the patient, it is vital that the therapist or the staff immediately make the move to direct the patient's attention toward the pre-3-steps and the 3-steps. Staff could say something to the effect, "It seems that this is an appropriate time for you to check the level in your cup. What number would you give the cup in the last few moments of our conversation? What was the level of the cup even before we entered into this conversation?" Often, the borderline patient appears to drain empty even as he engages in a conversation or interaction with another; this is an indication of the severity of the pathology and attest to the futility of simply filling the cup. A patient who is well versed in the work of DSA will instantly recognize that it would be crucial to do the 3-steps at this time and has the trust in staff that, once he has completed the first two steps, he will have an opportunity to meet with staff to process.

At times, the staff may have to be very firm about his request for the patient to implement the 3-steps given the natural tendency for the patient to resist the work in the initial phase of treatment. If necessary, the staff may have to make a physical move away from this patient while verbally making sure that the patient understands that this is a temporary break in their interaction and that the staff will resume contact in a given amount of time. The staff then returns in ten minutes (the amount of time elapsed is based on the patient's capability at that juncture in treatment) as planned and gives encouragement to the patient for the successful implementation of the first two steps and complete the process step with the patient. In so doing, step by step and day by day, the patient learns to feel more secure about this treatment method and his relationship with his staff.

When to Maintain a Watchful Distance

In the context of therapy, the inpatient milieu is very unique but not unlike the home environment for the borderline patient. On the unit, it is often difficult to determine when one episode of acting out behavior stops and another such act begins when viewed in the continuity of life in the milieu. Therefore, staff members frequently voice concerns about how best to implement treatment and support the patient as effectively as possible. "When should I keep a watchful distance and when should I step in to reinforce and encourage the patient on his positive behavior?" It can be very challenging at times to stay true to treatment boundary while providing compassion and support for the patient.

The key to this issue requires a great deal of individual staff and therapist assessment based on his or her keen observation of the patient. Referring to figure 8.3, after an obvious episode of acting out, when should the staff resume interaction as usual? How would such interaction be differentiated from general interpersonal interaction? An important point to keep in mind is to think about the borderline patient who has just recently turned to a round of drug or alcohol use and having had this "fix", he is rather satisfied for the moment and may not be interested in anyone else or anything else. If not for detoxification treatment, there is really little reason to believe that therapist intervention would be useful at this time. In DSA, the staff is best to stand back at a watchful distance between point A and B; staff will not directly interact with the patient at this time except to provide very brief cues to the patient to be mindful of the 3-steps.

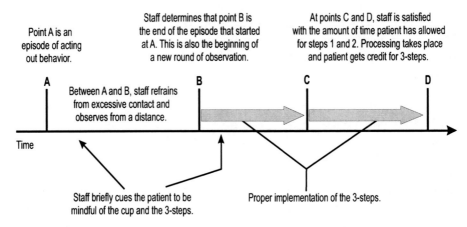

Figure 8.5 *Each episode of acting out behavior has its "acting out value" that is unique to the individual. Hypothetically, this value gives this individual a certain amount of "filling" expressed in terms of time. It is understood that by point B, he is empty once again. From B to C and C to D, the patient and the staff can mutually determine that sufficient time has passed for containment and meet with each other to check-in.*

The amount of time that should elapse between A and B is rather arbitrary and depends on the staff's discretion. While it is important to allow some time to pass, the essential action to take is to establish this period of time as a temporary break from interpersonal contact given that the patient has managed to fill his own cup with acting out behavior. The staff will then monitor for the beginning of a round of 3-steps, point B. Other than brief cues to do the 3-steps, the staff waits for a suitable amount of time to pass, and if the patient has not approached the staff to check-in, the staff can initiate proper interpersonal contact to complete the third step. Rather than specify a time for the staff to return, for a more initiated patient, the staff cues by stating, "I am looking for a chance to do the steps with you." Life on the inpatient unit should take on the rhythmic cycles of patient in un-therapeutic behavior and patient working in the 3-steps.

Figure 8.6 illustrates another clinical scenario frequently encountered in the acute inpatient setting. Working with patient's who are highly disruptive in the milieu, whether through aggression or self destructive behavior, the inpatient staff has few other choices but to engage the patient as therapeutically as feasible without introducing any anti-therapeutic stance or precedent in this interaction.

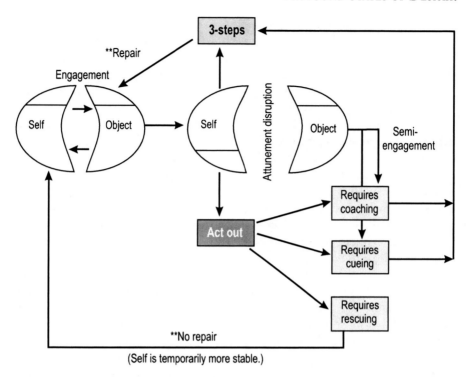

Fig 8.6 *This coaching, cueing and rescuing diagram illustrates the necessary steps to take in engaging a particularly difficult patient who is involved in severe acting out behaviors.*

In the engagement phase, the transference exchange between the self and the object flows smoothly and the core self of this individual can be felt as strengthened. Experiences of misattunement are inevitable and can manifest in a fragmentation of the self with the accompanying drop in the system level for the borderline patient. The patient who is actively engaged in treatment will realize the significance of this experience and knows to turn toward the implementation of the 3-steps to seek repair. The non-engaged patient may still turn to insipient ways of coping involving rescue or acting out behaviors. Certain manners of acting out can be especially disruptive and at risk in the inpatient milieu and must be contained for the safety of other patients and staff.

At the moment in which an angry patient is posturing to throw a chair or instigating a fight with another patient, responsible action on the part of the staff is required. When a patient has a piece of sharp object and gestures repeatedly to cut self or inflict injury on others, intervention must take place to assure the safety of all involved. This clinical moment is different from the repeated demand for rescue by the individual with chronic parasuicidal behavior. One family's acceptance of the risk of death of an individual patient does not translate to placing other patients or staff at risk.

In implementing semi-engagement (Fig.8.6), the staff can cue the patient about the 3-steps and other coping skills as well as set up a check back time with the patient. The staff can briefly discuss with the patient about his options for letting time pass/self soothe. In de-escalating a highly charged and aggressive patient, the staff may have to take the extra effort to coach the patient on how the 3-steps might look in practice while allowing for the patient to benefit from borrowing "ego" from his staff. If the inpatient staff elects to provide this degree of engagement, it is therapeutic to teach, demonstrate and extricate with an agreement to check back in a short period of time. At times, the reality of the moment may simply mean that the staff helps the patient achieve calm through any reasonable method and set the patient up for a 3-steps type of check-in shortly after. On the aggregate, all roads must lead to the 3-steps in order for treatment to be productive and to avoid another such episode.

On the frequent occasion in which a patient is perhaps new to treatment and is unable or unwilling to utilize coping skills, the therapist/staff may have limited options but to provide interpersonal rescue. Most times, even the most resistant patient can step up to treatment just enough to be given credit for the 3-steps. For the majority, interpersonal transference input is so valuable beyond belief that most borderline patient would readily opt for emotional rescue over that of acting out behaviors. In these instances, with patient and milieu safety in mind, the staff may elect to provide full care taking in order to avoid a dangerous confrontation with the patient or risk serious disruption of the environment. It is important for the therapist to understand that care taking can still be a final semi-therapeutic option for the extremely distraught patient. However, following such a therapeutic impasse, his staff must work diligently toward returning this patient to the treatment protocol as soon as possible.

A truncated exchange the next day between the patient and his therapist may look like the following:

Therapist, "How are you feeling today?"

Patient, "I feel pretty good but last night was something."

Therapist, "I am glad that you allowed me to talk with you. You seemed calmed by my being there for you."

Patient, "Oh, yes. I just needed someone to be there when I felt so lonely and could not stop crying."

Therapist, "You are now familiar with the cup and the 3-steps. How did your cup experience that episode of crisis last night?"

Patient, "Well, my cup felt fuller after you talked with me. I think it was good treatment."

Therapist, "I agree that both of our cups were probably filled up pretty well through that interchange. Is it your understanding that the cup would have gotten repaired in the process of our talking together?"

Patient, "Yeah. Sure. Why not?"

Therapist, "Did you experience yourself doing steps one and two?"

Patient, "No. I guess I didn't."

Therapist, "Although we both felt better as a result of that interaction, feeling good is not the same as getting better. You have indicated that it is healing that you want. In the future, we both have to work toward meeting in the 3-steps."

Patient, "I see. I think I would like to try to do that."

In summary, what is considered appropriate and normal interpersonal interaction found in the vicissitude of daily life has to be differentiated from that of a one way transference feeding of the cup as often practiced by the borderline patient. Guiding the patient toward a productive interpersonal interaction can be fraught with obstacles and challenges for the staff/therapist. Many instances of psychotherapeutic interchange that takes place spontaneously in the milieu may be deemed effective intervention in conventional thought although it is difficult to gauge the productiveness of such interactions. To address this, all interpersonal interactions in the milieu should be defined in the context of the 3-steps. The goal of de-escalation should involve getting the patient acquainted with the notion of the 3-steps. Because of the subtleties of differentiating normal from the pathological interpersonal exchanges, it is important that the team members provide feedback to help each other identify the presence of unhealthy interactions. The staff's willingness to confront this dynamic helps to keep the treatment team vigilant about one's boundary with this patient.

Confronting Resistance

Let us now consider patient resistance as the expected outcome of the initial introduction of this work. I would assert that most patients are quite compliant at the introductory family session to DSA. He may be quite enthralled at having the therapist place such emphasis on helping the family understand his emotional pain and the triumph of validation can be exhilarating. However, beyond the initial cognitive insight of the session, emotionally, he is likely to quickly return to the use of former coping. Although warned about the detriment of using people and acting out to fill the cup, he may become resentful that attempts are made to deter him from the familiar and easier methods of coping. This could result in an escalation of acting out behavior.

Many writers of psychotherapy advocate the importance of confronting resistance as a technique in treatment; it is especially true in working with borderline patients. "Historically, success in the treatment of the borderline personality disorder was long delayed. Chief among the many reasons was a failure to realize that, for the most part, the borderline patient does not come into treatment in order to "get better." Rather, he or she enters treatment primarily to "feel better" (Masterson JF, Klein R, 1989, p. 217). Resistance will be particularly strong in an individual at the stage of illness where he has discovered exceptional control over the people around him. In the language of DSA, this is the filling of the cup via source B in Fig. 7.1. As a result, it is understandable that he will be quite reluctant to give up this people input to the cup.

Abandonment Depression

Starting from the initial family session to introduce DSA as a method to understand the borderline dynamic, the patient will have to confront his fear of forsaking the unrealistic wish for all of his needs to be completely met by the hypothetical maternal object. "In the borderline patient, a move toward separation-individuation is always followed by or accompanied by anxiety and depression and/or defenses against them until the abandonment depression has itself been worked through in psychotherapy. Successful treatment occurs when the patient tolerates, manages, and works through anxiety and depression rather than retreats from efforts at separation-individuation in order to avoid the unpleasant abandonment feelings" (Masterson, Klein, 1989 p.173). Many writers of personality disorders points to the existence of abandonment depression at the juncture of separation-individuation, which parallels a phase of development from one to three years of age as described by Margaret Mahler. Relating the borderline defenses to this developmental phase is very significant to the work of treatment.

Developmentally, the elated mood of the toddler is dampened during the rapprochement subphase of separation-individuation. The false self of the borderline patient "consist of two coexisting, alternately activated, and equally unrealistic self-images: a helpless, compliant, dependent child who is rewarded for this behavior and an inadequate, bad, worthless person who causes others to withdraw emotional support at any hint of real self-activation or self-assertion" (Masterson, Klein, 1989 p.36). Abandonment depression can lead to a sense of anxiety and emptiness which then invokes the false self, a defensive self representation that is infantile and primitive and based on fantasy and distortion. It is worthwhile to remind the reader that the depression that is being discussed in this instance is a state of feeling resulting from the patient's general lack of self activation to recognize the true self.

Having developed a pathetically dependent affair with a married man, "She eventually brought herself to end the liaison. She became depressed and overwhelmed. Before this time, she had no awareness that her relationship had functioned as a defense against feelings of depression. *She seems to think that her emotional problems were a reaction to external circumstances.* Now she noted that when she began to explore her feelings and activate herself, she became more depressed" (Masterson, Klein, 1989 p. 175-177 italics are mine). In the language of the Masterson approach, behaviors that promotes the use of the "false, defensive self" will bring treatment to a stand still and no further activation of the real or true self in or out of therapy sessions. In short, her destructive behaviors were used in defense of existing emptiness and depression, not that external events lead to depression. The metaphor of the cup is to make this point absolutely clear.

Most patients who enter into treatment voluntarily want to demonstrate a willingness to make changes and show improvement to please his therapist. However, once the borderline patient finds that the application of focused treatment work demands an initial acceptance of emotional pain, he is likely to withdraw true investment in treatment. Rather than to directly reject treatment, given that he has voiced motivation for self preservation, he is more likely to sabotage treatment through other means. This type of resistance often takes shape as something that appears, on the surface, to be beyond his control. An example is the patient overwhelmed by such dysphoria that he is unable to function in treatment. In working with patients, I often use the analogy of an individual holding a dilapidated old ball aside with both hands while facing his therapist saying, "Sure, I am ready to pick up a new ball." His therapist might answer that, "As you hold on tightly to your old ball with both hands, it would be quite difficult for you to pick up a new ball."

Clinically, one often observes that the introduction of DSA can be intimidating for the borderline patient due to the prospect of change toward a more independent model of function. It may be difficult for him to grasp the fundamental idea that he will not ultimately be abandoned. However, just the switch toward independence and individuation can threaten his sense of self, in essence, the stability of the cup. He has the need to maintain his unrealistic self-image in order to parlay it into a satisfyingly dependent relationship with object figures. He may feel compelled to present as helpless in order to assure the constant availability of those around him. In DSA terminology, his maintenance of the false self will assure that significant others will continue to give to his very empty cup. The threat of not being able to maintain the usual homeostasis for the cup can rapidly reduce its level and trigger depression that leads to further anxiety. He can then become sullen, withdrawn, angry and rejecting. He wants to "sleep all day". He relates of feeling more depressed than usual. He has little energy to participate in life. On the ward, staff will note an up tick in his report of somatic symptoms. All of this may be an attempt to appeal to the empathy of others in order to restore the equilibrium as usual but often, the clinical observation is that of an individual who truly present sickly, depressed and withdrawn.

Confront with Compassion

Reflecting on the issue of resistance; let me cite a common scenario. A few days following a family session, the inpatient staff frantically reported that the patient had a difficult evening; he self-mutilated and attempted to tie a makeshift rope, made from some articles of clothing, around his neck. Although it is not possible to be predictive of suicidal behavior, in retrospect, he has many such attempts and gestures rooted in his helpless bid for emotional rescue. When staff intervened, he became combative and tried to prevent them from loosening the rope. This prompted the staff to step up their intervention to involve physical containment to assure his safety as well as others. He finally calmed and slept quietly in a monitored room until morning. As is usual practice, the attending psychiatrist is informed of such sentinel event.

At the team meeting the following morning, the decision was made that several of the key members of this patient's treatment team would sit down with him to review the cup and the 3-steps using this recent episode as subject of how he could better utilize treatment. The patient would be confronted with the reality that it was fortunate that he was discovered by staff but the outcome could have been easily tragic. The likelihood of death, as discussed in the family session, was reviewed. The patient was also informed that such events would have to be reviewed with the family and they too will be reminded of the discussion in family session about the ongoing high risk of death. When the opportunity is available, it is usually a good idea to bring the family back in to review treatment using recent events as points of discussion.

During a confrontation about his recent acting out behavior, I could now utilize some of the language of DSA in our conversation.

Therapist: "Could you tell me what you were feeling just before you attempted to strangle yourself? Were you having a particularly bad day?"

Patient: "I had a pretty good day but the feeling of sadness and emptiness just suddenly overtook me."

Therapist: "What were the events or triggers that led up to your feeling such emptiness?"

Patient: "I was watching and eavesdropping on some families visiting and I got to thinking about my own family. Then I just started to feel that no one really cared about me. I tried to look for a staff but it seems that they were more interested in some of the other patients. That was when I started to think about wanting to die and looked for a way to do that in the hospital. Working on that rope helped me to feel much better knowing that I was going to hang myself."

Therapist: "Can you recall what condition your cup was in at the time?"

Patient: "It was low."

Therapist: "Zero being the lowest and ten being the highest, what number would you give the cup?"

Patient: "I would probably give it a two."

Therapist: "Did you try to do your 3-steps?"

Patient: "No. I just wanted to die."

Therapist: "You put up quite a struggle with staff who tried to help you. How did you feel before you drifted to sleep eventually?"

Patient: "My body ached but emotionally I did not feel so upset inside anymore."

Therapist: "You seem calm this morning."

Patient: "I feel o.k."

Therapist: "I need to remind you that when you act out in this way to fill your cup, you are acting on the decision to fill the cup yourself in a way that is clearly not treatment. Given your familiarity with this work, I do not feel that it is necessary for me to review each episode of self-harm with you. It is important to review the chain of events that led up to you feeling increasingly empty in the cup but it is more useful to do this detailed analysis as part of your 3-steps rather than after an episode of acting out. When you cut yourself, you essentially fire everyone from your treatment picture for now."

An intuitive strategy by a staff, shortly after dealing with the acute outburst of a patient who then immediately apologized and wanted to process, was to make it clear to the patient that she could only process with him the next workday. She realized that following such an episode of intense intervention, she was not capable of the mindset to work with this patient immediately after and frankly, she may want to do her own 3-steps before she can be emotionally ready to work with this patient again. In her handling of this scenario, she was able to briefly address the acute acting out behavior of the patient but extricated herself as soon as possible (while other staff continued to monitored the patient from a distance). A therapeutic opportunity happens when the staff can demonstrate to the patient that she can integrate this experience, using the 3-steps, into her own emotional world without overt countertransference.

On confronting the extent to which one patient was fruitlessly resisting treatment, I used the analogy of a car that has sat corroding through much mistreatment. On each occasion in which this car was towed to the gas station to fuel up, it could only make it out of the station a few blocks before it's fuel gauge indicate empty again. Hence, this car would have to seek the closest gas station to refuel in order to continue; naturally, it was not going to travel far. Regardless of the manner in which it was abused in times past, it is pointless to discuss the cause of damage when repair is critical. Of course, understanding past damage can lend an understanding to best method of repair as well as how to avoid future harm.

Here I will provide another useful metaphor to help break through resistance by drawing attention to the fruitlessness of the borderline patient's incessant shortcuts to filling the cup. The therapist remarks, "The picture that comes to mind is that of you in a fast-food joint and the clerk has just handed you a broken cup along with your order of burger and fries. You set the food down and go to the soda fountain to fill up with your favorite soft drink. It seems that you are standing at the fountain a long time because each time you think you have filled the cup, it just all leaks out before you can take it back to your table. However, rather than get a new cup, you keep going back to the soda fountain to fill up yet again. But, as you get frustrated with not being able to fill it with your preferred pop, you settle for other flavors. As you repeatedly hit the various levers to fill your cup, you are momentarily encouraged that the cup is filling but nothing remains in the cup upon return to your table. In response to your frustrations, the clerk goes to make sure that the soda fountain has plenty of pressurized canisters connected to the soda fountain and you continue to push on the levers with your cup to no avail. What is interesting and disheartening about this scene is that I don't see you attempting to exchange the broken cup for a new one. As you know, I am not able to just hand you a new cup in this therapy work but I am trying to convince you that there are ways to patch the cup to make it more useful."

An acute sentinel event requires a review of treatment work with the patient but it should be done in a fashion that does not interfere with the overall goal of treatment. An appropriate timing would be point C in figure 8.5.

In this fashion, all of the staff are maintaining a good boundary and providing safe supervision of the patient without unnecessary filling of the patient's cup. The patient is assured that the staff will be taking time to regain composure and will return to help him complete the 3-steps at a later time. In the meanwhile, this patient, well versed in the work of DSA, understands that he could soothe himself through activities that are self rewarding as well as allowing time to pass before he could look forward to the step of processing with this staff. The staff's desire to delay the act of processing is a very natural consequence of this interpersonal interaction and an important dynamic in this patient's interpersonal learning.

External Contributors to Resistance

In order to resolve the impasse of resistance, it is important to keep in mind the role of the family system as well as all others involved. Interestingly, his resistance to change can be sustained by others with the conviction that they and they alone, can provide for and keep this patient happy. These individuals in his life may develop such transference as to consider their relationship with him as somehow special and exclusive. Granted, some of these individuals do play a special role in his life but the excessive development of this sentiment points toward enmeshment. This is projective identification of dependence at work, which will be further discussed in the following chapter, and given its bidirectional nature, should be monitored closely in therapy.

Using the cup analogy, every person involved with this patient should be confronted regarding his or her role in promoting his resistance to change. The therapist has to start with looking at whether or not there is an iatrogenic cause to this resistance. Inadvertently, the therapist or the inpatient staff can be seen by the patient as just another input to his cup. This type of dependence could arise out of countertransference or projective identification and render the therapist ineffective in guiding the patient toward change. As has been frequently encountered, whether in a therapeutic group home setting, a residential placement, acute inpatient milieu or the home and community environment, individuals around the patient may actively resist the treatment protocol due to his or her own misguided sense of interpersonal effectiveness.

Because the bidirectional transference filling of the cup can be so powerfully fulfilling for the moment, it can be intoxicating to the unwary and the uninitiated. This is an interpersonal scenario that could resemble compassion and empathy on the surface but it is in fact devoid of altruism. On review, this scenario is likely the most common reason that inpatient treatment fails to stabilize the parasuicidal behavior of the borderline patient. The therapist also needs to look at other concentric orbits around this patient and examine whether or not some individuals in these orbits are intentionally or unintentionally contributing to the patient's resistance. Confronting these individuals will not be easy, but the use of the cup illustration generally makes it more understandable and acceptable to the individuals involved.

DSA is a model of treatment that does not place blame but instead, is focused on insight development to correct the ineffective manner of interaction in which individuals in the family system are bound. When others see how their incessant input to the patient's cup will only leak out soon after, they would be more judicious and intelligent about how they would focus their effort in helping this patient. A picture is truly worth a thousand words. It is for this reason that I refer to the cup illustration each time I meet with the patient and his family to review his progress.

Three Steps for Supplying Compassion

Case 8.2: Madeline arrived on the unit after having metaphorically burned all of her bridges in her brief 17 year history. She is a tall and lanky teen with a casually tossed head of hair accompanying winsome good looks. She has a habit of looking at people as if glaring at them but most likely, she could just be studying others intently to learn of their intentions. There was actually nothing friendly about her on initial meeting. She seemed highly guarded and treated every question with suspicion. She made it quite clear that she has no reason to trust anyone. Furthermore, she stated that life has been frustrating and painful for her up to this point and that she just wants to put it behind her and move on. Her demeanor has a hint of defiance combined with a trace of frail vulnerability. Despite this declaration and the rather hostile initial façade, she came to display a very dependent relationship with all around her.

In time, she began to share some stories about her past and together with collateral information, a picture of abuse and emotional neglect built the foundation for understanding her development of the false self. She was the product of parents who were constantly embroiled in conflict with each other. Her parents suffered from their own mental illness and perhaps, coped by the use of alcohol. She often worked to keep her siblings from getting into trouble with the parents and made it her daily goal to do whatever it takes to avoid getting her father angry. Her father's episodes of anger outburst terrified and tormented her throughout her early childhood.

Having thus suppressed and denied her sense of self, she began to feel that she is not an acceptable person. She started to feel that there were reasons that her parents showed such explosive anger toward her and considered herself as unlovable and undeserving of love. Having denied her real self for so long, she can only recognize the aspect about her that seems to garner great anger and frustration from others. Soon after, she too began to dislike most everything about her. With this self hate, she discovered drugs and boys are a way for her to find temporary relief from her constant state of self loath and the incredibly negative internal feelings she was experiencing.

By the time of her first hospitalization, she was completely immersed in a very destructive life style. She frequently engaged in unprotected sex with near strangers. She incorporated self-mutilation and drug use into her daily routines. She ran away from home at every opportunity and when her father yelled at her on return, she left again.

In the hospital milieu, she presented as very aloof interpersonally and highly resistive to the treatment program. At every possible chance, she can be found voicing criticism of staff for not showing more care or compassion. She frequently points out that any attempt to explore issues related to her current acting out behavior constitutes a misattunement on the part of her staff or therapist. Appealing to the desire of staff to be helpful, she was able to mobilize this most basic of human instinct to her advantage. In a rather peculiar development, she began to turn the table around and placed responsibility on others to soothe and meet her needs. Some uninitiated and inexperienced staff quickly rallied to her aid despite the team's concerns about appropriateness of boundaries and consistency to treatment. At this point, she saw the "good" staff as individuals who were willing to lavish great amounts of attention on her when she experiences any distress. These staff felt that giving her the needed attention will appease her and calm her sufficiently to avoid any further escalation of her negative behavior at times of upset. As expected, her behavior and investment in treatment did not improve despite ever more attentiveness by staff members. In addition, she gradually evolved a greater dependency with a number of peers who were all willing to go to battle with staff to assert their proclaimed role of being a highly supportive friend.

The dynamics between this patient and her staff quickly degenerated to the establishment of "good" staff and "bad" staff. She harbored great animosity towards staff she perceived as being against her if they encouraged her to be mindful of treatment at times of mounting distress. What appeared to be some rudimentary acceptance of the treatment was then abandoned in favor of complete reliance on instant gratification through interpersonal fulfillment. What follows can be devastating to the treatment milieu as unskilled staff got more involved in care-taking and skilled staff became more rigid in trying to implement boundaries, countertransference became rampant. She became increasingly difficult to manage in the milieu. She presented as more emotionally fragile and acted out more aggressively toward others. Her demands of attention and support became increasingly difficult to satisfy. Her relationship with certain favorite staff also became quite unstable, and visibly, she appeared more frustrated and emotionally labile. At this juncture, she displayed a bewildering number of extreme demands or acting out behavior on a regular basis that keeps the team just dealing with crisis. Of course, the team is paralyzed in just doing everything they could to keep this patient safe and no treatment could possibly be delivered in this context.

The team then had to evaluate the situation at hand and come up with a synthesis understanding as well as a solution. When the team reflected on the issue, it was immediately apparent that staff morale was low and there were internal dissent about the direction that the team should take with this patient. The team was at odds with each other over how best to supply the empathy and compassion that most any mental health provider sees as a part of the job description. It was identified by the team that the tendency for some staff to offer interpersonal attention indiscriminately and outside of the context of treatment was eroding the opportunity for this patient to receive optimal treatment. This was probably the most difficult juncture for the treatment team in the course of working with this patient.

For a solution, the team came up with a compromise that worked surprisingly well in a less than ideal situation. It was felt that, while there was a lack of consensus amongst staff, getting the team to work consistently together in a timely manner could still offer this patient a productive treatment opportunity. The plan was for staff to provide the degree of interpersonal intervention they feel necessary to assist this patient through her difficult moments but to always approach these interactions observing the 3-steps protocol. The assumption is that this is obviously a very fragile and unstable patient; her ability to self soothe is very limited. She may not be capable of being mindful of the 3-steps at times of severe emptiness, but if we observe carefully, we could still pick out elements in her behavior that would be consistent with some degree of containment and letting time pass, the first two steps. The team will then allow her credit for doing an abbreviated version of the 3-steps. The staff would remind the patient that she has been observed to have performed the first and second step regardless of the brief period of letting time pass. The staff can then point out to her that their current interaction is consistent with the third step.

In this manner, those staff members who feel that the patient requires a greater amount of personal attention can do so without totally disregarding the treatment work of other members of the team. As a result, dissension within the team was resolved and treatment consistency restored. Subsequently, with a lesser degree of splitting, this patient showed greater calmness in the milieu. She may have learned that she can now access far more staff input as well as meeting her needs more successfully. Most significantly, on observation and patient self report, she can tolerate time alone and soothe herself far better now and does not require constant supervision from staff. In addition, she became much more willing to be mindful of treatment work and responded well to the requirement for her to check with staff a minimum of twice a day to report on the use of the 3-steps.

Prior to discharge, she was more trusting of staff members in general. She would no longer wave her past trauma in front of staff to demand special sympathetic treatment. She seemed satisfied in the overall attention she received from others but still required frequent reminders for maintaining appropriate boundaries with peers. She also ceased using self mutilation to ease her internal pain and to retrieve a sense of aliveness. At the time of discharge, the team felt pleased that treatment work had been rendered and were able to help this patient take the first step in therapy.

Discussion:
The treatment team came up on a major challenge in this case, although the degree of acting out on the part of this patient was not nearly a match for some that have been encountered. In part, the complication in this case was more iatrogenic than is strictly patient symptoms. From the staff's point of view, she quickly transformed, from a distrustful individual pushing others away, to that of a very vulnerable person who strived to engage others through her past trauma. Through her words and actions, she communicated that the world owed her greater kindness and care due to her unfortunate history.

Furthermore, a part of her subconscious metacommunication was that, through an intense relationship, she will make complete the person who becomes involved with her. This is projective identification and Cashdan suggests that there are four major projective identifications of dependency, power, sex and ingratiation (1988, p.71). This projective identification translates into a complex dynamic that drew her peers as well as unsuspecting staff into an interpersonal orbit that meets her demand for interpersonal input and defines the fundamentals of her relationship. In her interpersonal world is the metacommunication that she is very vulnerable and necessitates protection as well as using her sexuality to invite and involve others in a dependent relationship. For her, sex has ceased to have any meaning except when it is linked to risky circumstances or a context in which it brings her the thrill of doing something forbidden or nearly out of grasp.

In daily life, she is either exuding a great deal of seductiveness and dependence or when rebuffed, she will display tremendous anger and rage. One or several of the types of projective identification that Cashdan described can take place at times when she experiences increasing fragmentation of the self. When her "cup" is near empty, she is at a primitive level of functioning with the release of *original anger* (see chapter 9) which enhances various types of projection. Thus, one can observe that she uses different types of projective identification with different levels of cohesion of the self. At times of immense crisis of emptiness, her projection of anger combined with splitting can set her up to push all others away and becomes exceedingly self destructive.

Every team member knew how fragile she can be and no one wanted to see her decompensate. Combine this anxiety, on the part of the team, together with her seductiveness and neediness, it was all too easy for some members of the team to be drawn into the dynamics of the projective identification and feed into her demands for emotional rescue; this is paralysis. Once this occurs, the team could no longer maintain good treatment stance with this patient. It is only through a thorough and honest self evaluation could the team recognize this dynamic and take uniform steps to correct the inconsistencies and discrepancies within the team.

Maintaining Consistency

In classic behavioral management, the therapist understands that a worsening of the target behavior could occur as a result of any attempt to contain it. The period of increased challenge is generally said to be up to about six weeks; although this length of time varies as to the consistency of implementation of the technique. I generally find that the period of challenge can be a great deal shorter than six weeks given good implementation. One must keep in mind that the key to success in implementing behavioral management is consistency as well as persistence.

Resistance should be addressed early in treatment once the patient and his family have been formally introduced to DSA. In some sense, DSA is about the interpretation of the behavior of the patient and others in order to confront, perhaps subtle but, ineffective interpersonal dynamics. If the preparatory work in the initial introduction to DSA has been undertaken adequately, the patient should feel validated and understanding of the ferocious leakiness of the cup and motivated to make the repair to the self. Once the motivation is in place, it is far easier to help the patient analyze his behavior and DSA becomes a powerful tool for confronting resistance.

By maintaining the prescribed course in treatment, providing highly appropriate boundary and gently encouraging pro-treatment behavior, the patient will gradually transform from his false self and start to exhibit more independent and self-activating internal function. This is achieved through purposeful assistance from the significant people around him; assuming that his family or significant others are working in conjunction with his therapist through DSA. Understanding his initial dysphoria and fear of abandonment, he will need careful assessment as to his current needs. On the ward, the staff will carefully measure out the appropriate boundary to maintain while still encouraging him to exercise the 3-steps. At times, staff may present him with material reward as motivation to draw him closer to the treatment experience. Once he has a taste of the joining with his selfobject without evoking the false self, (he does not have to be dependent to be loved and he does not deserve to be attacked due to his feelings of worthlessness) he can then function as himself, the real self.

Experiencing less abandonment anxiety and depression, one young woman emerged from self imposed isolation and self pity to report feeling much less depressed, more energetic and feeling physically well, no further medical consultations had to be obtained for her for the rest of the hospitalization. In the treatment of individuals with BPD, it is essential to pay attention to the defenses arising out of his reaction to treatment maneuvers. Implementation of treatment can often bring about such reactions as anxiety, depression, anger, aggression, suicidal acts as well as self-mutilation. Anxiety and depression arise from separation-individuation while anger and aggression arise from the need to act out to fill the cup. Without anticipation of the patient's reaction to confrontation, one can not fully prepare to adequately and therapeutically deal with the fallout. Responding to the borderline patient's depression with an increase or dramatic change in his medication may only contribute to unnecessary medication complication as well as missing critical psychotherapeutic opportunity.

The 3-steps

On the whole, the 3-steps are a reenactment of the developmental relationships in the context of therapy, like a bridge that momentarily allows us to tap into the past and make a corrective action. Therefore, the recapitulation of the parent-child relationship is played out whether he is interacting with his parent, his therapist or an important other. It is a powerful vehicle in capturing the individual's behavioral tendencies through heightening of his transference with selfobject figures in his life. The 3-steps inevitably interfere with the patient's previous habits of interpersonal interactions. In her resistance to the work of the 3-steps, one patient angrily stated, "You are just like my Dad." She expressed feeling angry that her therapist and staff on the unit are not intensely engaged in soothing her when she signals distress through various unskilled behaviors. A common misconception in treatment is that of trying to make up to the patient what he has been deprived of in his past; the truth in treatment is that no amount of direct compensation will replenish what he has missed. Although her staff did not neglect her, they simply had no effective way of interacting with her until she came to realize that she can get her needs met and do the work of healing through the work of the 3-steps.

All of our daily interactions with the patient, whether in the hospital or the home, are always in the 3-steps manner. Whether our interaction is regarding a major event or minor event in the patient's day, it is always done in the context of the 3-steps. This is based on the assumption that the patient is constantly in or near crisis and is in need of being mindful about treatment. "We have had a good conversation and I just want to give you credit for doing the 3-steps and thank you for allowing me to process with you." "I just wanted to check in with you. You seem to be doing well lately. You have helped me to understand that your cup can often be nearly empty; therefore, I appreciate the way you try to do a good job of containing and letting time pass. You have just completed another round of the 3-steps." In a typical quick check-in, I would ask the patient to assign a number to the level in the cup and talk about his recent activities. It is important to realize that the 3-steps can be accomplished multiple times a day and in the context of very simple and brief interactions. The 3-steps are about living daily life in a structured, predictable and validating environment.

The 3-steps achieve the following dynamics:

1. The 3-steps interfere with instant emotional gratification which can bring about the presence of *original anger*, discussed in chapter 3. When the patient is resistant to the work while those around him are adhering to the 3-steps as a guide to interpersonal interaction, the patient will experience a precipitous drop in the content in his cup. This can then evoke the surfacing of the original anger, a state that should be addressed directly in treatment rather than kept hidden or ignored. This is accomplished through addressing the original anger as the sedimentation in the cup.

2. The hastening of the development of *transference*. Transference in the classical sense of inducing feelings from one's past or transference in terms of interpersonal giving, the 3-steps invokes both.

3. It re-enforces the experiencing of the *here and now*. Whatever may be the state of the patient's readiness to do the work of the 3-steps; these states represent the interpersonal negotiation between the patient and his therapist. As such, it is a very rich source of discussion regarding his anger, disappointment, loss or perhaps, joy, pride and accomplishment in relating to the 3-steps.

4. As part of the structure of the 3-steps, one is reminded of the importance of regarding life through the concept of *person, place and time*. There is an appropriate time for most everything in life.

5. The 3-steps are about *handling disappointments*. In reality, all human interactions are based on the fundamentals of contain, let time pass and then process. "Daddy, Daddy, can we play?" "No, not right now. Let me finish my work." A while later, Dad says, "Gee, you have been doing such a good job waiting for me. What did you do while you were waiting?" "I was playing with Legos." Father and daughter can now play together.

6. The 3-steps as a *"corrective emotional experience."* Authors have advocated that the therapist "actively promote a 'corrective emotional experience' by deliberately relating to the patient in a manner that dramatically refutes the latter's transference expectations." (Strupp 1984) The borderline patient often feels that his interpersonal needs are not being fulfilled; the 3-steps assure that his needs are met in a fashion that is both surprising and satisfying.

Through *micro-corrective reenactment*, this patient transforms his transference expectation via repetition of a corrective emotional experience. Metaphorically, within the 3-steps, one reaches into the muddy bottom in the recess of our psyche, scoop up a small handful, shape it, pack it and return it. Through repetition, one becomes familiar with this material and extrapolated to realize that the whole of this pond is made of this same material that holds no threat to our being.

7. The 3-steps represent the most fundamental of *structured interpersonal interaction*.

8. The achievement of being able to adhere to the work of the 3-steps brings the individual a sense of greater *independence*. In addition, the steps foster the confidence that, "I can be independent and still feel loved."

9. The consistent meeting with the selfobject on the playfield of the 3-steps allows for the growth of trust.

10. Selfobject validation based on empathic connection through the mutual awareness of core emptiness is a much more sincere form of validation than the superficial recognition of external affect expression.

11. Validation by the selfobject, when offered in an authentic and consistent fashion, optimizes idealizing and mirroring transference. This selfobject experience strengthens one's inner experience and accomplishments. Being recognized and appreciated by someone we value can provide the additional level of soothing, guiding and protecting that are not available to us at that moment. Functionally, through the 3-steps, a larger number of selfobject representations become available to us.

12. Most of all, the goal of the 3-steps is to bring the patient an improved *self-concept*. He comes to realize that he can experience the self as a more consistent entity that remains stable regardless of the whims of his environment. In his writing, Meares spoke of an individual's act and ownership in play (like that of the second step) as conducive to the growth of the real self (1993).

Summary

The 3-steps are simple in concept but demanding in practice. They are designed to overcome some of the common obstacles in the treatment of BPD while providing a central focus in the continuing development of object constancy in the lives of all people. Most people do instinctively gravitate to the practice of the 3-steps out of their original growth and maturational experience with their selfobject. For them, the 3-steps would just be a way of life. For the borderline patient, it is a way of maturation and growth that has to be taught. The 3-steps can seem overly simplistic at first glance but the developmental implication is critical to treatment. Consistent deployment of the 3-steps can be very challenging but the persistence and conscientious involvement of the therapist and other selfobjects in the patient's life have the primary role of keeping the patient on the path of treatment.

·IX·
FURTHER DISCUSSIONS ABOUT TREATMENT

From Theory to Clinical Cases

Translating a model of therapy for a way of working with BPD into a practical modality of treatment is highly challenging. Furthermore, implementing a system of treatment in real life clinical scenario and attempting to obtain consistent results time after time pose an even greater challenge. Whether one is a student of psychoanalysis or a disciple of CBT; it is always going to be a challenge when one attempts to practice the discipline in actual patient care. In clinical care, there are an infinite number of wild variables. This follows the common adage about how "disorders don't read textbooks"; this is very true and to be expected. In this chapter, I will draw attention to the usage of psychological defense mechanisms in the context of DSA to help us develop better insight into clinical challenges. An integrated understanding of the important defense mechanisms with that of the psychodynamics of the internal emotional system as described in DSA will help the practitioner better formulate a synthesis understanding and treatment plan.

Of course, learning a treatment method does not mean following a rigid recipe in hope of success. Doing psychotherapy is a very personal endeavor for each therapist and any new concept and model of treatment has to be integrated with the therapist's existing skills as well as philosophy and style. It is my hope that due to the compactness of the concepts involved in DSA that it lends itself to rather straightforward rendering of important DSA protocol. This would allow for individual therapists to adhere to the key areas of DSA work while still able to inject a good dose of the therapist's individuality.

Three Steps for Consistency and Persistence

Case 9.1: Casey is an 18 years old female with an extensive history of severe trauma. She was born to a mother who was only 14 at the time of Casey's birth. As a young child, she was often left unattended or in the care of strangers who came in and out of her home. As she got older, her mother would leave to go on alcohol binges while leaving her in charge of her younger siblings. Along the way, she was severely abused physically and sexually by multiple adult figures in her life. By the time she was a teen, she had already started to experiment with alcohol and street drugs. She started to spend more and more time away from home. She was finding comfort and solace in mere acquaintances and strangers. She became a victim of rape. She felt very lonely and lost in her daily existence. She never had an interest in or the stability in school. She could not focus her mind or energy in anything productive. She could be easily swept off her feet by passing fancy and momentary thrills but these interests all seem to reflect her desire to escape the harsh reality of her life.

Soon, she abandons all hope of finding happiness and ceased to have any dreams of a future. In fact, it seems that nightmares are about all that will accompany her loneliness. She felt increasingly aimless in life and sank into deep depression. With this additional level of pain in daily existence, she began searching for further relief. What follows is a long list of very self-destructive behavior that landed her in inpatient treatment settings repeatedly. Interestingly, she never quite got to the point of feeling suicidal; at least, she was not intentionally or purposefully suicidal. However, she placed herself in precarious situations with casual sex and drug use. Afterwards, she would always lament her actions saying that these activities only bring traumatic flashbacks from her past. She talked frequently about not being able to trust. Yet she seems unable to keep away from people who are sure to hurt her. Despite this awareness, she would repeatedly find herself in dire predicaments.

Over time, all these high-risk behaviors became less efficient in filling the persistent loneliness and emptiness within. Her behavior has long since alienated any remaining supports she may have in life. Very soon, no matter what she does, she simply could not find sufficient gratification in life to fill the deep void within. At this point, she began a journey into gory self-mutilation. In the next few years, in and out of various hospitals, she continued a masochistic journey into a world that few could comprehend. Her self-mutilation took on such intensity that people who have tried to help her could only look at her with aghast and sickening wonder. She would cut so deeply and repeatedly rips out her sutures to the point that emergency room physicians no longer want to suture her wounds. In the psychiatric hospital, without access to sharp objects, she would open up existing wounds and insert a variety of items as well as her own finger deeply into the wounds as if she was fishing for something inside the tissue.

In response to inquiries about such severe self-mutilation, she would flippantly answer that it feels good and that everyone should cope just like this. She sarcastically said that she would recommend it to close friends and family. This single minded resistance to treatment represents the collective clinical picture of all of her previous hospitalizations here as well as at other psychiatric facilities. She maintained a "love / hate" relationship with staff; she obviously craved a high degree of interpersonal care taking but the slightest disappointments would cause her to unleash tremendous wrath upon all those around her. When angry, she posed a high degree of physical threat toward others and responded poorly to any attempt by staff to intervene in these situations. Observing her tearful tirades at such times gives the impression that it is a form of self flagellation and a confirmation of her very negative self worth although it is also a victim stance that seemingly satisfies the need for filling an internal void with an intense activity at this moment of fragmentation of the self.

Her hospitalization came at a time when this hospital was in the midst of evaluating and incorporating the best de-escalation programs popular across the country. Trauma informed care was the catch phrase for all staff on the unit and every effort was made to avoid seclusion and restraint with this patient. Frustratingly, seclusion and restraint occurred just about daily and not even the aggressive use of medications changed the statistics. Repeated reassessment of her symptoms presentation still precluded consideration of mania or psychosis, although these are often the diagnosis such symptoms would garner. In her case, aggressive medication usage were targeted at addressing symptoms of depression, anxiety, explosive outbursts and lability of mood. Interestingly, she was quite compliant with all her medications despite the fact that she was starting to experience increasing side effects. All the while, her clinical presentation was unchanged.

Unfortunately, her family remained very scarce during this period of her treatment. Without the involvement of family, the treatment team made the decision to carry on with the treatment staff in place of her family. She has a rudimentary relationship with numerous staff as a result of the staff's ongoing compassion in working with her. She was in the hospital for about a month this time and the team felt that we should make the best of it before she was transferred to a step down program at another facility. The treatment team followed the guidelines in DSA closely in developing some degree of treatment rapport with her and then helped her to explore and put into words some of the painful emotional feelings she likely constantly lived with. Instant familiarity with the presence and feelings of emptiness is a prerequisite to beginning treatment. She was asked, "Are you able to tap into that feeling or sensation you get just before you have the urge to cut yourself?" From this preparation to treatment, the team held a "family conference" and introduced the cup and the 3-steps to her. During this session, she listened with focused curiosity and showed appreciation for the validation of her pain.

As treatment followed, she flailed about like a fish out of water, struggling to regain some former control and coping. The treatment team met frequently to provide moral support for each other in maintaining the courage to sustain the momentum in treatment. It was difficult to maintain adequate empathy in the daily work with someone who can be so angry, aggressive and self-destructive but the team managed by drawing on compassion. Team members used the analogy of the porous cup to help us locate the compassion within each of us for the suffering of this patient. Everyone tried to maintain appropriate boundary, monitoring closely from an appropriate distance and remained vigilant for any semblance of the 3-steps on the part of the patient. We did not allow her to paralyze the team through her high risk behavior.

On the surface, unit staff maintained a cordial, caring and appropriately interactive stance in the everyday interpersonal interactions with her. If normal everyday routines are somehow interrupted by her emotional escalation, staff will cue her to do the 3-steps and remind the patient that the appropriate time to process is the third step. Not long after, she started to develop some rudimentary motivation for this work and began to pay more attention to the completion of the 3-steps as a way of coping with distress. Within a few weeks time, she was able to demonstrate improved management of her urges to act out. Her arms began to heal and she seemed more content in her life on the unit without excessive staff involvement and input.

Soon, her time at my particular acute psychiatric care facility came to an end and it was time to transfer her to a residential treatment center. She did not resist the transfer of care although she hinted at feeling abandoned by this team since she wanted to stay on for treatment but we were not able to keep her. It was sad for the team to discontinue our work with her at this stage but we also understood that our purpose was not to do long term work with her. Instead, all through treatment, we made it clear to her that we were here to teach her a method of treatment work that she can then take with her to whichever facility awaits her next. Along this theme, we continued to remind her of our stated goal and encouraged her to be mindful of this work regardless of the treatment setting. She understood that DSA is a method of work that can easily integrate with any type of therapy that she enters into in the future.

Discussion:
Invariably, self-mutilation in a hospital setting would draw some intense response from nursing and therapy staff. No one wants to stand by and watch someone perform severe self-mutilation. Likely management of such behavior would include the use of seclusion and perhaps, restraint for the safety of the patient. This can quickly set up a very problematic dynamic between this patient and her providers. Firstly, staff may feel confused as to whether they are simply keeping her safety in mind or that they are in fact responding to projective identification and countertransference. Secondly, the staff's use of force could only confirm in her that they are indeed angry and aggressive toward her even though she could well be using projection and not recognizing her own projected anger. Thirdly, in the language of DSA, staff's use of force can reinforce the intensity and extremeness of her acting out behavior, which fills her cup. Fourthly, within the DSA protocol, even the attempt to de-escalate and head off a showdown without force can turn out to be rather un-therapeutic given the propensity for such actions to just fill the patient's cup. This is not to say that such de-escalation programs are never effective but one has to be cautious about the potential of the patient's pathological reliance on such interventions. Generally, the goal of crisis intervention is to do what it takes to quickly calm the patient and reach a point of safety for all involved. There are times when safety is the only consideration. However, treatment providers have to direct the patient toward therapeutic work whenever possible.

In addressing safety, medications are invariably involved or perhaps, at times, excessively involved. Determining the role and use of medication should always start with an accurate assessment of the patient and the formulation of a reasonable diagnosis. In the case of this patient, she presented with neurovegetative symptoms and signs of depression but there were no clinical evidence of mania. In clinical practice today, many mental health providers would likely argue that the history presented here contains elements that should be considered as mania and there-fore, the diagnosis of bipolar disorder should be considered. No doubt that some borderline patients also suffer the co-morbidity of bipolar disorder as well as a number of other psychiatric conditions but caution must be heeded in regards to the emotional balance in a "cup" that is just as "up and down."

Medications have generally played a major role in her life, having been on them for the majority of her teen years. Through the care of multiple providers over the years, she has experienced medication effects ranging from antidepressants, anxiolytics, mood stabilizers and antip-sychotics. One has every reason to believe that medications have little impact one her long term treatment outcome despite some short term stabilization. Such stabilization has been so limited that scarcely anyone expects much from medications in her treatment. One remark worth mentioning regarding medication is the possibility that, with proper and appropriate expectation, she can benefit from a mild stabilization of the worst of her internal pain. During the course of this treatment, she contin-ued on an antidepressant, a mood stabilizer and an antipsychotic medica-tion; a combination that she remained on for the duration of this hospital course.

Three Cheers for the Three Steps

Case 9.2: Elizabeth is a late teen who has been repeatedly hospitalized in recent times due to her increasing aggression at successive foster homes. She has suffered much physical abuse in life and as a result, has been separated from her abusive family for some time. Intellectually, she meets diagnostic criteria for mild mental retardation but more than make up for it by her charm and intuitive awareness about her surroundings. Socially, she can be blunt and demanding; and often suffer the frustration of not understanding the nuances of how to navigate a social setting. As a result, she would often become the scapegoat and victim of her peers. When angered or frustrated, she can display tremendous demonstration of physical strength; it would take several strong male staff to contain her at that point. She exhausted all the conventional methods of behavioral management and therapeutic measures while still posing as a high-risk threat to all on the unit. De-escalation management with a focus to an-ticipate common frustrations were minimally helpful. Various attempts to teach her coping and problem solving skills were beyond her cognitive ability to grasp.

Even though she has been unable to articulate her internal emotional pain, given her history, one might expect that she suffers the dynamics of a very leaky cup; she is unable to sustain the self. However, the team questioned her ability to comprehend the complete discussion with the cup and the 3-steps. As simplified as the treatment concepts involved in DSA, it does require a certain degree of cognitive savvy to fully understand the significance and importance of looking inwardly to recognize the need to repair the cup. On first glance, most people comprehend the need to avoid acting out behaviors. However, on introduction, many individuals fail to understand that many interpersonal care taking types of behaviors are indeed rescue seeking behaviors that does not truly contribute to their long term well being. As a result, individuals may continue to rely heavily on others to rescue them from the pain of emotional fragmentation.

The team identified her strength as someone capable of making good interpersonal connections and is willing to please her staff. In addition, her tendency to be rather concrete is also strength in treatment using just the 3-steps; this was an occasion to forego the metaphor of the cup. The team felt that, with this strategy, we can easily meet her demands of attention while setting up a good structure to encourage a degree of independence. She was then placed on a behavioral management program emphasizing the 3-steps. She remained on the levels program utilized in the milieu but had to earn her level through the implementation of the 3-steps.

Once introduced to the program, she accepted it immediately and although she still exhibited occasional outburst, she was involved in fewer conflicts with others and when upset, did not go directly to physical acting out. For her, the satisfaction of having a simple structure to follow in the face of anger and frustration appeared quite calming. The 3-steps program allowed her to have a sense of control over the chain of events. She has control over the amount of time she wants to spend on her own in self-soothing as well as the control over the selection of staff to seek affirmation. In so doing, she can also truly claim credit for having resolved the conflict on her own without assistance from staff. Initially, her tolerance of letting time pass may be rather brief, but she is still given credit for any amount of time she allows to pass. Therefore, she can achieve success in treatment very easily. For many, achieving a modicum of success and enjoying an opportunity to complete any one thing in life is so rare that they relish their ownership of the 3-steps. Within a short period of time, she was no longer the explosive individual that terrified milieu.

Discussion:
The 3-steps program by itself is very similar to many behavioral management protocols that are widely used. Described in different terms, many methods and techniques are indeed about the use of contain, let time pass and process. Some of these protocols are not explicit about how this sequence should best be used, or that the patient may be encouraged to do part but not all of the steps. In DSA, the 3-steps can be used independently from the rest of the model of treatment but these steps have to be carried out in a linear order. Elizabeth accepted the program quickly because it did not place blame on her. It was not necessary for her to perform any intricate chain of event analysis of what happened and what went wrong. The analysis can be done at a later time when she is able to rationally process with someone.

In her case, the act of self-observation is for her to simply notice that she is getting angry. Once she is aware of this, she is asked to contain, meaning that she is not to act out. Secondly, she is asked to let time pass, meaning that she has to manage her anger for a short period of time on her own. This reduced her tendency to constantly approach staff for emotional rescue or to save her from yet another conflict with others.

This in effect removed any secondary gain that may be the result of her frequent conflict with others. She is willing to comply with the demands of this program because of her therapeutic relationship with the staff and because she is aware that there will be an opportunity to process with staff following the first two steps. This is a very crucial piece of this program that works to encourage her willingness to cooperate. She will quickly learn that the attention that she will earn from staff as part of the third step will be far more rewarding than the attention that she could get by any other means.

To make sure that the staff is consistently available for processing, as part of the third step, a simple worksheet was developed that allows her to check off the first two steps as she accomplishes them and then approach the staff to complete the third step. The staff then signs off on one round of the work completed. The use of the 3 steps was effective because it is easy to understand and to remember. She is quickly rewarded for accomplishing the first two steps which is highly reinforcing for her. She is able to rapidly feel a sense of accomplishment in this work. For this teen, completion of anything at all is a foreign concept given her unfortunate circumstances in life. She beamed with satisfaction at the accomplishment of each round of the 3-steps. Importantly, this work also kept the staff working in a consistent fashion that was critical to reinforcing her positive behavior. The 3 steps gave the staff a sense of boundary and structure in working with this patient. It prevented staff from feeling overwhelmed by the patient and feeling resentful about interacting with this patient each time she misbehaved. Interactions at such times could be misconstrued as reward for negative behavior by the patient. Now, staff is generally quite happy to work with her. The milieu became a more positive place with this patient working toward a specific goal to do the 3 steps. This protocol is highly suitable for the patient who requires a simple and straightforward behavioral management program.

Hospitalization as a Treatment Option

Hospitalization has been viewed as the bane of borderline treatment. However, high numbers of borderline patients continue to be admitted to inpatient treatment. If hospitalization serves only to safeguard the patient at times of crisis, it would have only achieved half of its potential to help this individual. A common concern about hospitalization involves worries that the borderline patient may develop greater dependence on the artificial milieu offered in such a setting. It has been thought that, given the prospect of long term therapy work required in treatment, the borderline has little to gain through inpatient care except to somehow "stabilize" and return to the community for ongoing care. However, a valuable opportunity could be lost if hospitalization is simply seen as a stopgap measure in the worse case scenario. Inpatient care should offer a degree of observation and insight development regarding an individual that may not be easily achieved any other way. It is an opportunity to confront the borderline patient's unskillful coping with his internal pain and bring about greater insight about the needs for treatment.

There are instances in which a borderline patient has to be hospitalized due to court order or that the patient is simply not invested in an outpatient setting and has suffered repeated failure to maintain safety in the community. The patient who is unable to discontinue substance use due to dependence or overwhelming internal emotional distress will be unable to contain his acting out. The severely depressed and emotionally empty individual may seem very insightful about the need for change but voice his inability to resist his impulse to self-mutilate. This intensity of emotional dysregulation is best understood through the metaphor of the "bone dry" empty cup. Severe symptoms of anxiety, depression, paranoia, obsession, compulsion, impulsive urges, anger, aggression, psychosis, envy, jealousy as well as a variety of physical complaints escalate when the cup is empty. Hence, it is reasonable to consider external containment in the form of psychiatric hospitalization or chemical dependency treatment at times of increased acuity.

When DSA is implemented in an inpatient setting, it brings about a very powerful set of structure for the patient as well as staff. It places strong emphasis on the respect of interpersonal boundary. It gives clear guidelines about how to access the attention of others. In this fashion, it reduces the constant attention seeking behavior of borderline individuals. "Attention seeking" or "rescue seeking" should be understood through the compassionate view of an individual striving to fill a painful internal void. This model of treatment helps the staff to understand that their role is not to provide unlimited content for the empty cup of the patient but to be a consistent "object" in predictably returning to validate and support the patient following the first two steps. In this respect, this patient is made to feel secure with the sense that his staff is to be trusted and will predictably return once he is able to contain and allow time to pass. Through this experience, he will intrinsically be reinforced through building trust for his treatment providers and strengthens his commitment to treatment.

DSA clearly labels the types of behavior that constitute overt and covert acting out. Some borderline patients frequently entertain the thought of suicide even though he may be uncertain about taking such a step. This type of thinking can evolve toward a type of covert acting out in an attempt to fill the cup. Eating excessively or severe restriction of food is acting out. DSA confronts many types of behavior as acting out. DSA also realigns certain types of acting out behavior as stemming out of individual internal emotional pathology, thus, confronts the patient's incessant denial of internal tension. In this manner, an individual could no longer retreat behind the rationalization of acting out for acting out sake. Instead, every act of acting out is examined in the light of one's inner pathology of the self. Additionally, the inpatient setting allows treatment providers to make observations about a patient's tendency for covert acting out. In so doing, one is confronted in having to take responsibility for this internal pain and to take steps for its healing.

This model of illness explains how the use of inappropriate interpersonal attention and other acting out behavior can have short term function but undermines treatment. By constantly calling the patient's attention to what constitutes acting out behavior, he is being made aware of how important it is to be mindful of how such behavior can easily sabotage his treatment. Most times, people are not aware that covert acting out is directly hurting his progress in treatment. By calling attention to this issue, which can best be achieved in a supervised inpatient setting, he will come to understand that hospitalization is hard work and he can not go about coping with life oblivious of how his acting out is counter productive to treatment.

The traditional view of psychotherapy consists of the therapist playing the role of a consistent, non-judgmental, and supportive other who renders the corrective experience for the patient. Often, this lone advocate for the patient is not sufficient to sustain the patient in the early phase of treatment. It is most effective when a patient has willing family to work through this process of healing. However, not every patient has the fortune of a family that is sufficiently insightful and willing to participate in this work. In such a case, it would be beneficial for the patient to start treatment in an environment that could support this work. The inpatient environment can serve as a corrective emotional experience for the patient when such opportunities are not available elsewhere.

An argument can be made for substitution of treatment providers as temporary selfobject representations when steady consistent objects are missing from the patient's realm. Looking toward the patient's lack of selfobject constancy, this individual is likely to require rapid intense intervention for him to achieve some semblance of object stability. It is only after the ability to internalize some degree of proper selfobjects could this individual reach some reasonable stability that can possibly have a longer term benefit. Through the accomplishment of numerous individuals who were fortunately able to reside in inpatient treatment for an extended period of time, despite the trend for brief inpatient stays of today, it is evident that the realization of some measure of object constancy has allowed these individuals to experience improved long term stability in outpatient treatment.

Addressing the Revolving Door

The subject of inpatient hospitalization brings about heated debates about an artificial environment that could potentially foster greater patient dependency. One in ten patient's with borderline personality disorder complete suicide. "Hospitalization is of unproven value in preventing suicide by these patients and can sometimes have negative effects" (Paris 2002). In order to have an impact on this outcome, this very critical issue has to be addressed from the start of each hospitalization as part of the treatment plan. Inpatient treatment work must be lateralized to implementation in the home and outpatient therapy settings. If this implementation through DSA is successful, the patient should be able to achieve a sense of being able to have his needs met in a consistent and therapeutic fashion outside of the hospital milieu. Despite the best of preparation, some patients may still require multiple hospitalizations before achieving sufficient stability to function in further treatment in the community setting.

Multiple factors are at play when certain patients seem to make quite a concerted effort to seek repeated hospitalizations. It is obvious that the inpatient environment is a highly restrictive setting in comparison to life as usual in the community. However, for many borderline patients, the inpatient milieu offers a higher degree of shelter that can not be found elsewhere. For some, the hospital appeals to his flickering desire to remain living, while others find this refuge to temporarily distract from the apprehension of death. For others, the inpatient milieu promises to fulfill the needed interpersonal connection and emotional rescue at times of perceived abandonment. Regressing to an infantile wish for complete merger with the all powerful selfobject, fragmentation of the self brings about that temporary belief that the ideal mother figure can make one whole and complete once again. For yet others, the psychiatric hospital is held as the hope for seeking the still elusive medication combination to resolve the chronic sense of unwell whether that be labeled as depression, anxiety and so on. On occasion, a borderline patient addicted to prescription medications may include the hospital in his network for seeking drugs.

The aforementioned issues are only a few of the examples in which the borderline patient could inadvertently rely on the inpatient setting. It is commonly recognized that the interpersonal empathy and validation offered by healthcare personnel in emergency rooms, medical wards as well as psychiatric units, play a sizeable role in drawing the borderline patient towards the inpatient milieu. Inasmuch as some borderline patients require such interpersonal emotional input that few can meet his needs, while others might be leery of closeness to others, the inpatient environment can appeal to his deep desire to be at least understood. Medical personnel and mental health providers tend to be highly empathic in the treatment setting, somewhat contributed to by working in shifts or by appointments, and less overwhelmed by the patient's behaviors.

The treatment approach discussed here was developed with respect to the complexities of hospital treatment of BPD. Bearing in mind the great propensity for the borderline patient to become overly dependent on the inpatient milieu, many of the strategies of this work focuses on the ever important interpersonal boundaries. Based on the concept that respectful interpersonal boundaries is one in which the patient is allowed sufficient independence for growth, the therapist and patient interaction becomes a central strategy for healing. In this work, the patient and his world sphere receives a renewed model of meeting each other's emotional needs. Additionally, the inpatient staff works in an empathic and compassionate manner without overextending their interpersonal reach. Through idealizing and mirroring transference, the patient learns to be highly selective in meeting his needs; through the work with his own family, he now has a concept of how he can achieve emotional equilibrium. The outcome of maintaining good boundaries through the practice of the 3-steps means that the patient is encouraged to meet his emotional needs in the community the same way he would obtain it in the inpatient milieu. By adhering to the principles of this work, the issue of repeated hospitalization can be assuaged.

Day Hospital Programs can be Highly Efficient

In between the acute setting of the inpatient unit and the lesser structure of outpatient care, lies the often under utilized modality of care in the form of the day hospital program. In the state of Washington, most private insurance cover the option for day hospital care while the state offers no such coverage. This manner of coverage is inconsistent with the philosophy of prevention but rather, in line with salvaging the aftermath of acute illness. This is reflective of a system of care that is highly skeptical of mental health treatment and sees no value in higher levels of care. The reluctance to utilize the higher or more restrictive levels of care is unfortunate but the mental health community is partially to blame for the general perception of ineffectiveness in inpatient and day program for those with the pathology of the self.

There is a lack of good data about the efficiency of day treatment programs. However, clinical experience would inform us that good inpatient and day hospital program starts with a combination of effective didactic teaching, contributing to insight development, in conjunction with an opportunity to repeatedly apply the work learned. Repetition is the instrument for turning the blossoming insight about one's pathology into true healing. Too often, patient's leave a treatment setting full of excitement about a newfound personal discovery that could not be translated into solidifying ongoing treatment work and stability. Wherefore, the presence of such factors as a compact and rapidly teachable model that can encourage the patient's self understanding of the real purpose of therapy and provides the initial treatment experience in supervised setting, would allow for a highly productive and efficient use of the day hospital milieu.

It has been my clinical experience that a course of day hospital treatment, in line with the work discussed here, can be highly efficacious in initiating a patient into therapy or as a reinforcement of ongoing therapy for a patient struggling in outpatient treatment. For the uninitiated patient, the intensity of the day hospital milieu can be a powerful setting to help the patient to address the true issues of his seeking help. For the seasoned therapy patient, the day hospital is an opportunity to examine frustrations in his current modality of treatment. DSA is often useful as a tool to help clarify issues obstructive to general treatment. Those patients familiar with DSA through their outpatient therapy work may also benefit from a DSA day hospital exposure. The benefit of intense emersion and focused application of DSA can not be over emphasized. Rarely can insight development or transference interpretation in therapy work stand alone without heightened experiencing of object relatedness to bring about true healing. In this setting, patients can rapidly learn or review DSA, observe the modeling of the 3-steps and become immersed in repeated practice. Therefore, rather than see day hospital program as an absolute last resort in treatment, it could be a very appropriate use of treatment resource to strengthen DSA therapy to improve productivity of work.

Our program offers intense group didactics, process groups operated in the context of DSA and ongoing reinforcement of the practice of the 3-steps in group as well as individual sessions. Experiential groups to emphasize the need to recognize the degree of one's emptiness within has been an important component of this work. Bringing together many elements of our interpersonal world, such as peers, authorities, friends and foes, makes for a heightened dynamic in which to work out our deepest emotional troubles. Confronting the borderline patient on his incessant intense focus on others in the milieu and in group work brings his issues to the forefront in the here and now. Pointing out the multitude of ineffective and inappropriate filling of the cup in the treatment milieu can be a powerful learning experience for the patient seeking to understand the didactic discussions of his emptiness.

We will need to pay some attention to the borderline patient with the great tendency to cling dependently to the security of the hospital milieu that time away from the program can be experienced as excruciating emotional pain. Similarly, a patient may resist the change of unit within the hospital with the stated complaint that only a specific environment provides him the sense of security. In careful review, it is apparent that there is indeed emotional attachment to the environment while it is quite clear that the dependence is an interpersonal need. On the hypothetical note that the inpatient staff maintains an excellent treatment boundary with this patient, it is unlikely that this stance will greatly reduce his reliance on the hospital milieu. One has to keep in mind that the borderline patient can often be truly lacking in support in the community. Therefore, any sense of safety and security in the hospital is valued by this patient.

In DSA, this dynamic has to be understood through the patient's requirement for filling of his cup. Without some repair to his leakiness, he has little chance of maintaining a sense of the self. What miniscule sense of wellness can quickly disappear due to a lack of object constancy, the ability to hold steady the sense of the selfobject. Since just filling his cup is not therapeutic, we have to allow for filling of the cup while encouraging the patient to achieve object constancy through the introjection of the selfobject in the context of the 3-steps. Once again, the patient has to have a clear understanding of the objective of treatment being that of the repair to his leakiness and that his urge to return to the hospital milieu for filling of his cup should not overshadow the emphasis for repair. Thus, dispelling emptiness and obtaining object constancy are tasks that are one and the same. Independence in function can only be obtained through a greater sense of the self when important selfobjects are able to reside within.

Putting Treatment Pieces Together

Case 9.3: Sandra is 16 years old. She is dressed very plainly and looked thin and fragile but carried an air of defiance that conveys years of experiences in the streets. She is at once a hardened street kid while still a lost child pretending to be in charge of her life. She has stories to tell as well as secrets to keep. Whether truth or fabrication to elevate her status amongst her peers, the known facts suggest a young life already full of tragedies and trauma. All of this came about while her mother was inebriated with alcohol to numb her own pain while the father abandoned the family long ago to face his own demons.

As a pre-teen, she moved around with her mother and several younger siblings in search of any tenuous stability that is afforded a family of such misfortune. As the eldest of her siblings, she tried to help out but admits to always feeling helpless. She has commented that the focus on caring for the younger siblings and the needs for basic survival may have allowed her to feel a sense of control in life. It also kept her mind off the very sad and dire situation at home. She knows no other life and had a naïve belief that others suffered as she does and therefore, the hardship is something to be handled as opposed to something to be wished away. As the years passed, she was both more mature and more immature than her peers. Her maturity came from having taught herself the toughness to survive; and her immaturity came from living in seclusion within an unhealthy environment. When she faced abuse and molestation from seemingly total strangers, she took it in stride and treated it as if it is just a part of her very harsh life that she has to cope with. In some ways, she had a great deal of control in her life running the household and caring for her younger siblings while her mother was emotionally removed in her struggle with alcoholism. This measure of control probably hid any insecurity she had about life and her poor sense of the self.

The trouble for her came on the day that her mother became sober. Having gained this nascent sobriety, her mother immediately tried to regain her parental authority and displaced the patient from her responsibilities in the family. The aftereffect of this change in the family dynamic was profound for this patient. She became even more disenchanted with life. She found herself in daily conflicts with her mother and much of this was due to her continuing attempts to interfere with the mother's attempt at parenting. She encountered great resistance when she attempted to rule over her siblings, which resulted in her feeling left out and intensely alone. Feeling thus dejected, she began to experience increased sense of disquiet from within; this she later described as a feeling of emptiness.

In response to this pain, she began to seek a sense of belonging from people who were willing to offer her companionship and instant gratification; in exchange, she pays with the remnants of respect for herself. What followed was a trail of drugs, alcohol and promiscuity interspersed with several psychiatric hospitalizations. In between the hospitalizations, attempts were made by family and providers to involve her in outpatient therapy. She was tried on many psychotropic medications to no avail. She was in constant conflict with her family and would run away for days to weeks at a time. During such times, she would repeatedly come into conflict with the law and placed on probation. Her outpatient mental health team and even her probation officer can only watch helplessly while she spirals into increasingly more severe self-destructive behaviors. By this time, she had all but given up on the taking of medications and of course she was non-compliant while on the run. She now returns home full of new superficial scars that she has created or in fact has gotten others to perform on her. There are cigarette burns, lighter burns and the usual multitude of cuts. We met after a particularly severe set of such self-mutilation.

In this set of hospitalizations, she was admitted several times in a row and was now on an involuntary hold for treatment awaiting a residential hospital placement. Managing her behavior and safety on the inpatient unit was no less difficult than the task in the community. Beyond the initial weeks during her first stay on the unit in which she basked in the light of the novelty of being in a brand new environment, she began to steadily demonstrate her tumultuous inner life. With each re-hospitalization, she became even quicker to resort to superficial self-mutilation. It was as if the attention from all the people around her was not nearly enough and she supplemented it with all kinds of acting out behavior. She was so self-destructive that the emergency room physicians no longer wanted to stitch her up because she would simply remove the sutures on her own and tease the wounds open. Any attempt to monitor her more closely brought a new round of highly creative methods of self harm. It was as if any increase of attention only caused her to be hungrier for attention. As if developing tolerance to medications, she develops tolerance to attention from others just as quickly and demands attention of escalating intensity.

On those rare moments when she actually spends a small amount of time on her own, she wanders the hallway chasing after invisible demons. Perhaps as a ploy to engage others but at least a demonstration of the internal torment that she suffers, these times are fraught with dramatic and disruptive behaviors in the milieu. She seems to select the most inopportune times to begin such disturbance. Most often at bed time, her demonstrations of auditory and visual hallucinations can be very frightening and unsettling for all others. When ignored, she will generally escalate the ordeal to include physical acting out that would certainly prompt staff to resort to stronger measures to bring about calm and safety for the milieu. It would not be uncommon for her to be physically contained and/or be given sedative medications.

Finally, the treatment team convened and met with her to discuss DSA and set the ground rules of her new treatment routines. Given that her family was not available to participate in her treatment, the treatment team served as her surrogate family to encourage the introjection of the selfobject in this developmental work. This initial meeting serves to confront her behavior as well as an attempt to help her to develop a psychological understanding of her emotional pain. If she is already aware of the aversive inner tension, this series of talks can help in comprehending her internal dynamics of filling and leakage. If she lacked true awareness of a psychological pain, this discussion can serve to help her redirect her attention to the repair of her internal wounds rather than forever blame others for a life that is rarely satisfying. For the borderline patient, being validated for one's external affect feels satisfying temporarily but receiving validation based on recognition of one's core sense of emptiness is a greater therapeutic empathic connection. (Refer to fig. 5.1)

In initiating this work, it is imperative that all staff in contact with this patient should be well versed in the treatment model of DSA. Every staff should be utilizing the same treatment language and carefully mindful of treatment boundaries. At our treatment facility, the adolescent program is divided into treatment teams consisting of a psychiatrist, case manager and a primary staff or a program therapist in addition to her milieu staff. This patient is assigned to primary contacts within the core team as well as a designated milieu staff. When her team is not available, she also has access to a designated milieu staff for each shift. Working off our ongoing conversation pertaining to the state of emptiness, she was readily able to relate to this treatment discussion. She had no trouble grasping the analogy of the cup and appeared relieved that others could understand some of the pain she is experiencing. Her initial openness to the treatment plan may be more motivated by the curiosity for the attention she hopes to garner through engaging staff. Thus, the team must be prepared to weather the stage of resistance to treatment and the evocation of defense mechanisms that will derail treatment course. In very little time, she returned to frequent self-mutilation and aggressive posturing toward staff. She appeared to hallucinate even more intensely.

This is the most demanding and challenging juncture in treatment. In the hospital, much of the work of implementing treatment according to DSA protocol rests on the one primary staff with the greatest amount of treatment contact with this patient. The primary staff has a special challenge in this work; the job of encouraging the patient to do treatment work without losing compassion and empathy in this therapeutic relationship. She tends to shadow her staff very closely and demands near constant attention, resulting in the need for her staff to work diligently at maintaining proper therapeutic boundary. Even though every member of the team works at adhering to the protocol, it is the core staff who may feel that the patient is excessively demanding of his or her input into the patient's cup. At times, the staff feels the patient is overly dependent on others to fill her "cup" and finds this familiar scenario to be frustrating. Each staff member must be mindful of our own vulnerability through countertransference as well as respect for the influence by which projective identification and splitting can act upon us.

One evening, frustrated at the lack of easy access to others for emotional rescue, she told her night staff that her mother was dying of cancer. Most staff familiar with his treatment plan took the news with appropriate compassion but refrained from overt engagement through being aware of her tendency to falsify information. Besides, the team was used to confirming such issues with family before taking action. However, the rumor of this development spread through the hospital quickly and a non-team staff assigned to another unit abandoned post to console her on this late evening. They spent an exorbitant amount of time together that evening while other staff looked on with unease. The next day, her mother informed the team that she is in fine health. There are therapeutic issues related to Sandra's choice of declaration that evening but the staff clearly needed to be admonished for abandoning both team and treatment protocol that fed into this patient's plying for unreasonable interpersonal input.

At team meeting each morning, such issues are discussed and processed. It became clear that routine, daily interactions with the patient constitute low level and low intensity interchanges. These types of filling of the "cup" would only be of value when her cup is relatively full. Inevitably, she will exhaust the good grace of others around her and come to find herself alienated from staff and peers. With the onset of solitude, she will quickly decompensate toward the feeling of profound emptiness once again; at this point, low level, low intensity interactions of daily routine may not be sufficient to refill the cup. She has to act out in extreme to meet her greater needs of that moment.

What follows is the opportunity for treatment. The team reminded her of the non-therapeutic choice she is making by saying, "You have made the choice to reach out to extreme, high risk and intense behavior to fulfill your needs for the cup. This effectively is a choice to distance yourself from everyone on your team. You are quite aware that this is only going to help you feel good temporarily. I will be waiting to work with you again when you enter into the 3-steps for treatment. I'll be back." With this message, the team, including the primary staff, set off to monitor this patient from a short distance. The routine interaction in this regard is low level and low intensity; therefore, this type of interaction does not sabotage treatment and is therapeutic in the context of DSA. There were times when she wants to indulge in self-mutilation but also demanding of attention from her staff and team without applying treatment protocol. With experience, her team was able to maintain good treatment boundary without becoming enmeshed in her cycle of self destructive behavior followed by engagement of others in a rescue role.

Upon realizing that she will not be able to obtain extra attention from staff without the 3-steps, she may attempt at doing the "pseudo-3-steps." Her staff then looks for any opportunity to reward her for the methodical completion of the 3-steps. At first, the staff will give her credit for doing anything that even resembles the 3-steps; sometimes, this could really take some imagination on the part of her staff and team. We call this the "spirit" of doing the 3-steps. In offering assistance to the 3-steps, her staff would demonstrate the completion of the steps to include "processing." This positive reinforcement can be a powerful motivation for her further engagement in treatment.

Her cognitive comprehension of the cup also played a crucial role in her daily work. Through the primal human desire for self preservation as well as an exposure to an easily accessible manner of understanding her exquisite internal pain, she was able to arrive at improved motivation to engage in treatment. The illustration of the cup became an important part of her daily treatment. She was encouraged to be highly mindful of this internal space and all types of daily issues were also examined through the metaphor of the cup.

Shortly after, she began to complete the 3-steps without prompting and the majority of her meaningful interpersonal interactions with her primary staff and core team members were in the context of the 3-steps. Along with this observation, she stopped all apparent self-mutilation and maintained a good standing in the level system of the milieu, indicating good functioning in coping with daily life. She managed to achieve this level of improvement within a month of treatment. A few weeks later, she was discharged to a therapeutic group home to continue in treatment. Before leaving the hospital, she gathered together all her program didactic hand-outs and promised to continue to do this work at the group home. At the follow-up, seemingly, her "revolving door" of acute hospitalizations stopped.

Discussion:
Here is an illustration of a dire situation with a teen girl who could not have been able to tolerate and eventually benefit from longer term, more complex psychotherapy. Without treatment, her life seems headed straight for a literal dead end or something worse. Whether one views her issues as related to the emotional/physiological dysregulation or a consequence of developmental frustration, treatment has to be precise and concise. In her case, treatment using the general milieu program popular amongst most inpatient psychiatric facilities and incorporating variations of CBT did not yield any discernable improvement despite several rounds of such work. Perhaps the use of conventional treatment is indeed very short term in benefit and can possibly augment her dependence on others for critical soothing. As Masterson suggested, the borderline patient enters into treatment with the sole purpose to "feel good"; this priority has to be confronted. On the other hand, confrontation is not so easy to do, especially when this is likely to be interpreted by the patient as blame and invalidation, leading to the breakdown of open communication and formation of distrust in the therapeutic relationship.

A lack of steady family involvement and stability in life contributes to another area of challenge in her treatment. "In contemporary society, therefore, the shrinking importance of the family results in a gradual impoverishment of the self-sustaining aspects of the selfobject experiences that the child has. This may be one explanation for the apparently increasing morbidity of narcissistic disorders, that is, disorders of the self" (Wolf 1988). DSA encourages the involvement of multiple object figures in the patient's life and treatment, she has none. It is unlikely that she would have sufficient support in the community to get her to treatment sessions and to remain compliant with medications. Despite these issues, treatment has to be attempted and an inpatient milieu incorporating DSA can be a highly effective introductory treatment avenue.

In preparation for treatment, her psychotropic medications were stabilized as much as feasible and held as consistently as possible through the course of this treatment. Lessons learned from her previous hospitalizations would suggest that anxiolytics, mood stabilizers, antidepressants and antipsychotic medications help only marginally but can still be a valuable edge in treatment. Maintaining consistency in the use of medications has the added benefit of reducing confusion regarding whether or not a set of symptoms or issues is related to the treatment work or the medications. As discussed in the pharmacology chapter, one must be vigilant to the possibility that medication side effects can exacerbate the patient's experience of inner tension.

Borderline patients experience a mountain of unusual symptoms on a daily basis. Symptoms attributable to the emotional pain of emptiness can often be confused with symptoms of side effects related to complex medications at use. The psychiatric practitioner has to carefully balance appropriate pursuit of medication trials with that of an attempt to hold steady the use of medications in order to better discern what the psychotherapeutic treatment issues are. When the psychiatrist and the patient are overly focused on finding pharmacologic solutions, it is easy to overlook the manner in which patients can often turn to excessive medication concerns to obtain the desperately needed caretaking and rescue. Such scenarios will frequently result in the patient being prescribed more medications or higher doses of medications inadvertently.

For the treatment team, maintaining compassion and empathy with this patient was not always easy, but the diligent effort by all involved was rewarded by the rather rapid stabilization of the worst of her acting out. This stability also allowed her to become more involved in the interpersonal, psychodynamic and dialectical behavior therapy work also offered in the program. She remained quite stable through the course of this hospitalization spanning about two months while awaiting a less restrictive treatment setting. This degree of stability was never achieved through previous stays of similar length; many youth experience similar predicament in repeated hospitalizations. Despite the statistics of such discouraging results, DSA offers such youth the hope of treatment in the context of inpatient care. Inpatient hospital care may be contrary to conventional wisdom about the treatment of borderline patients, but I would urge the reader of this work to remain open minded about this option. Hospitalization is the most expensive and restrictive option in treatment, but the benefit of effective hospital care can easily outweigh any negative detractors to inpatient care.

External Containment in Treatment

The course of psychotherapy can be full of both progress and setback. The therapist can at most hope for an essentially upward moving trajectory. Whether doing treatment on an outpatient basis or inpatient basis, there comes a time when the borderline patient may require greater external containment which could encompass hospitalization; in the case of a patient already in a hospital milieu, external containment could mean seclusion and restraint. Many "best practice" initiatives have looked at how to reduce seclusion and restraint in inpatient settings. Most of these protocols take a pragmatic look at the inpatient psychiatric environment and analyze the top reasons that seclusion and restraint happen. Risk assessment is then used to identify the specific behaviors that are likely to require the use of seclusion and restraint and a treatment plan is developed to help the patient and the staff focus on early intervention. These approaches generally advocate a problem solving and focused attitude toward milieu management. There are clearly advantages and disadvantages to this category of approach to avoidance of seclusion and restraint.

Interestingly, the inpatient environment is often witness to a high number of seclusion and restraint despite a more restrictive setting. Patients who have not exhibited the intensity and frequency of self-harm may actually escalate such behavior in the inpatient milieu. Group dynamics and psychological defense operations may play a role in encouraging some individuals to test the limits of their acting out behavior. Splitting and projective identification can quickly set up two camps over how to best manage a patient. These defense mechanisms can cause the borderline patient to experience more intense feelings of rejection. Certain authoritarian dynamics of staff as well as the pragmatics of managing the milieu can also contribute to tensions that can cause some patients to act aggressively. For example, the staff's need to implement rules rigidly can easily pit staff against patients.

On the issue of seclusion and restraint, the state of Pennsylvania has been collecting information since 1985 in a system called Exclusion, Restraint, Protective Restraint and Seclusion (ERPS). It was found that many justifications for seclusion and restraint have nothing to do with behaviors posing an imminent threat of serious bodily harm to the patient or others. Instead, there was a culture of milieu management that emphasized certain expectations. Often, banging, pacing, running, restlessness, disruptive behavior, urinating on the floor and fecal smearing were not tolerated and were justifications for seclusion or restraint. Logical and natural consequences were generalized to the idea that "people must learn that bad behavior has consequences; therefore, punishment is necessary for effective learning." Furthermore, "Staff are in control- Do what we say and show us respect." In this survey, less restrictive measures to avoid seclusion and restraint, surprisingly, did not involve listening to how the patient felt, what happened and what the patient wanted or needed.

Frighteningly, as is often the case, staff members quickly realize that the patient seems to be intentionally provoking others or induce self-harm in order to trigger external containment from staff. In so doing, the patient appears to relish the physical hands-on containment that is required at such moments. In our model of understanding, the individual is acting out through the need to instantly supply filling to the desperately empty cup and the intensity of physical containment serves to fill the cup temporarily. The reader needs to keep in mind that when the borderline patient becomes self destructive, he is filling his cup; when he gets others to help him contain, he is filling his cup. In effect, all of his actions are focused with cup filling in mind. As one can see, external containment, especially physical containment and close personal observation by staff, another act of filling the cup, may not further treatment and can often make worse what is already a difficult clinical situation. External containment is not often effective unless it is kept to a minimum and a path transitioning back to general milieu has been established.

Physical containment is often a very traumatic aspect of patient care for both the patient and the unit staff. Once hands-on physical containment is utilized, there is invariably an escalation of behavior that maintains this negative interaction. Interpersonal respect, boundary and compassion for all involved can quickly deteriorate. The treatment team often turns to one on one direct observation to keep this patient safe. Just as quickly, the team will realize that, once again, this level of direct interaction with this patient is not going to be effective and in fact, likely to bring about greater number of seclusions and restraints. The reason is very simple, the treatment team has now become ineffectively enmeshed with this patient's attempts to fill his cup by means of negative acting out. The affinity for the borderline patient to experience physical restraint as effective filling of the cup becomes a compelling reason for him to repeat such interactions.

After repeated scenarios using physical containment, the treatment team nearly always acknowledges that the safety of the patient has not been advanced. In short, the team says, "It has occurred to us that we have been doing a very poor job of keeping you safe despite following you around all day and being vigilant about keeping dangerous material from your reach." Furthermore, "When we attempt to keep you safe at the moment of your acting out, we often end up hurting you and you often fight so hard that some of us inevitably get injured." This is an opportunity for the team to involve the patient in the DSA model of treatment. The team should involve the "family" whenever possible. Once the treatment parameters are set up with this patient by delineating clear treatment boundary, the team conveys, "Death and serious injuries can certainly happen in your daily struggle with life, however, seclusion and restraint is not therapeutic, therefore, treatment must carry on without the use of extreme containment." At this point, the patient would be informed that the treatment team would no longer be dependent on the use of seclusion and restraint as part of his safety management. One on one observation as a way of keeping him safe would no longer be a treatment option; although the team would do everything possible to make sure that the inpatient environment is reasonably safe. Reasonable safety in this case is what is achievable without infringing on human dignity and done with compassion and respect.

The acutely suicidal patient has to be taken seriously. The therapist has to be familiar with one of the numerous suicide assessment protocols in order to be able to perform the very challenging task of evaluating suicide risk. Detailed discussion of suicide assessment is not within the scope of this writing. I would highly recommend that the therapist review suicide assessment with a separate resource. Despite the best of preparation and experience, suicide assessment is still an incredibly challenging task and at best, one could only take the path of excessive caution keeping in mind that none of us can predict or anticipate suicidality. If containment for the highly suicidal patient is required, much consideration must take place as to how best to implement this while maintaining treatment course.

The reader should note that this model of treatment is very much based on relationship and empathy; it is not about abandoning the patient at a time of crisis. When appropriate, it is important to provide the support and compassion that the patient requires at such times. If the patient is found to be acutely suicidal, all else should be on hold and the patient has to be monitored in a safe setting, which could involve hospitalization. If the patient is in a hospital setting, a higher level of supervision and monitoring of the patient could be warranted. However, the patient should be made aware that the *treatment is now on hold* pending further stabilization.

When it is time to implement external containment, this has to be done in a consistent way in accordance with our model of illness and treatment. One is always concerned that such "reinforcement" in the traditional hospital setting would further regress the patient and increase his reliance on others to help him contain his self destructive urges or to overindulge him with the much needed content for his cup. In keeping with DSA, the external containment should not contradict our attempt to avoid indiscriminate interpersonal filling or allow the patient to access filling through acting out. In the outpatient setting, external containment could mean hospitalization. In the inpatient setting, external containment could involve temporary issuing of greater staff intervention. Of course, some degree of interpersonal support is unavoidable in any effort at external containment and perhaps needed at such times of absolute crisis. When hospitalization becomes unavoidable, it is generally hoped that hospitalization would not reinforce the patient's dependence on others for critical soothing.

The therapist or the treatment team has to be vigilant about whether the external containment implemented to avoid imminent self harm will, at some point, contribute negatively to the overall course of treatment. Good treatment approach necessitates a sensitive balance between safety and healthy treatment boundaries. A patient who is prone to make frequent statements of suicide may be communicating a sense of hopelessness as well as a need for the alleviation of an internal emotional pain. Some patients are quite aware that the threat of suicide can become a desperate way of connecting with others but knows of no other way. "What do I do? It is all I really know." External containment may seem the only option to keep this patient safe at times but the chronic nature of this patient's emptiness and hopelessness must be considered in order that an efficacious treatment plan can be devised.

When the patient exercises the choice to consider death as an option, this decision, communication or act toward this end can set into motion reactions from others that can ultimately hinder treatment. As discussed in an earlier chapter, the high risk of death and severe injury can often bring about a paralysis in treatment as therapist or staff pursues every means possible to insure safety, although this approach tends to set an unproductive tone in treatment. Of course, the balance between sustaining life and productive treatment progress is delicate. This work favors the approach described in chapter 6 on dislodging the paralysis while maintaining a respectful emphasis on safety.

External Containment without Dependence

Case 9.4: Jennifer is a young adult who has been in therapy for several years. She sees her therapist on a weekly basis but her progress in treatment has been fitful. She has periods of doing fairly well and feeling fairly content in life. This is interspersed with periods of feeling very stressed and depressed. When feeling down, she has frequently resorted to superficially cutting herself on her thighs. On this day, after having had a difficult evening with her most recent boyfriend, she is feeling particularly dysphoric about life. She called her therapist and asked to come in for an emergency consultation.

In the session, she divulged that she has been cutting severely and has had moments of feeling suicidal. The disappointments from tumultuous relationships have increasingly caused her to feel emotionally labile. She has suddenly felt that her depression, for which she is taking an antidepressant, is worse than usual. She feels as if she has no one to turn to. Through her successions of relationship disappointments, her family remains distantly involved but are emotionally detached in their support for her. She thought out loud that, perhaps, no one really cares about her anymore. She appears to be in a great deal of inconsolable pain. In turning to her therapist, she seems to be asking for more than the usual support that her therapist has offered at such times in the past. As she came to face the reality that her therapist could not offer more than the usual solace, she became increasingly agitated and was unable to contract for safety. Her therapist then made the decision to contact the local psychiatric hospital and inquired about admitting the patient for stabilization.

Given the number of severe emotional crisis in recent time, she felt that hospitalization is the only way to get anyone to take her sense of crisis seriously. She hoped that her family would come to visit. In the hospital milieu, she initially felt a sense of warm support from the staff and the patients on the unit. It even appeared that she has quickly stabilized and is no longer feeling suicidal. She says, "I talk to people here and they understand and it makes me feel better." As a result, this newly found comfort and connection lowered her need to inflict self-injury.

However, this stability was short lived. Her sense of overwhelming emptiness began to overtake her superficial sense of connection and novelty with her new environment. Soon, she began to make more demands of the people around her. She also found herself in competition with the other patients on the ward for attention from the staff. Not long after, she was found to self-mutilate, and when confronted by staff, she would become enraged. Due to this behavior, she was viewed as a risk to self as well as others. Her ongoing acting out behavior started to consume a great deal of time and attention from unit staff. She could not be left alone because of the risk of severe self-mutilation. This clinical situation became quite a dead lock in her treatment and management. The team was aware that all they were doing in support of her had no lasting therapeutic value.

The team's decision was to remove her from the milieu programming and utilize a degree of one-to-one monitoring. Within the milieu, she was making such tremendous demands of the others that she was quickly alienating her peers and it was encroaching on their ability to do treatment. The team realized that any management strategy would need to address the need to discourage this cycle of meeting her needs temporarily through the others or through her acting out behavior. A program was set up in which she was separated from the general milieu as long as she is meeting her internal pain through the act of engaging staff by her provocation or through self-injurious behavior. Staff felt that her extremes of acting out constitute a type of emotional assault on the others on the unit and it is not fair to the other patients.

Because of her unwillingness or inability to contain her severe acting out behaviors, it became necessary for others to exert external containment. Physical containment is fraught with complications. Aside from the obvious safety issues, physical containment is intense and extreme, which then contributes to the risk of propagating unacceptable or unsafe behaviors through the filling of the cup. Even though staff attempted to separate her from the milieu and monitor her from a distance to reduce her impact on others, without a cohesive treatment plan, she was understandably confused and upset by this sudden arrangement.

Her team then looked for a "window of opportunity" to bring in her family as well as significant other for a conference to discuss the treatment using the DSA model. In this introductory family session, she was able to make some astute observations about her inner tension by describing the emotional flux as "exhausting and draining." One highly essential component of the family conference is the review of risk, sometimes referred to as the death talk. (See Chapter 6) This is an often ignored segment of this work but generally an important component to revisit when treatment is not going well. Once the cathexis of energy is removed from the issue of self-harm or suicide, she is less likely to hold the family and the team in paralysis.

From this point forward, every effort was made to help her regain some independence of function while rewarding her with positive con-

nections with others upon her successful completion of even brief periods of containment and letting time pass. These would be the first two
steps of the 3-steps program. Eventually, every interpersonal interaction
was in the context of the 3-steps. Through family work, her pain of emptiness was highly validated, her fear of functioning on her own was challenged and she was able to enjoy a much higher quality of interpersonal
relatedness.

Gradually, she was encouraged by the conceptualization that her
advancing ability to accept the internal emotional pain, contain the
impulse to act out or seek rescue, will be rewarded by obtaining selfobject introject through the connectedness of the 3-steps. What appeared to be her initial quiescence in the milieu turned out to be
short lived but her eventual adoption of the 3-steps brought about
a more consistent sense of wellbeing. A brief time later, she no longer required external containment and was better prepared to benefit from further psychotherapeutic exploration in the community.

Discussion:
In this case, there is the demonstration of two examples of the use of
external containment. First, this patient was admitted to the inpatient
hospital setting after failing to contain her suicidal and self-injurious impulses. The second example is that of the need to contain her still strong
impulse to cause self-injuries in the hospital milieu. This could be a patient
who has never been inducted to the treatment method with DSA or this
could be a patient who has not been able to fully adapt to the treatment
method with DSA. In either case, this would be a candidate for temporary
external containment for further stabilization.

External containment such as hospitalization is a common practice
in the treatment work with BPD but it is generally viewed as a short term
measure that is not necessarily therapeutic. The consensus concern about
hospitalization of individuals with BPD is that of the issues of dependence.
It is well known that many individuals with BPD tend to overly rely on
such external containment. In the language of DSA, this patient can easily
become dependent on the hospital setting if the indiscriminate filling of
her "cup" occurs. In a world in which she may encounter ever greater difficulties in meeting the requirements of her cup, it is all too easy for her
to turn to an environment that provides the potential for endless filling of
her cup through highly empathic staff staggered in shifts.

Hospital settings are naturally more interpersonally intense due to
the nature of the work done here. Nurses and hospital staff are more inclined to dispense the attention and care that fits in well with the needs of
an empty cup. Additionally, she is likely to encounter many patients with
their own dependency needs in this environment and this is all thrown
together in a tight space with many hospital workers. Because of this concern about dependence, many treatment programs advocate admitting
the patient for only a few days. This rational is based on the idea that this
patient's needs are ongoing and predictable; and scheduled admissions
prevent over utilization of hospital as a resource. There is often a subtle
secondary message in the design of such a short hospital stay, "We really

don't know how to help you and don't want to habituate you to this help-less situation."

In DSA, inpatient hospitalization does not have to be viewed as the antithesis of treatment. As a microcosm of the larger world outside of the hospital, the inpatient milieu can be a stable environment for the bor-derline patient to begin to grapple with his or her developmental issues that result in his emotional pain and make the discovery toward thera-peutic repair. With trained and experienced staff, the hospital milieu can be highly conducive to the meaningful practice of this work. Once the pa-tient develops some rudimentary insight about the benefit of this work, he can then move on to the longer term psychotherapeutic treatment in the community.

Working with Defense Mechanisms

Understanding and taking into consideration Freud's conceptualization of the warring factions within our psyche as well as Klein's emphasis on the develop-mental importance of the death instinct, will now help us to better comprehend the dynamics of the cup. It is through the theoretical understanding of the early frustrations that one can then arrive at the idea of an innate, inborn existence of original anger. This then gives rise to the hypothesis that healthy resolution of these primitive emotions is required for the proper development of a healthy self. Numerous complications and frustrations can jeopardize early develop-ment and interfere with proper introjection of early selfobjects. Therefore, one can suffer developmental hurt without explicit abuse or neglect. It has been suggested that poorness of fit or lack of attunement may explain the resultant pathology in later life. Hypothetically, this would account for the high number of individuals in our society who suffers from character pathology. Hence, in our work, one has to be particularly appreciative of the intense manifestations of defense mechanisms in any treatment subject.

In chapter 2, the concept of projective identification and splitting were discussed, and in this section, I will address the understanding of these defense mechanisms within the model of DSA. The consideration of maladaptive de-fenses in the context of the work with DSA is a more in-depth and challenging exploration of the pathology of the self. In further illustrating the dynamic role the cup plays in daily life, I will take the reader through a more advanced view of the cup involving defenses. It is possible to conduct treatment with the fundamentals of DSA described up to this point, but the consideration of projective identification and splitting will further enhance our understanding of the dynamics of BPD as well as conditions related to the self. Repeatedly in this writing I have emphasized the importance of understanding the function of the cup and the role it plays in driving and motivating many of our behaviors in everyday life. Of the defense mechanisms, splitting and projective identification hold the most significance in understanding the psychic complexities of our inner world.

Projection, as with all of the defense mechanisms, is a part of the subconscious. As such, no one ever says that they intentionally project their anger onto someone else. Yet, in daily life and clinical situations, the therapist can often witness how the patient displaces his anger, dependence and insecurities onto others as well as experiencing the patient's projection. "Typically, a therapist who 'receives' a projective identification from a patient may develop a new set of feelings, and only during later self-scrutiny come to understand that they, so to speak, 'belonged' to the patient" (Migone 1995, p. 627). It is useful to mention that some writers in this area take into consideration defensive projective identification and adaptive projective identification. "I consider that projective identification works in two ways: a normal way, in which the analyst-mother takes into herself a part of the patient-child's emotional identity in order to return it to him in a detoxified and hence assimilable form, and a pathological way in which the negative aspects are so plentiful that projective identification operates to excess" (Doucet 1992, p. 657).

In the work of DSA, I attempted to describe the fundamental representation of the emptiness of our inner world. Now, I will utilize our analogy using the cup to further understand the concept of projective identification and illustrate the role this defense plays in our everyday life, especially in the world of the borderline patient. To truly understand the impact of projective identification, one has to first comprehend the power of the emotions that drives it. DSA draws upon the parallel between the clinical symptoms of BPD and the metaphor of the cup. It is suggested that the fluctuating level in the cup can leave one in predictable emotional pain. The cup is not always empty, and when somewhat full, the individual can experience the self as perhaps pleasant and calm. The self may even take to feeling that it not only feels good but that the self is good. On the other hand, when the cup is at a low level, the self can be experienced not only as painfully empty but that the self is bad.

Mud as a Precursor to the Defense Mechanisms

Here is a simple visualization to the formation of original anger. It is helpful to think of early frustrations as contributing to the malformation of the cup as well as leaving the first layer of tenacious sediment that continues to build over the years. Although it is most likely that the earliest frustrations caused the holes in this cup, there continues to be muddy sedimentation that further settles to the bottom of the cup. In choosing the source of input into the cup, one can invariably obtain material of questionable quality and the resultant impurity in the substance settles as sticky mud around the holes at the bottom of the cup. Conceptually, the source of the mud can be conceived as coming from chronic misattunement with important selfobjects as well as acting out behaviors that brings us a sense of guilt and shame.

Once the self is experienced as empty and "bad", it then uncovers the original anger that lays dormant in the deeper recesses of our psyche (visualize this as the sediment at the bottom of the cup). Original anger, whether arising out of nature or nurture, is the collective anger and frustration that might have formed in the earliest developmental stages in life. One might suggest original anger as the nails that punched holes in the psychic vesicle or otherwise, prevented the normal formation of the cup. Original anger, as the sediment at the bottom of the cup, exist as a baseline and therefore, far more constant and consistent in nature as compared to the pain of emptiness which fluctuates inside the cup. One can hypothetically view original anger as the cause of the malformation of the cup and the constantly changing level in the cup today in turn affects the uncovering of original anger.

In clinical observation, the characteristic operations of the borderline patient reverberate with the existence of original anger. These individuals experience a pervasive sense of anger and frustration that belies the ups and downs of daily life. There is a general view of life as highly unsatisfying and rejecting. As a result, the borderline patient may maintain a pernicious notion of the world as hostile. This individual is likely to hold very strong and unwavering opinions of others based on original anger as evoked by the emptiness within. This manner of experience is especially prominent when the emotional system of the cup uncovers the sediment. Because of the covert and insidious nature of original anger, a set of feelings often hidden in the deepest recess, therapy has to address the fundamental hurt rather than focus only on external frustrations.

In practice, the fairly healthy cup is one that is predominantly full and rarely reveals the full wrath of original anger. This emotional system maintains reasonably good boundaries with selfobjects and others in the near orbit. Therefore, his selfobject introject is better integrated with his experiences of the self. In this respect, negative projective identification is kept under check and less likely to evoke the sort of negative transference that would interfere with giving to his cup. (Fig. 9.1) Keep in mind that in an optimally positive environment, this individual is also reciprocating by giving to the selfobject. Projective identification has been referred to as "reciprocal role procedures" described as bidirectional communicative process that organizes interactions with others (Ryle 1994).

In the case of the individual with a highly porous cup that is conducive to frequent emptiness, his emotional pain is often compounded by the turmoil of interpersonal conflicts. Others around him find themselves experiencing confounding emotions. Whether it is a sense of dependence, power, sex or ingratiation, the resulting metacommunication from his projective

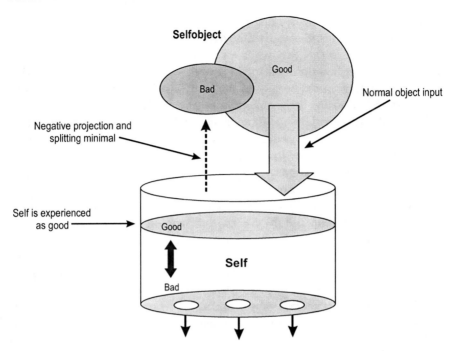

Figure 9.1 *In this diagram, the content of the cup is high and the self is experienced as "good". In this case, there is inherently less negative projection by the self toward the selfobject. As a result, the selfobject is felt as providing plentiful "stuff" to the self (cup).*

identification may work in tandem with splitting to give rise to very intense interpersonal interactions. In the more direct type of projection, the individual making the projection assumes that others are angry or aggressive through his own use of the projection of hostility (Cashdan 1988 p.55). Regardless of the type of projection, these dynamics induce in others an intense response that may seem bewildering, threatening or confusing. Once the others become aware of what is taking place, the typical response may be that of feeling used, manipulated and react with anger or withdrawal. This would serve to confirm to the self that part of him is bad or undesirable.

One young woman pertinently reported that when she becomes upset in one arena in her life, she can often come to feel that the whole world is against her. It turns out that she has a hostile projection towards the selfobject. The projection of anger can quickly take hold in the recipient or recipients in a subtle and subconscious fashion. In addition, a strong transferential response can take place if the recipient combines projective identification with his own history. Either way, the selfobject's experience of projective identification is clearly going to interfere with his ability to provide positive cup input for the individual in discussion here. (Fig. 9.2) In a patient who is prone to be frequently empty in this emotional system, projective identification is a mechanism that can cause havoc by reducing the number of transferential input from available selfobjects.

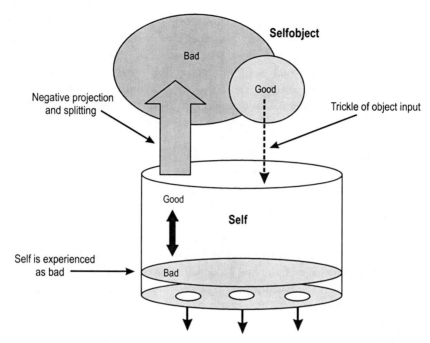

Fig 9.2 *In this diagram, the content of the cup is low and the self is experienced as "bad". In this case, there is a great deal of negative projection and splitting from the self toward the selfobject. As a result, the selfobject can experience negative projective identification and selfobject input toward the self (cup) is significantly reduced.*

Here, I am reminded of a young girl who holds the greatest disdain for one person, her father. Although there is some degree of truth in her remarks about him, as best that I could put together for my own understanding, her revulsion toward him seemed unfounded. Session after session, she berated him mercilessly. Even after conferring with other family members, it was difficult to comprehend her wrath. However, what was revealed in our work was the very insecure and fearful core of her internal self. Then we established through ongoing work her experiences of a profound sense of emptiness throughout much of her daily life. Although not one to act out overtly or aggressively, she seems to bicker and whine incessantly and when all else fails, the tears come streaming down. By any measure, she probably cried more than most people. By crying, she was able to draw the pity of others but it is also a behavior that was intense and extreme enough to be categorized as a covert acting out behavior; it was a perfect acting out tool.

No matter how she coerced and fought through daily life, she could never get enough lasting satisfaction or calm. Her immediate and extended family has become quite exhausted in their care and support of her; in this desperate search for content for her cup, she continues to alienate one important person in her life, her father. Why is it that she has the need to maintain such animosity toward one person who could have been one of the major sources of input into her cup? The key here is the understanding of the pain of emptiness and the mechanism by which ***original anger***, like a precursor to the defense mechanisms, is brought to the surface where previously it could be hidden out of sight like a shameful and dirty secret. Through splitting, she manages to intensify her object relations world into the extremes of good and bad. Additionally, this split allows her to exercise projective identification of dependence and ingratiation with the "good" objects. In this fashion, the void of emptiness can be filled through the rescue seeking projective identifications as well as through the covert acting out behaviors of splitting.

Splitting comes into play early in life as part of the infant's attempt to address satisfying and unsatisfying basic sensations of fullness, emptiness, coldness and warmth etc. as well as, perhaps, the death instinct. As some maturity takes place, the constant frustrations with the good and bad breast becomes coalesced into the image of the good and bad mother. At this stage, abnormal splitting can occur if the bad mother experiences are extreme or rejecting and the seeds of interpersonal pathology are planted (Cicchetti 1987). Through a process Kohut termed, "transmuting internalization", the young child constructs the sense of the self by engaging others. Now the differentiated self consist of "good me" and "bad me". As an adult, *identity splitting* is embedded within the various identities such as sexuality, career, marriage and parenting (Cashdan 1988, p.52).

Splitting separates the object world into those that are "good" and those that are "bad". One has to keep in mind that each selfobject and each self is subjectively composed of both good and bad; it is a matter of an object or self being mostly good or mostly bad. This serves to protect the good objects from the anger, hatred, aggression and contamination from the bad self (empty self). Now that the good objects are protected, the self can perhaps "safely" project his anger and aggression toward the bad object.

Projective identification when viewed as an outgrowth of the dynamics of splitting, attempts to manipulate the external world through interpersonal relationships. The projective identification of ingratiation involves eliciting appreciation from the recipient. The individual who uses this projective identification came to believe that he is unlovable unless he gives to others. The sexualized projective identification establishes and maintains relationships through sexual means.

In concert, splitting and projective identification helps the borderline self to achieve a semblance of better functioning. Splitting emphasizes the all good or the all bad in various selfobjects. Subsequently, projective identification can be implemented more effectively with specific target recipient for the projection. Thus, it is far more effective to induce sexual arousal from a "good staff" once the dynamic of splitting is activated in the milieu. The display of helplessness is more likely to garner caretaking from the recipient staff if splitting has already set up the stage for the "good" staff to be highly empathic to this metacommunication.

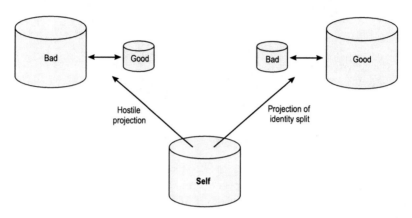

Fig. 9.3 *Diagrams the splitting of each selfobject in to two portions consisting of good and bad. With hostile projection, the bad object garners fear. In identity split, the self projects a stance to induce a predictable response from the selfobject.*

In DSA conceptualization, splitting and projective identification brings about transference input to the cup through manipulating interpersonal relationships. In emotional emptiness, this pain has such magnitude that even temporary input is welcome. Splitting and projective identification effectively provides input to the system although this filling to the cup is short lived due to its inherent leakiness in the borderline individual. The need to exercise these defenses most often peak and troughs with the needs of the cup. Emptiness continues to be a trigger for original anger and this in turn activates the defenses to better guard against the pain of emptiness. (Fig. 9.4) Gratification through this mean tends to be unidirectional toward the self and ultimately, quite unsatisfactory to the selfobject.

On the other hand, hostile or negative projections, in the presence of splitting, will intensify the magnitude of the "bad" object. As splitting takes place, the selfobject that takes on the "bad" self representation and labeled as a bad object will reconstitute toward becoming more threatening due to the cathexis of affective energy. The resultant split of the selfobject creates a large and

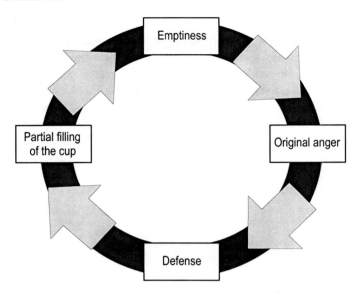

Fig. 9.4 *This cyclic dynamic of emptiness has influence over ineffective coping through the use of the defense mechanisms.*

prominent bad object while the good object separates to become rather anemic although there is generally a preservation of a vestige of the good object in the dichotomy of the split. (Fig. 9.2 and 9.3) This effectively causes this particular selfobject to become useless as well as unwilling for transference input to this patient's cup. What follows is often the development of excessive anxiety in connection to the threatening selfobject. (Fig. 9.5)

The selfobject world of the borderline patient is in a constantly fluctuating state. Whether the self experiences the object as good or bad often depends on the efficiency of transference or emotional reciprocation between them. The object is good when all is well and the self is enjoying a flood of input. The object is bad when the self is projecting negatively toward the object or when the object fails to respond to the projective identification. Thus, one observes that projective identification arising out of identity split appears to have the purpose of bringing transference input to the cup unless the selfobject sees through this projection and refuses to comply. In such a case, the self then experiences a sense of rejection that quickly turns the object toward bad. Thus, the selfobject can easily switch from good to bad based on whether or not it is providing positive transference input or not. The hallmark of severe borderline pathology resides in the tendency for this patient to be unable to entirely recognize that the object can consist of both good and bad characteristics concomitantly and integrate these opposite representations into one cohesive whole object.

In the case of this young girl, through subconscious means, splitting and projective identification work in tandem to allow her to preserve some sense of organization in her frustrating world. The good objects are supposed to fill her cup and the bad objects, mainly her father, are to be the receiver of her negative projections. This brings us back to a point discussed in Chapter 6 about the role of each member in a family system. In an established family system, one that has had the time to settle into a semi-homeostatic state, each member has a specific role to play even if some roles seem particularly unfair and traumatic to that individual; same can be said of sibling sequence within a family. Having made the distinction between the good and the bad, the latter is likely to remain the recipient of her angst and anger. She will continue to see her father as unfair, targeting and aggressive towards her. Sadly, one would expect that her father is very unlikely to behave in any way supportive or comforting to her given that he is at the receiving end of her projective attack. His experience of projective identification will confound and baffle him to the point of feeling true anger toward his daughter. Once this occurs, it would be simple for her to justify the "anger" that she harbors for him.

Effective treatment has but one goal at this juncture; it is to bring forth this young girl's awareness that the nature of her suffering is directly connected to the emptiness within. I wish to point out that this foregoing statement is not fundamentally identical to telling the patient that she should take more "responsibility" for herself or that she should examine the different sides of these issues. Furthermore, engaging the patient in interpretive activities, therefore, avoidant of the relational implications in the projective identification is also counterproductive in this treatment. "If the true benefits of object relations treatment are to be realized, the therapist needs to send an unmistakable, unambiguous signal regarding an unwillingness to participate in the patient's pathology" (Cashdan 1988, p.121). The challenge to the therapist resides in how best to prepare the borderline patient in facing the inevitable confrontation about the defense mechanisms. However, without addressing the core issue of the patient's own defective self, any attempt to help the patient process about the frustrations of everyday life runs the risk of fault finding or problem avoidance.

Practical Lessons from Projective Identification

I have proposed the use of the cup in the DSA model of treatment to help bring the patient better awareness of the defect of the self in an understandable and ego-syntonic fashion. DSA is grounded in the belief that the overwhelming majority of the patient's behaviors can be attributed to his emotional pain of emptiness. For the teen girl in this discussion, DSA help the therapist to convey an attempt at understanding the patient's internal experience and acknowledges the patient's emotional pain. Hence, she is more willing to explore the possibility of original anger and the resulting projection. At once, when she is able to accept the fundamental deficit of the self, she can then overcome the impasse of her treatment and become productive in therapy.

In the case of a young man with a history of school refusal, video game addiction, substance use and "extreme mood swings", projection of power and control was his way of feeling accepted and valued. Within the setting of the day hospital milieu, he can present as tolerant and helpful to some while belittling and critical to others. He wants to be highly regarded by those that he respects and can be outright cruel to those that he sees as in lesser position of power. His metacommunication around the stance of control was so effective that it brought numerous staff to tears in feelings of ineffectiveness and incompetence. In the milieu, his projective identification of power was quite pervasive and it was apparent in the obstructions that his projection created in his treatment.

Confronting this narcissistic projective identification has to be done with consideration for the delicate ego state at task as well as the need to make certain that this patient realize that his therapist is not ready to accept this projective identification as the basis of their relationship. It is especially challenging to confront this patient's needs for power and control. Classic transference interpretation may only serve to calm and diffuse the intensity of the situation when such play of projection has to be strongly addressed. This model of treatment approaches this issue through preparing the patient to better visualize his internal emotional world and recognize the pain he suffers here before attempting to help him to see the problems related to his projective identification.

Understanding compulsion and control

Case 9.5 I first met Derek, a late teen, when he became quite suicidal due to the stresses going on in his life. On initial meeting, he presented as cordial, articulate and seemingly confident but unable to hide a nervous edge to his overall demeanor. He politely accepted a quick handshake, offering a sweaty palm, before sitting down. In the weeks to follow, he came across as guarded and resistive to detailed discussion of his current troubles. He can be charming and talkative about everything else in the world except for his personal difficulties in life. Finally, with some corroboration from his mother, a rudimentary picture of his life came together. It seems that he is full of guilt for the anger he harbors, most of which pertains to his father, long ago divorced from his mother, an individual he sees as cold, aloof, critical and unkind. He admits to feeling powerless in the dramatic conflicts between his parents while secretly aligned with his mother, with whom, he has a very close relationship. As for his father, he would not even allow for any contact in the context of treatment. Eventually, it was revealed that he has not been able to attend school for some time and in addition, he has a severe case of obsessive worries about germs and dirt. In this regard, he has involved his mother in an elaborate ritual to clean his sheets, his bath, the carpet and even the air in the house.

As the picture further unfolded, it revealed an individual who is highly anxious in the social arena and never had a close friend. His social difficulties seemed related to his propensity to hold very high expectations for those around him. He has no traditional hobbies and detests any type of sport. Although a very intelligent individual and tests extremely well, he has gradually lost all ability to attend school. Reluctantly over several sessions, he shared that there is one male teacher he finds particularly unsavory. It has gotten to the point that he does not want to go near any place that he imagines that the teacher might have been. When asked why he finds this one teacher so intolerable, he was unable to answer except to raise the suspicion that this teacher has something against him. When he comes home, he wants to practically decontaminate any piece of clothing and material that has been to school.

In treatment, it became readily apparent the tremendous resistance building up. The work of therapy became increasingly burdensome for the patient and the therapist's experience of resignation was a signal to seek consultation and examine the psychodynamics at play. Even though this patient attends sessions compliantly, he does so because it is his nature to be externally compliant, but how he feels internally about the work of treatment is a different matter. With tangential and irrelevant distractions, he sidestepped and dodged issues like a football quarterback, at once trying to maintain control and maintain survival. In the meanwhile, he is failing school and his controlling behavior with family has paralyzed everyone's ability to function in life.

Finally, in seeking a different approach to traditional treatment for obsessive compulsive disorder, his therapist turned to DSA. The therapist's argument for doing so was centered on the concern that despite intense supportive psychotherapy and cognitive behavioral work, it was felt that this patient still has not reached sufficient insight about his need for change. Without reaching a true motivation for change, it is easy for him to blame his fear of germs on germs and blame his revulsion for his teacher on the teacher. While skillful psychodynamic exploration and interpretation to his resistance took place, he maintained a controlling stance in this treatment, effectively stonewalled any chance of progress. Through the introduction of DSA, with the goal of exploring and validating his very deep internal pain of emptiness, it was then possible to convince him of the dire internal emotional condition that demands his immediate attention.

As to the effectiveness of this work, Derek was able to stabilize quickly once he was confronted with a way to understand his pain. From his initial description of the void within, he was able to grasp the significance of this pain as a primary driving force in all of his needs. "I feel empty inside, hollow, like I am just a shell." "This feeling makes me feel weak all over." He now understood the source of his great anxiety and able to see the ineffectiveness of his former ways of coping. By referring to the illustration of figure 7.1, he was able to work with his therapist to analyze his interpersonal dynamics with the people in his life and came to understand not only the source of his anxiety but his anger as well. He then came to recognize the "beast", that entity with a very primal need like that of an infant, seeking only to meet basic survival. Once this degree of insight was achieved, he made fairly rapid progress in the reduction of his compulsive behavior and seemed more prepared to explore issues related to his school refusal.

In gaining further insight into his illness, he understood how the defense mechanisms played a role in the manner in which his eventual anxiety regarding the bad selfobject evolve to such a proportion that only an act of extreme compulsion could appease. He now has good reasons to view his selfobjects differently than from the past and would be more conducive to involving them in the 3-steps which further their role as selfobject introject. As he accepted the principle of projective identification, he was then less compelled to experience his teacher and a few others as antagonistic. Believing that important others in his life are not out to destroy him, this was sufficient for him to feel less anxious and thus, his obsessive/compulsive symptoms were much reduced. I might here venture to suggest that his symptom improvement did not rely on a direct attack on the compulsive behaviors but rather, a comprehension of his emotional emptiness.

In the case of this young man, it is immaterial as to how much of his school refusal is related to actual incidents of being victimized, this is certainly to be true to an extent. For progress in treatment to be made, he has to be made to understand his own role in provoking the reactions of others. For him, the use of traditional chain analysis of events did not seem to impress upon him the significance of his individual responsibility in external conflicts. In addressing this dilemma, his therapist again turned to DSA, using fig. 9.5, to help him understand the chain of events. As he goes about visualizing the tremendous propensity for his "cup" to be so extremely empty, which he can readily relate through his own increasing awareness, he admits to feeling highly validated by this analogy. He then came to realize the significance of feeling empty and the tendency for this state to trigger *original anger*.

Armed with improved insight through the cup analogy, he is now prepared to better understand and accept the existence of original anger in addition to the painful state of the emptiness of the cup. Being aware of the source of the powerful drive to his strenuous urge to exercise his compulsion, he can now be assiduous in the treatment work. His ability to relate to the "cup" also allowed him to comprehend the possibility for the existence of splitting and projective identification, defense mechanisms that are readily discussed with the patient when possible. Progression to this stage of cognitive understanding of his illness followed a natural path starting with his acceptance of the pathology of the self through the model of the cup that culminated in his fervent attempts to cull his compulsions through the practice of the 3-steps. Furthermore, through the work of the 3-steps, he began to experience greater authenticity of the self in the context of interpersonal engagement. We may conclude that this insight about his illness then allowed him to experience rather rapid improvement of his obsessive/compulsive symptoms.

Discussion:
As has been suggested by Kernberg, "borderline personality organization", if viewed as a broad range of pathology of the self, should encompass many

other commonly encountered psychiatric diagnoses. Here is just one example of an Axis I diagnosis that is generally not thought of in the same formal framework as borderline personality disorder. In working backward from the external to the internal, one should realize that this patient sees his world through superstition, phobia and magical thinking, which are inconsistent with his culture. This type of thinking seems to have its roots in emotional survival. This likely arrived from experiencing of life as strictly black and white or perhaps, splitting his object world into distinct good and bad. It is nearly magical in which his selfobject world is separated into such distinct pockets of good and bad. As a defense mechanism, splitting allows him to deal with the unacceptable anger and aggression within, the likes of which can generate overwhelming anxiety. A lack of integration of the disparate parts of the self is a natural part of infancy, but if splitting is utilized and persisted from an early age, it then interferes with the proper integration of the self. The pathology of his "cup" and the development of his "original anger" likely arose from early frustrations of having to modify his self in conformity to an environment that somehow brought about a developmental distraction. In another word, a lack of appropriate mirroring and idealizing transference may have taken place and his true self had to be placed on hold. This obstruction to the internalization of the selfobject may have roots in his inherent temperament or contributed to by conflicts with the external world.

Carrying forward, splitting continues to play a major role in his life as he grew older. It is natural for the infant to experience frequent frustrations in connection to feeding, elimination, sleeping and safety, due to the limited ability he or she has to fend for the self, but one might be puzzled as to why the older individual should face such frustrations. Many writers of classical analysis point to overwhelming anxiety as the drive behind a defense mechanism such as splitting. An infant may utilize splitting as a matter of survival, and in classical understanding, pathological coping seems to involve splitting as part of this individual's permanent ego function beyond infancy. As the individual grows older, he should generally be able to acquire better survival capability, but it seems that the insult to the self is so severe that the infantile ego function continues to exist in teenage and adulthood.

Perhaps anxiety and frustrations are handled differently by infants and young children or possibly, rudimentary mirroring and idealizing transference allows the young to vicariously obtain adequate transference input, but in this dependent state, children are traditionally not viewed as very individualized. As one approaches the teen years, the stage of greater independence and individuation prompts the activation of the cup to provide better individual function. It is at this juncture that many come to realize the emotional pain of emptiness and experience the drive to neutralize such tension; an instinctual strategy is to evoke the defense mechanisms. Ironically, this action places the individual back into a developmental realm of the infant.

Naturally, the splitting of the selfobject into good and bad is then incorporated into the dynamics of the cup; this results in a reciprocal interaction between the cup and the defense of splitting. Thus, in our illustration, when the cup is low in content, the self is viewed as bad and when the cup is full in content, the self is viewed as good. Having a picture of how one can understand the maintenance of splitting, we can now consider how Derek's emptiness and defense mechanism play out in his daily life. As would be expected, his emptiness drives his fear of the original anger which is comprised of anxiety, anger and aggression. In this empty state, he experiences himself as bad, which brings fourth another defense mechanism, projective identification. "The anxiety which provoked the projection of the impulse onto an object in the first place now becomes fear of that object, accompanied by the need to control the object in order to prevent it from attacking the self when under the influence of that impulse" (Kernberg 1985, p. 56).

Here is a young man trying to juggle a number of very difficult demands placed upon him by the dynamics within. Firstly, he has to find a way to fill the hollow emptiness within. For this, he reaches for the few select people he has identified as being good. Secondly, he is given to see the self and the world around him as distinctly good and bad; therefore, he has to be very cautious about who and what he turns to for filling. There are portions of the world that can be very dangerous and to be avoided at all cost. Through projective identification, his negative affects, such as original anger, is projected outward in an indiscriminate manner like the scattering of dirt. Effectively, this is like an insidious contamination of the world around him. Anything that he has not identified as good can then fall prey to this massive contamination. There is a double dose of contamination in this case. Due to his perception of the self as being very bad at a time of severe emptiness, and that the good self is very minimal, he will feel fearful that the bad self will contaminate everything good outside. At the same time, all of this negative affect within will bring about projective identification which then scatters more negativity all around in a mostly subconscious fashion. Hence, he now experiences the world around him as a very negative space that is angry, aggressive and possibly dirty. What are contaminated could be animate as well as inanimate objects, which could include people, places and things.

Understanding his emptiness via the analogy of the cup allows us to be able to empathize with the existence of splitting and projective identification in this individual's internal dynamic. This understanding then paves the way for us to see how he copes with anxiety by using intense, extreme and controlling behaviors in order to deal with an interpersonal world that is experienced as highly dangerous and negative. This is how he came to experience several people in his life as very negative but is then unable to justify why he should feel so negative about them. This also help us to understand how such a seemingly logical individual should be so fearful of germs, to which, he too has a hard time explaining why he has such extraordinary fear of them. Because of splitting, he has effectively reduced the number of possible good objects around him. This would lead to a shortage of people who can provide filling to his cup. With the cup running so chronically empty, he has to turn to acting out behavior, such as intense compulsive routines and battles to maintain control over others as an alternative way of filling this cup. With the horrific leaks of the cup, he will never be able to reach any equilibrium through any means, thus; he is stuck in a perpetual negative state of emotion and pain. Due to such urgency, he will have a difficult time making sense of conventional therapy work until he develops sufficient insight about his emptiness and the work needed to gain a more cohesive representation of the self.

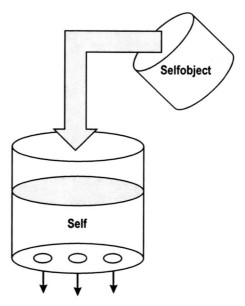

Fig. 9.5 (A) *The selfobject is viewed as whole when transference input is uninterrupted.*

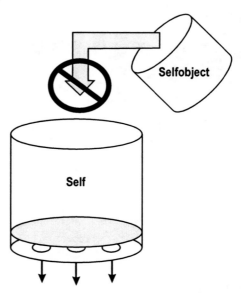

Fig 9.5 (B) *Once the transference input from the selfobject is discontinued or disrupted, the content of the self is reduced rapidly.*

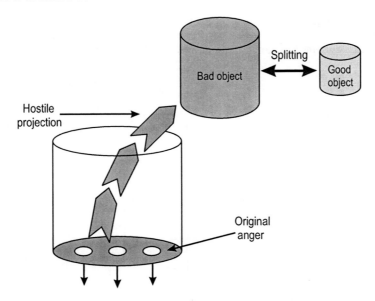

Fig. 9.5 (C) *Severe emptiness results in the revealing of original anger dormant at the bottom of the cup. Original anger then contributes to the hostile projection to get rid of the bad parts of the self.*

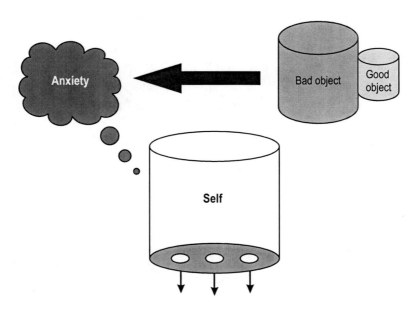

Fig. 9.5 (D) *Upon experiencing the selfobject as bad, anxiety is generated and the self sets out to seek some sort of relief from this emotional discomfort.*

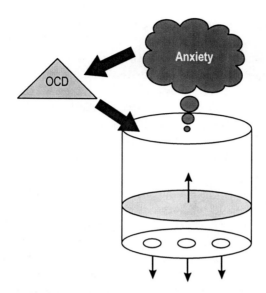

Fig 9.5 (E) *Obsessive compulsive symptoms can be viewed as a type of covert acting out behavior that can ultimately provide for temporary filling of the emotional system and return the cup to a sustainable level.*

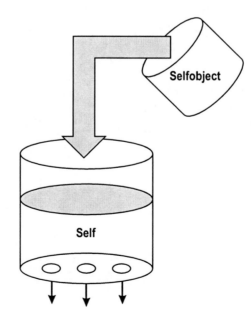

Fig. 9.5 (F) *On recovery from fragmentation, anxiety and projective identification are reduced, the selfobject can be invited to provide further transference input. The self can now be experienced as whole, as can the selfobject.*

By far, hostile projections are easier to detect. Projective identification in which other metacommunications are being used can be more covert and often engages the selfobject undetected. The narcissistic individual with a hankering for power relates through control and induces a sense of incompetence in others. In a projective identification of dependency, the individual relates a stance of helplessness which then induces caretaking from others. To truly comprehend the clinical symptoms of the borderline patient, we should best recognize that defense mechanisms are not at play continuously; this is a controversial conceptualization but it is critical to the principle of treatment in DSA. For example, the dependent person is more likely to activate the projective identification of dependency at times of severe emptiness. (Fig. 9.6)

One might propose that projective identification and transference are linked because it takes a particular character background of the recipient to herald the types of response that reverberates with the projection. Transference, as a dynamic in DSA, is a material that one exchanges with others depending on our relationship with them but the quality and quantity of this transfer depends on how our own history mingles with the present projection identifications being experienced. The mother of a severely abused child will respond excessively to the child's plea for caretaking due to her guilt related to not having protected the child from past perpetrators. We thus see how an individual with co-dependence issues can inadvertently react to the projection of helplessness by the borderline patient with a care taking stance (Cashdan 1988).

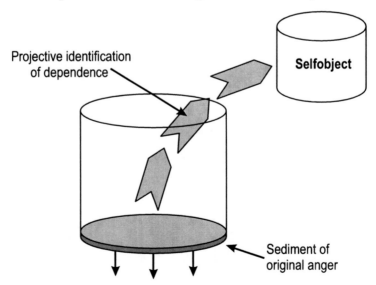

Fig. 9.6 (A) *Following severe loss of content, projective identification of dependence can be especially prominent. This induces a response of caretaking by the selfobject.*

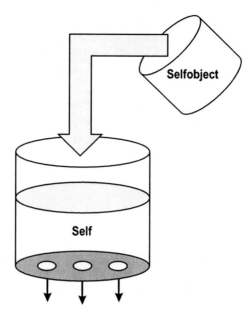

Fig. 9.6 (B) *The dependency plea for caretaking will result in the transference input by the selfobject, thus, restoring some essential functions to the self.*

Another Look at Projective Identification

Another look at projective identification is warranted here. As a defense mechanism, its presence and impact on the daily life of every person, individuals not traditionally considered to suffer from BPD, has been poorly recognized. This work is based on the fundamental hypothesis that the pathology of the self is more pervasive than those meeting DSM IV criteria for BPD. It is my belief that any fundamental characteristics of an individual that can potentially interfere with basic trust and interpersonal connection, can contribute to a defective development of the self. Hence, the inherent temperament and developmental frustrations of an individual could intensify the developmental pathologies of the self. There is much compelling evidence of such pathology in the clinical histories of patients presenting with frustrations in relationships, work and school.

Disorders that Disrupt Healthy Development

It has been suggested that ADHD and autism spectrum disorders are associated with an increased risk of personality disorders and deficits in character maturation. Individuals with personality disorder often demonstrate neurocognitive problems (Burgess 1992, Dinn 2000, Bazanis 2002). Furthermore, personality disorders are common in follow-up of subjects with neuropsychiatric disorders (Rasmussen 2000, Fischer 2002). "Hypothetically, neuropsychiatric diagnoses designate dysfunctional extremes of normally distributed abilities, such as attention and impulse control; adaptive decision-making strategies; adequate perception and control of voice, posture, mimicry, and interpersonal skills; and mentalizing. The variation in such abilities is partly constitutional and may influence personality development to a greater extent than recognized in current personality theory." "Considering the high rate of clear-cut neuropsychiatric disorders in childhood, and considering the evidence for 'broader phenotypes' or 'shadow syndromes' of these disorders, a reasonable hypothesis would be that neurocognitive skills including attention, impulse control, empathy, and communication are of general importance in the development of 'personality' (Anckarsäter 2006)."

Perhaps, similar to neuropsychiatric disorders, anxiety spectrum of disorders can effectively contribute to a hindrance in the healthy development of the self. Picturing anxiety as a shroud that surrounds the developing cup provides the sense that such neurosis can lead to a frustrated developmental process. Anxiety contributes much preoccupation and can potentially distract the individual from critical developmental task in the early life. Furthermore, this veil of anxiety continues to function as a filter and therefore, reduce the amount of transference input available to the cup. (See illustration in case 9.6) Developmentally, the cup is unable to reach healthy maturation, illustrated by the leakage. Interpersonally, the veil of anxiety prevents sufficient input. Yet, many individuals enter into the world with just such a temperament and perhaps, carry this trait into adulthood.

As an older teen and adult, this individual may not suffer the severe pathology of the individual with BPD, but it is likely that at times of personal crisis, he too can experience the painful emptiness of the cup just as the borderline patient. For instance, his anxiety can isolate him from much social interactions outside of the family; he becomes highly reliant on just a few members of his family. As a result, he is highly vulnerable to even minor interpersonal upheaval in his world and this can lead to profound changes in the level of his cup due to decreased input. Even without a great deal of original anger, he can still suffer the tremendous pain of emptiness. It is conceivable that this pain is sufficient to bring about the need to exercise splitting and projective identification.

Another interesting clinical exercise to consider would be the case of a patient with mild to moderate pervasive developmental disorder (PDD). This is an individual with an inherent challenge in the interpersonal arena; unlike the fully autistic individual with little awareness of the world outside of his mind, the individual with PDD may desire interpersonal attention but lacks quality reciprocal interpersonal interactions. One might speculate as to whether this patient suffers the anger and frustrations of early infancy and childhood that could lead to the development of pathology of the self. The detailed discussion of PDD is not within the scope of this work but the further understanding of this disorder could perhaps shed some light on our understanding of the pathology of the self. Children and adolescents diagnosed with PDD represent a significant subgroup (14 percent) of patients with serious emotional disturbance referred for psychiatric treatment. This study also suggests PDD can be easily missed because it can be mild and associated with co-morbid psychiatric conditions (Sverd 2003).

As has been suggested by Anckarsäter et al (2000), autistic temperament comes with increased risk of personality disorder. It is my clinical intuition that original anger and the accompanying disability of the cup exist in the individual with such neuropsychiatric disorder. The mechanism by which development is frustrated also applies to the individual with PDD. The leakiness of the emotional system should appear no different from others who are similarly affected. The individual with PDD can be thought of as experiencing an interpersonal filter that screens out a portion of the positive transferential input from potential selfobjects. (See illustration in case 9.6)

Neuropsychiatric Root to Pathology of the Self

Case 9.6 Mark is a 35 year old Caucasian male. He turned to psychiatric treatment when his wife threatened divorce if he did not get help for his temper, which was increasingly more focused on his two young children. He is prone to suffer short periods of unexplained trembling combined with a sudden overwhelming sense of restlessness. When these episodes occur, he also feels "drained" and wants to go to sleep; on awakening, he would usually feel improved and refreshed. These episodes were frequent enough that it was very difficult for him to concentrate and interfered with his ability to do work. Extensive medical work-up yielded no further leads to these mysterious symptoms. On the surface, he is a successful researcher in technology. Having both financial stability as well as the recognition of his colleagues as a promising star in his field, he was, nevertheless, insecure and depressed.

Throughout his childhood, he was generally described as shy and tends to live in his own world. Yet, he was stubborn and outspoken in familiar settings. He did not have friends growing up but instead, spent most of his time with his books and comics. The world of his comic heroes seemed nearly real and tangible to him, the world outside just seemed surreal and incomprehensible. Even the world right outside his bedroom door seemed foreign at times. His father, an engineer, was more adept at the math equations for airplane construction than any casual conversation with a son. Despite such communication and relationship chasm, he had great respect for his father as a person who cherished intellect and logic. They had a simple relationship based on the world of numbers. His mother, a kind, caring and attentive person, has learned to compensate for his interpersonal deficits and comes across as overly caretaking.

In high school, he excelled in math as if following in his father's footsteps but lived a very lonely existence at the periphery of an environment that seemed distant as well as bizarre to him. He felt curious about the social scenes of his teen years but kept a distance and occupied himself with books, comics and math puzzles. Although he loved math and tolerated school, the humanities classes were a nightmare for him. He often failed to see the relevance of topics such as civics, politics and history; creative writings were simply missing assignments for him.

In college, he had no trouble with the select math and physics classes for his majors, once he struggled past the freshman level humanities classes. He still did not make any inroads into the interpersonal arena but had a good mentor who guided him through his studies. Hesitant to enter into the job market after graduation, he decided to work toward graduate degrees. Obtaining his masters and doctorate degrees were simply extensions of his talent. He published some landmark papers and thought that he fell in love with a graduate music student he heard in concert on campus. In his very unique way, he pursued this relationship for a year before accepting the rejection of his overture. At which point, he left academia suddenly and moved to a lonely small town. There, he spent the next few years in self imposed solitude. In retrospect, he described those years, without many of the amenities of modernity, as somehow easy and pleasant without the hustle and bustles of everyday modern society. He supported himself with an occasional odd job and lived off his earlier savings. In most everyway, this would have been an ideal existence but for one thing; he began to experience periods of distress that felt like the pang of existence. His attempts to write and contemplate mathematical enumerations were becoming increasingly difficult and without inspiration; this is coming from someone who has always taken pride in his creativity.

His decision to return to civilization was motivated by the desire to seek help for his perceived physical distress. Upon return to his hometown and becoming reacquainted with the family that he left behind, he got a good job with a technology company that utilized his talents with numbers. He underwent repeated examination by various medical specialists to determine the cause of his physical distress but found himself to be an enigma in the eyes of the experts. He realized that he was different but since he had no explanation as to the source of this difference, he felt defective and inferior. In this self pity, he used his substantial intellect to essentially revamp his whole being and this remaking of himself allowed him entry into the greater society around him but at the cost of having to keep his true self hidden. Through this period of time, he tried everything he could think of to become just like everyone else around him. He tried to be funny, entertaining, helpful, kind, generous and sincere, but all of this just eventually left him feeling very empty and still very lonely.

During this period of time, he met a woman at work and found a thread of connection with her through their mutual needs for each other. She took responsibility for handling the external social aspects of their life together. His job was to be a good provider and a reliable husband and father. As his "episodes" increased, he was no longer able to maintain sufficient concentration for the demanding work at his job, and at home, he was often so irritable that the kids kept a distance. Finally, due to persistent symptoms resembling anxiety and panic, his primary care provider prescribed a selective serotonin reuptake inhibitor (SSRI) type of antidepressant for him. He experienced some initial symptom improvement with decreased irritability and anxiety. Curiously, the SSRI seemed to have helped with affording him greater flexibility in the vicissitude of daily life but his social and interpersonal ability did not improve.

Eventually, his family physician referred him to psychiatric care and there, he was told that he presented with very classic characteristics of Asperger's disorder, consisting of mild autistic like symptoms. He came to embrace this diagnosis following some further research as well as a soul searching of sort and began a journey of discovery about himself. Somewhere between the therapeutic effects of his medication and the new insight about Asperger's disorder, his mysterious "episodes" became less noticeable for a time. He continued to be diligent in pursuing a better understanding about his life long difficulties through psychotherapy and made notable progress. He began to notice the fervor in which his mind raced about the work he is doing. He started to entertain many ideas that intrigued him. He related of feeling more creative in his work than he has ever felt before. Frequently, he felt the difficulty of being able to contain his excitement about an idea or a thought. He extolled of his new found impetus to think more broadly about his work. There were times when his therapist worried that he seemed to be a bit manic in the excited state of his creativity. It was not mania. He explained that he felt a tremendous sense of freedom once he understood the fundamentals of his being. Until this point, he never understood the reasons behind why he felt so differently from others and why he was treated so differently by others; he just thought that it was somehow his fault.

In psychotherapy, he was able to identify a sense of emptiness from time to time in his life. He also recognized that he is prone to be exquisitely sensitive to interpersonal frustrations. He frequently feels that people simply do not like him and do not want to be around him. Possibly due to his own lack of conversational skills as well as his tendency to be an observer rather than a participant in interactions, he would quietly take note of other's seeming lack of interest with great pain. He came to recognize that it is during such times that he is prone to these "episodes" of profound distress. At this point in treatment, he was introduced to DSA.

Through this therapy, he came to be more aware and familiar with the rousing pain of the emptiness within. Recognition of this emotional state means that he can now take full responsibility for all of the feelings that accompanies his daily life, whether it is a positive or negative feeling. He came to realize that happy external events can contribute to even greater sense of fulfillment when his "cup" is already fairly full. Conversely, he also realized that external disappointments can be even more emotionally painful at a time when his "cup" is rather empty already. Following this very critical evaluation, he was less likely to blame the outside world for all of his anger and frustration; he now possessed true insight about the need for the treatment of the self.

As he embraced the use of the 3-steps, he became quite adept at meeting his needs in a socially and treatment congruent manner. Working with his therapist, he indentified appropriate selfobjects with whom he actuated transference reciprocation. Within a short period of time, he was free of the "episodes" and he continued to be creative and productive in his work. He reported of feeling much more fulfilled in his life as a husband and father. In addition, he also expressed feeling that he can continue to be highly creative without the desperate sense that he has to depend on the intensity of the whirlwind of creativity to feel adequate.

Discussion:
The importance of recognizing and accepting the existence of a fluctuating internal emotional state is at the center of the work with DSA. Self psychology suggests the dependent relationship that exists between the self and the object throughout the life cycle. "Proper selfobject experiences favor the structural cohesion and energic vigor of the self; faulty selfobject experiences facilitate the fragmentation and emptiness of the self" (Wolf 1988, p.11). I must comment here that one would certainly expect that selfobject experience has to have an impact on early development, as suggested through object relations hypothesis. Subsequently, any hindrance to good object and self relationship in early life has to create a difficult environment for the proper development of the seat of the self. Whether this hindrance to relationship has its source in the external (environmental), such as abuse or internal (genetics), such as autism, the end result can be quite remarkably similar.

The belief that every human being has the fundamental requirement for selfobject experience is at the cornerstone of our understanding of the pathology of the self. In this regard, the individual with pervasive developmental disorder (PDD) will face exceptional challenge in meeting his selfobject needs. PDD or Asperger's disorder appears to be a good example in helping us to understand the developmental needs of the self. "Lack of social or emotional reciprocity" as described in the DSM IV is the central issue in our concern about the healthy development of the self. This lack of quality reciprocal interpersonal interaction for the infant/toddler with PDD is likely to contribute to the same anger and frustration that a non-PDD counterpart would face when exposed to extreme emotional challenges early in life. In DSA, this developmental aggravation is described as a malformed cup with excessive leakage. If one accepts the existence of original anger, one has also to recognize that this obstacle to normal development exist for all people. As a hurdle to overcome, it has to be successfully traversed by all, regardless of medical disability, neuropsychiatric illness or interpersonal frustrations.

The individual suffering from PDD has to make allowance for a degree of resolution of original anger; to the best of our knowledge today, this is a process that requires adequate selfobject experience. "Gratifying experiences reinforce basic trust, shape the expression of libido, and influence the relative balance of life and death instincts" (Kernberg 1980 p.23). Any hindrance to sufficient reciprocation of mirroring and idealizing transference could result in the pathologic development of the cup. Thus obstructed, the cup takes form incompletely and results in high capacity leakage. In addition, the characteristic of poor interpersonal connectedness is akin to a cloud or filter that reduces a large percentage of the input from selfobjects and all others. Note that this hypothetical filter is likely to obstruct interpersonal and selfobject transference but would not interfere with gratification from rewarding activities and even those from acting out input.

Complications related to his reduced ability to fully benefit from common selfobject interactions can theoretically lower his emotional payoff in working with others in the 3-steps. One may ask if this means that he is less likely to benefit from the work of DSA. To answer this question, one must refer back to the central concept of understanding one's emotional system via the metaphor of the cup. We shall assume that the fundamental structure and operation of the self is identical in all human beings regardless of physical or neurological illness. The natural expectation of such a system is exercised unless the organic component overwhelms the emotional in the case of severe anxiety or neuropsychiatric conditions. The possibility is quite high that the cup of the individual with mild PDD operates under the same rules of development as all others. For the patient to fully understand the self through the various inputs and losses is to evoke his sense of self preservation. Thus is he able to find the motivation to partake in this process of healing.

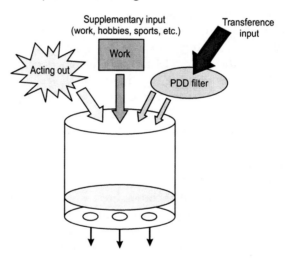

From these remarks, the reader will no doubt sense that this patient's progress in psychotherapy did not amount to true improvement in function until he began to comprehend his internal emotional life and in DSA terms, started to address it through the use of the 3-steps. One of Mark's initial improvements came about through the interruption of his use of the "extremes." As a result of his treatment work, he was improved in his balance of work and life as well as equilibrium between high intensity events and the commonplace events. As he became more cautious about the use of acting out behavior to fill his cup and recognized the limitations of his interpersonal filling of the cup, he was able to focus on rebuilding his fundamental connection with others through the use of the 3-steps. Within the 3-steps, he found the valuable selfobject experience that he needed. This simple strategy in interpersonal connectivity paved the way for the much needed integration of the self. Over the course of treatment, he should hopefully experience increasing sense of self contentment, better self-esteem, improved interpersonal confidence and decreased anxiety.

Similar to the case of the patient with anxiety disorder, the individual with PDD faces the challenge of obtaining sufficient content for a leaky cup. He starts with difficulties in the interpersonal arena, which is one of the key deficits of PDD relating to his lack of reciprocal interpersonal interactions. Even with the appearance of having people around him, he has insufficient quality of connectedness to make efficient use of these relationships. Positive transference, that warm sense of attunement resulting in a bidirectional feeding of the cup is only a vestige of its potential. He is likely to rely on just a few people in his life who are exceptionally committed to him. However, even the most committed individuals in his life may have difficulty in providing adequate transference input. Consequently, he has to cope with a chronically lower level of content in his cup and having to adjust to this condition.

PDD is like a filter over his cup that can potentially reduce the amount of available input. When he reaches the pre-teen and teen years, a time when many individuals start to awaken to a discriminate age in which the cup now demands differently, he began to sense an increasing difficulty in getting the cup filled. A hypothetical model for the experiences of the extreme emptiness in this individual with PDD perhaps resides in his very specialized neurological makeup and perceived as a matter of norm. Alternatively, it may be his never having experienced an internal emotional world any differently that shapes the interpretation of his sense of emptiness. Stated another way, the level of fluctuation of his cup is likely narrow and this is his relative reality. It is my clinical experience that many individuals suffering from PDD also endure the pain of emptiness.

One would anticipate that the slightest trouble in the interpersonal arena can set off a chain of negative events for this individual. When others pull back in their input into his cup, in a classically borderline fashion, he is likely to experience the emptiness of the cup as a sense of the "bad" self. When the self is perceived as "bad", projection takes place to eject the all-bad, aggressive self and object images. This then results in his experiencing the selfobjects as dangerous or aggressive, while the object experiences a sense of feeling aggressive toward the patient. Unless the selfobject figure is able to understand this dynamic, he or she will be less inclined to provide reciprocal transference input into this patient's cup. Given that this patient with PDD suffers from chronic lower levels in the cup to begin with, once projective identification takes place, his cup will now easily run dry.

In considering the substantial challenge facing the individual with neuropsychiatric conditions, one is unlikely to dispute the humanistic needs for object relatedness, the usage of the 3-steps serves to simplify a treatment plan and propose an achievable method of relating to this patient. Beyond the fundamental understanding of this work, the 3-steps can be implemented in a highly structured and scripted fashion or if feasible, carried out in a general pattern with daily living. Either way, these steps then form the groundwork for the connectivity that allows for introjections of selfobject representations; this makes possible the repair of the leakage.

DSA for Daily Life

On a less austere note, DSA is a way of life. Being aware of the developmental needs of the self is valuable whether the issue is related to parenting, educational pursuit, professional productivity, relationship satisfaction, leisure quest or retirement. The central concept of emphasizing the 3-steps in DSA lends itself to easy implementation in the structures of daily activities. As has been discussed earlier, life is essentially based on the immutable concept of person, place and time; a natural extension of this simple rule is the 3-steps. I believe that these precepts are an integral part of everyday life and growth in the lives of most people. Hence, healthy development in general can be achieved without intense therapeutic intervention.

Alternately, some individuals can be identified as being more at risk of developing greater issues related to the self. Pediatricians, parents and therapists frequently have questions regarding the prognosis of a child with behavioral or temperamental concerns. These could be youngsters with a shy and anxious temperament. Some of them could simply be quiet and introverted in nature; others are rambunctious and spirited in nature. One child could be overly cautious and another could be exceedingly adventurous. Such temperaments or behavior may not necessarily bring about development of character pathology, but for some, these types of behaviors likely contribute to frustrations in development and interfere with the growth of the self. Through temperament or behavior, some of these individuals may face challenges in interpersonal connection with important selfobjects. If appropriately identified, such individuals may benefit from earlier interventions in therapy, at home and in school.

In the case of an individual who may be rather reserved and introverted, possibly described as shy, the challenge to the parent and the teacher is often the decision of whether to intervene or not. If this is the natural disposition of this individual, would he require any special attention regarding this temperament? The reality that faces this individual can be that of a debilitating disability in a complex world that favors people who are charismatic and forward. In our culture, many parents are quite alarmed by the quiet and shy offspring. Some parents look upon such a child with dismay while others encourage their child to be aggressive and rambunctious. Taking the opposite notion to "boys will be boys", the expectation becomes, "boys should be boys." Often, this misguided attempt to shape a child without the awareness for supporting the true self of the child can result in psychopathology.

The 3-steps, as naturally encountered in daily life, can be instrumental in good parenting. Often parents instinctively offer these steps to the child in their routine interpersonal interactions since infancy. The father who praised his son for containing his anger after he was ridiculed by a peer at school is teaching his child about the 3-steps. The boy refrained from acting out in retaliation and managed to focus on the work of school by putting in some extra effort to master a particular set of information in his science class; he has essentially allowed time to pass while taking ownership for his excellent work in school that day. Upon return home, he is familiar with the importance of relating his feelings to someone meaningful to him. In so doing, his father realized that his son has handled the situation in a responsible manner and can simply listen or perhaps, offer some mature advice. A mother working in the garden asked her 7 year old daughter to find something to do for herself while she finishes her planting. On conclusion of her work, the mother approached the child and praised her for handling her feelings of boredom and her attempt to find something productive to do while waiting for her mother. Her mother then rewards her by lavishing some well deserved attention for a successful attempt to soothe herself.

Recapitulation and Conclusion

It could be said that the helping professionals are not always helpful. It could also be said that the patient is not always seeking to get better. Stories abound with individuals who enter into treatment with all of the intentions of getting help only to frustrate their therapist with poor compliance. It must be understood that, regardless of the modern emphasis on individual responsibility, the patient's lack of insight is generally not to be blamed for his poor treatment compliance. Most patients do not have a clear idea of what treatment is all about and what will be expected of him in treatment. He may come into treatment to feel better but not necessarily to get better. The therapist, generally someone who wants to help and is actually under a great deal of pressure to produce some results, can easily become an accomplice in the patient's quest to feel better and therefore, achieve, at best, status quo.

In this work, I have emphasized the importance of differentiating between just feeling better and that of getting better. For many suffering individuals who enter into psychiatric treatment, the ability to retain the good feelings from meaningful interactions is lacking. Insight development is of course the tenet of good psychotherapy, but the achievement of insight about the powerful drive of emptiness and defenses of projective identification and splitting is unfortunately a rarity in psychotherapy patients. Lack of insight about the representational world of the self and the object contributes to a disproportionate amount of preventable human suffering.

DSA makes use of a simplified model of pathology to convey the dynamics of complex defense mechanisms. It is the analogy of pointing out to someone that, when there is a large puddle of oil underneath your car, it is not wise to attempt to start this car. Without making a repair to the leakage, the engine will be unable to run for long and adding oil to it will only prolong its misery and would not solve any problems. One has to accept the inconvenience of not being able to drive the car in order to begin the process of making plans for repair of the car. Furthermore, when one steps out of the car to find the surrounding air chokingly acrid (hint: projective identification), it is not the fault of others when it originates from one's own car.

·X·
Pharmacotherapy in Borderline Conditions

"If I had a pill... for every time that I said I wish...
I would have cured all of the world's ills."

–Anonymous

Adjunctive Role of Medications

A comprehensive discussion of medication treatment of borderline personality disorder is not within the scope of this work. However, given the complexity and severity of borderline conditions, it is crucial to plan for the adjunctive use of psychopharmacology in stabilization as well as ongoing care. Although a review of articles published before 2003 found limited evidence supporting any agent or class of drugs for the treatment of BPD, it does suggest that antidepressants, antipsychotics and mood stabilizers may all be useful in certain patients (Binks 2006). There have been some studies suggesting that combination of medication treatment with some form of therapy, in this case dialectical behavior therapy, constitute effective treatment of BPD (Soler 2005).

In determining a medication approach to the treatment of BPD, one has to bear in mind our earlier discussions regarding the broad expanse of the borderline condition. In the view I have propounded through DSA, borderline characteristics can be conceived as a manifestation of deeper underlying psychopathology of the self; a pathology that, to a degree, exists in each and every person. Therefore, this perspective of the pathology of the self is going to have a strong bearing on how psychopharmacology is utilized in the treatment of borderline personality and related disorders. Additionally, understanding emptiness as the core pathology of BPD means that a realistic comprehension of the treatment of a certain aversive inner tension has to be taken into consideration.

It should be observed that, with the ever expanding gamut of psychotropic medications available today, pharmacologic treatments have become more therapeutic as well as increasingly more complex. Many patients are exposed to a multitude of medications with ever more confounding side effect profile from drug interactions. To be fair, the majority of psychiatric providers do due diligence in introducing patients to the safest and most efficacious set of medications for the symptoms at hand. However, it is still quite common for many patients to experience persistent symptoms despite complex and long term medication trials. The really surprising answer to this common dilemma may actually reside in understanding the pathology of the self.

To be frustrated by what appear to be fairly straight forward cases of depression is not uncommon in the chronicles of psychiatry and applies to many other conditions in the field. Encouraged by the myriad of drug studies touting the ever expanding possibilities for the use of each drug, most providers feel compelled to explore new territories of pharmacotherapy for their treatment resistant patients. The consequence of this trend is many fold. Most obviously, patients are perhaps exposed to unnecessary trials of medications. Secondly, doctors and patients lose faith in what previously were highly respected medications for specific purposes. The problem may not be a lack of efficacy on the part of the medication; the issue could well be a lack of recognition of the fundamental pathology of the self beyond the superficial presentation of the symptoms such as depression. In accordance with the particular nature of antidepressants, its benefits can easily be overshadowed by aspects of borderline pathology.

The role of medication stabilization hinges on our understanding of the nature of emotional dysregulation and symptoms that can contribute to further exacerbation. Additionally, the borderline patient's tendency toward self-mutilation and suicidality will account for much of the planning in medication use. It is commonly recognized that the disorder of the self does not fully respond to existing pharmacological means. With current pharmacological armament, we have to accept the limitations of medications and understand that it is symptom management that is at the core of our use of medications in the treatment of BPD. Symptom management is the basis of treatment in any psychiatric disorder today. It is generally accepted that medications help in assisting a patient to "stabilize" sufficiently to be able to take on the work of psychotherapy.

Although with limitations, pharmacotherapy can be an indispensable part of treatment for most individuals with severe pathology of the self. Borderline personality disorder is characterized by pervasive psychopathology of affective regulation, impulse control and aggression (Zanarini 2003). The severity of emotional dysregulation of the borderline patient can give rise to further suffering by way of extreme anxiety, irritability, agitation, as well as a certain amorphous unease that resides somewhere between panic and extreme boredom. In certain cases, as we have discussed in case 9.5, the symptoms of borderline condition results in the manifestation of compulsions; such symptoms of obsessions and compulsions can often meet criteria for obsessive compulsive disorder as described in the DSM IV. In such a case, pharmacologic intervention should play an integral role without overt complexity.

The borderline patient's anxiety and depressive symptoms will often meet criteria for disorders in the DSM IV. Although, most commonly, these symptoms appears to have a long term, chronic characteristic with a waxing and waning course. These patients will often describe experiencing "mood swings", a description their families will readily concur. On closer examination, the upper end of these moods do not usually meet strict criteria for mania, and the lower end of these moods do not usually meet strict criteria for major depression. From an object relations perspective, these moods often coincide with cohesion and fragmentation of the self. In the language of DSA, cohesion is maintained when the cup is reasonably full, and fragmentation occurs when the cup is rather empty as a result of interpersonal ineffectiveness or inability to self soothe.

Medication usage is strictly about symptom management. On the contrary, many patients go about taking their medications as if it was the mainstay of their treatment. Often, family members also look upon medications with false hope. No less often, the psychiatric provider conveys the false impression of pharmacologic solution through the fervent trials of a cornucopia of drugs. Unfortunately, iatrogenic complications can worsen an already complex clinical picture. Both the borderline patient and the psychiatric provider need to accept the limitations of pharmacology through judicious use of medications in order to truly benefit from this branch of psychiatric treatment. An insightful patient once suggested that successful medication usage conveys the metaphor of placing some rocks inside of the cup so that, despite the leakiness of the container, there can still be the appearance of some fullness as the rocks takes up space to raise the level. He recognized that authentic repair of the emotional leakage will still require earnest psychotherapy.

Risks and Benefits

Treatment of borderline patients is almost always a tenuous undertaking. As discussed in chapter one, the rate of suicide attempts by individuals suffering from the borderline condition is such that inaction is not acceptable. Without enrollment in effective treatment, which should generally include both psychotherapy and pharmacotherapy, the risk of death or severe injury will be high. Moreover, even for a borderline patient in treatment with medication and psychotherapy, the risk of death can still be quite high and the complications of medication, another concern.

In addition, there is the distinct possibility that medication side effects can contribute to exacerbation of the patient's sense of emotional dysregulation. Often, the central nervous system and autonomic nervous system side effects can bring about palpitation, anxiety, sedation, tiredness, mental dullness and dis-connectedness that can heighten the borderline's sense of emotional emptiness. Periodically, a patient on a psychotropic medication will comment about feeling that his medications seem to cause him to feel "numb." One such patient on an antidepressant attributed her suicide attempt to the taking of an antidepressant she was taking. She described the feeling as neither a sadness nor happiness but it was this aversive tension that caused her to act impulsively. As in most cases, her clinical history suggests the great possibility that her "numbness" was a preexisting condition that has already contributed to frequent acting out behaviors. It is for these reasons that such risks should be made clear to the patient and his or her family before the task of treatment should begin.

"Most studies show a positive effect of medication on at least some mea-sures of borderline psychopathology. The most consistent results have been improvements in affective dysregulation and impulsive aggression" (Zanarini, 2004). Medication treatment itself has certain risks. The psychiatric provider should be mindful of the frequency in which prescribed medications are utilized in suicide attempts. However, pharmacologic treatment can be an important cornerstone to the stabilization process and long term treatment outcome for a variety of pathology of the self. In this regard, DSA recognizes the pathology of the self as ranging from mild to acute severity and pharmacologic management has to be titrated to each individual. In addition to targeting medication treat-ment toward "affective dysregulation and impulsive aggression", selection of medication strategy should take into consideration the total symptom picture presented by each patient. Very often, symptoms of anxiety, depression, obses-sive compulsion, post traumatic stress, sleep difficulties, appetite irregularities, manic episodes and psychosis have to be addressed.

Pharmacologic Strategies

By our definition of the borderline condition, as broad spectrum pathology of the self, the role for medication involvement actually becomes quite broad as well. This means that medication usage is likely part of the majority of patients undergoing treatment using DSA. For medication to enhance and not detract from treatment, the provider must be mindful of the borderline's tendency of worsening his experience of emptiness by interpreting medication side effects as a part of his ongoing internal experience. Given the developmental com-plexities of the self and the varied descriptions for the symptoms of emptiness, it is not surprising that even drowsiness and hunger can potentially enhance the pain of fragmentation. Furthermore, borderline patients often request ever more psychotropic medications to help distant themselves from the pain of emptiness. One has to balance what is adequate symptom relief from that of excessive reliance on medications.

Pertaining to affective dysregulation in patients with BPD, an algorithm based on current clinical literature recommended by the International Psychopharmacology Algorithm Project (Jobson 1995) suggest starting with a selective serotonin reuptake inhibitor (SSRI) or related antidepressant and if lacking efficacy, try another SSRI or related antidepressant. Following the second attempt with an SSRI, the addition of a low dose neuroleptic for symptoms of anger or add clonazepam, if symptoms lean more toward anxiety, to enhance efficacy. It then suggests a switch to monoamine oxidase inhibitor (MAOI) as the next step and if still lacking in efficacy, switch to or add lithium, carbamazepine or valproate. For impulsive-behavioral dyscontrol symptoms, the algorithm starts with an SSRI and low dose neuroleptic is added after which lithium or MAOI can be added or switched to; with further lack of efficacy, atypical neuroleptic can then be added. In this report, treatment for symptoms of paranoia, depersonalization, referential thinking and hallucination-like symptoms starts with low dose and then higher doses of neuroleptics followed by SSRI or MAOI. Authors of this report emphasized that there are no empirical trials of the complete algorithm and recommendations may not be applicable to all patients.

Benzodiazepines

Although benzodiazepines can be effectively used in the management of anxiety with the borderline patient, caution should be taken regarding the optimal use of such an approach. As a class of medications, benzodiazepines are also highly sedating and this can be both beneficial as well as detrimental in its use. Many individuals taking a benzodiazepine mistakenly accept the sedation as part of the efficacy of the medication's anti-anxiety effect. As a result, these patients continuously request a higher dose as sedation is reduced due to physiological tolerance. Very soon, the patient finds himself in a pattern of addiction. Hence, it is critical to make certain that the patient comprehends the need to separate the anti-anxiety effect from the sedation of the benzodiazepines.

Some patients with chronic sleep challenges may be prescribed long acting benzodiazepines. The differential diagnosis of insomnia can be many and the suffering immense. Whether dealing with a sleep disorder or one of many psychiatric conditions conducive to disturbance in sleep, many patients try multiple sleep aids without consistent benefit. At times, benzodiazepines can be helpful as an aid for sleep but this use has severe limitations due to the propensity for physiological tolerance and the tendency for addiction. One young woman with persistent initial insomnia was tried on various medications for sleep including a non-benzodiazepine short-acting hypnotic (an imidazopyridine) to no avail. Eventually, it became clear through her therapy work that her pervasive sense of loneliness and emptiness is likely worse at bedtime and she needed more medications at such moments to escape this pain at the end of the day.

The use of benzodiazepines rarely reduces the aggressive acting out behaviors of the borderline patient and could potentiate disinhibition in an individual already prone to impulse. One also has to be concerned about the excessive sedation in a person already complaining of numbness and lack of appropriate experiencing of life. Furthermore, the short half-life of benzodiazepines raise concerns regarding the potential of developing withdraws. Here again, physiological withdrawal is a complex set of symptoms that may have an emotional component. This combination of symptoms can bring about an unpleasant physical experience as well as possibly exacerbating the borderline patient's feelings of emotional dysregulation.

Conventional wisdom regarding benzodiazepine would dictate its use in a precise and limited fashion. Use of klonazepam takes advantage of its long half-life in order to reduce the potential for addiction by avoiding the frequency in which another dose has to be given to maintain continuing efficacy. This would also discourage the patient from continuingly trying to anticipate the timing of the next dose. The use of a mid-range anti-anxiety agent such as alprazolam can be therapeutic if the patient is educated about its potential problems and the proper therapeutic strategy. Lorazepam, a very short acting agent has therapeutic uses in acute, short term intervention of a highly agitated individual in a closely monitored environment.

Foregoing remarks about benzodiazepines should not preclude this class of medications from the treatment plans for the borderline patient. Short term use of these agents following a stressful life event to provide rapid relief run little risk of dependence and withdrawal while extended use of greater than 4 to 6 months for general anxiety disorder, panic disorder or anxiety associated with depression increases the risks of dependence and withdrawal greatly. Such treatments should best consider the other available therapeutic interventions. Antidepressants are now considered the first-line treatments for both depression and anxiety disorders (Stahl 2000, p.305-323). However, there are schools of thoughts in which benzodiazepine can be safely used in a carefully selected and well educated patient to treat a limited set of symptoms. A properly educated patient who is adequately dosed on a select benzodiazepine could have his anxiety symptoms well managed while maintaining a consistent dose over an extended period of time without the risk of addiction. This degree of medication consistency allows the patient to become well acquainted with any side effects that may accompany his medications and recognize them as separate from his core symptoms of emptiness. He now knows that drowsiness is not a part of the desired effect of this medication and therefore, not prone to ask for an increasingly higher dose to maintain a degree of sedation. He will also become familiar with the anti-anxiety effect of his medication and accept the limit of this class of anxiolytics.

Antidepressants

Insecure attachment (Kenny 1993), dysfunctional family patterns (Rapee 1997), stress (Compass 1994), neuroticism as a heritable trait (Costa 1980, Larson 1992, Levenson 1988) have all shown empirical evidence of contributing to depression. Drawing upon our collective awareness suggesting that all of the above factors also underlie the hypothesis of early developmental hurt contributing to the formation of character pathology; now, this may inform us of the pervasiveness of depression in individuals suffering emptiness, including the borderline patients. It has been shown that combination treatment using medication and psychotherapy was more effective than psychotherapy alone in recurrent or severe major depressive disorder (Thase et al. 1997).

Many patients undergo treatment with antidepressants without adequate response or recovery. Often, individuals with convincing neurovegetative symptoms and signs of depression are treated on a series of antidepressants with minimal improvement. Complete symptomatic remission is difficult; the existence of residual symptoms, especially when the first episode occurs in adolescence, is the best predictor of relapse or reoccurrence (Keller 2003). It is assumed that individual biological differences account for this variability. There is accumulating evidence that drug efficacy of antidepressants results from the combined effects of genetics and single nucleotide polymorphism to explain the variability of antidepressant effect in the population as well as sex differences in drug response (Serretti 2004; Lin 2006). Nevertheless, there may be another very notable reason for the existence of so many non-responders to conventional antidepressant treatment. Individuals suffering from severe pathology of the self are unlikely to fare well on just antidepressant treatment alone. It is important for the psychiatric provider to search vigorously for any underlying pathology of the self when confronted with the frustration of a patient who is not readily responding to pharmacologic treatment.

In the pharmacological armament, antidepressants play an important role in the treatment of depression and anxiety spectrum of disorders. It is the preferred class of medications for generalized anxiety disorder, panic disorder and obsessive compulsive disorder. Antidepressants are selectively used in the treatment of depressive symptoms in bipolar disorder. It is generally agreed that antidepressants should only be used in combination with a mood stabilizer for the treatment of bipolar depression (Thase 2003). Anecdotally, small doses of a selective serotonin reuptake inhibitor (SSRI) are also used to bring about greater flexibility and decreased perseveration in individuals with PDD, as discussed in an earlier chapter, a neuropsychiatric condition likely to contribute to borderline pathology.

Antidepressants include the tricyclic antidepressants (TCAs), monoamine oxidase inhibitors (MAOIs), selective serotonin reuptake inhibitors (SSRIs), selective serotonin and noradrenaline reuptake inhibitors (SNRIs) and the novel compound, bupropion, which acts by blocking noradrenergic and dopamine reuptake. Whether used as monotherapy or in conjunction with antipsychotic medications or mood stabilizers, antidepressant medications often play a pivotal role in treatment of borderline symptoms. In a study of women with BPD, it was found that fluvoxamine significantly reduced mood lability but no other symptoms (Rinne 2002) while a review turned up that fluoxetine was superior to placebo at controlling anger and MAOIs were better at reducing hostility (Binks 2006).

Symptoms of mood disorders can often be difficult to distinguish from symptoms of BPD. Treatment resistant depression may have distinct biological basis but the clinician should be mindful of the impact of the pathology of the self. For an elegant discussion of drug combinations for treatment resistant depression, I would urge the reader to peruse "Essential psychopharmacology" by Stahl (2000). There has been some evidence that combination of antipsychotic medications with antidepressant medications can be useful in treatment-refractory depression (Shelton et al. 2001). In a review of papers, authors in one study found that lithium augmentation is the best-supported strategy for treatment-resistant depression (Barowsky, Schwartz 2006).

Mood Stabilizers

Since the advent of lithium as a mood stabilizer, a number of other classes of medications have been found to have mood stabilizing effects; notably, the anticonvulsant and antipsychotic classes of medications. These medications are of particular interest to the clinician working with the borderline patient because of their particularly robust effects in clinical care. The severity of affective dysregulation, impulse control, aggression and disruption in interpersonal relationships are frequently associated with suicidal behaviors. In meta-analysis of suicide risk, lithium is the only pharmacologic intervention that shows consistent anti-suicidal effects (Tondo et al. 2001a, 2001b). A related meta-analysis suggest that lithium has antisuicidal effects in recurrent major depressive disorder similar in magnitude to that found in bipolar disorder (Guzzetta 2007).

Thus it is, lithium, valproic acid, carbamazepine, oxcarbazepine, lamotrigine and topiramate are the generally recognized mood stabilizers utilized today. In most cases, psychiatrists select the medication according to the patient's clinical profile as well as side effect profile of the drug. In a placebo controlled study, lamotrigine reduced aggression in women with BPD (Tritt 2005). Similarly, topiramate also was shown to reduce aggression in female (Nickel 2004) as well as male borderline patients (Nickel 2005) in which further improvement took place at 18 month, beyond the initial 8-week acute treatment evaluation (Nickel 2007). In another study, topiramate appeared to improve interpersonal sensitivity, anxiety, hostility, somatization and phobic anxiety in borderline women (Loew 2006). Interestingly, topiramate has been used in the treatment of sexual addiction, eating disorders, pathologic gambling, alcohol addiction and kleptomania (Shiah 2006), (Marazziti 2006), (Khazaal 2006). Is this not really about the treatment of an aversive inner tension? Further studies regarding the connection between medications and the treatment of emptiness would be warranted.

Antipsychotics

A review of pharmacotherapy for BPD found the most commonly use intervention was antipsychotic medications (Binks 2006). These authors felt that antipsychotic drug therapy for BPD is not based on good evidence but it may be helpful and there is not evidence it is harmful. A 2004 review of literature found atypical antipsychotics reduced a wide range of symptoms and improved psychosocial functions although changes in aggression, anxiety and depression were not consistent across studies (Zanarini). Nevertheless, a 2006 study with aripiprazole found significant improvement than did placebo on obsessive-compulsive, insecurity in social contacts, depression, anxiety, hostility, phobic anxiety, paranoid thinking and psychoticism scales (Marius). Olanzapine has also shown statistical significance in improvement of depression, anxiety and impulsivity/aggressive behavior in BPD (Joaquim 2005).

Although dysfunction of serotonergic and dopaminergic systems have been implicated in the pathology of BPD (Friedel 2004) (Hansenne 2002), the clinical applications of these theories to patient care have not consistently brought about notable improvements in patients suffering from severe emptiness. It is possible that improvements in impulsivity and hostility do not generally contribute to easing of the aversive inner tension of emptiness.

Attempting treatment with an antipsychotic medication may be a sensible tactic but most clinicians are quite aware of the need for additional assistance to these patients. Many of the recent studies in drug treatment of BPD included patients enrolled in some form of psychotherapy. Treatment of the pathology of the self is an elephantine endeavor, what seems to work in a study does not always translate to good result in general patient care. From looking at the available results of recent drug studies, one would likely make the conclusion that antipsychotic medications can play an important role in the treatment of BPD but the clinician must balance the risk and benefit of a class of medications with notable side effects.

Other Considerations

Some interesting treatments for BPD are coming from less commonly considered class of medications as well as non-traditional compounds. Omega-3 fatty acid has shown promise in treating women with BPD (Zanarini 2003). This is supported by a preliminary study suggesting that omega-3 fatty acid improved antidepressant response in a small group of patients (Su 2003). Based on indirect evidence supporting increased noradrenergic activity in patients with BPD (Southwick 1990), one research group looked into the use of clonidine in a sample of female inpatients already enrolled in dialectical behavior therapy (Philipsen 2004). Patients in this study experienced a significant decrease in aversive inner tension, self-injurious urges, dissociative symptoms and suicidal ideation.

Summary

The pharmacologic strategies discussed here focuses primarily on the more unique symptoms often encountered by the borderline individual. Many patients expound on the difference between the symptoms of mood disorder from that of the aversive inner tension or emptiness within. Psychological emptiness is difficult to portray and even more difficult to study; most pharmacological studies have focused on symptoms such as interpersonal sensitivity, anxiety and hostility but it is questionable whether these symptoms represent the treatment of emptiness. However, intense pharmacologic management of depression, mania, obsessive compulsions, anxiety and so fourth should take place in parallel with serious psychotherapeutic work. Hence, a familiarity with the broad expanse of literature in this regard is important for the clinician working with this challenging segment of patients.

Many who seek mental health treatment are vaguely aware of their inner sense of feeling unauthentic in their everyday self. When one feels compelled to act bravely, focusing on physical illness to garner care, forcing a smile in order to feel deserving of love, will inevitably feel empty and false. While feeling emotionally empty, the prospect of a medicine that could make you feel upbeat and more cheerful seems even more insulting than to just wallow in the pain. Perhaps, many who suffers from the psychological pain of emptiness realize that this distress within is more than a sadness, anhedonia or irritability; thus, the idea of taking a medicine to treat depression seems somehow incongruent and particularly invalidating. Discussion of pharmacologic treatment with the borderline patient is a delicate matter requiring that the psychiatrist demonstrates sensitivity and understanding of emotional emptiness.

REFERENCES

Alhanati S (2002) Primitive Mental States, Volume 2 Psychobiological and psychoanalytic perspectives on early trauma and personality development. Karnac Books, New York, p. 9, 11-12.

Als H, Tronick E, Lester B, Brazelton TB (1977) The Brazelton Neonatal Behavioral Assessment Scale. Journal of Abnormal Child Psychology, 5:215-231.

Anckarsäter H, Stahlberg O, Hakansson C, Jutblad SB, Niklasson L, Nydén A, Wentz E, Westergren S, Cloninger CR, Gillberg C, Rastam M (2006) The impact of ADHD and autism spectrum disorders on temperament, character, and personality development. Americacan Journal of Psychiatry, Jul 163:1239-1244.

Baker HA, Baker MN (1987) Heinz Kohut's self psychology: an overview. Am J Psychiatry, 144:1-9.

Barowsky J, Schwartz T (2006) An evidence-based approach to augmentation and combination strategies for treatment-resistant depression.Psychiatry, (July):42-61.

Basch MF (1980) Doing psychotherapy. Basic Book Inc., New York, p.45.

Bazanis E, Rogers RD, Dowson JH, Taylor P, Meux C, Staley C, Nevinson-Andrews D, Taylor C, Robbins TW, Sahakian BJ (2002) Neurocognitive deficits in decision-making and planning of patients with DSM-III-R borderline personality disorder. Psychol Med, 32:1395-1405.

Beck AT (1976) Cognitive Therapy and the Emotional Disorders. New York, International Universities Press.

Beck AT, Rush AJ, Shaw BF, et al. (1979) Cognitive Therapy of Depression. Guilford, New York.

Beck AT, Freeman A (1990) Cognitive Therapy of Personality Disorder. Guilford, New York.

Beck AT, Rush AJ (1992) Cognitive therapy, in Comprehensive Textbook of Psychiatry. 6th Edition, Edited by Kaplan HI, Sadock BJ: Williams & Wilkins, Baltimore MD, pp 1847-1857.

Binks C, Fenton M, McCarthy L, Lee T, et al. (2006) Pharmacological interventions for people with borderline personality disorder. The Cochrane Database of Systematic Reviews, Issue 1. Art. No. CD005653.

Black DW, Blum N, Pfohl B et al. (2004) Suicidal behavior in borderline personality disorder: prevalence, risk factors, prediction and prevention. J Personal Disord, 18(3):226-239.

Blehar MC, Oren DA (1995) Women's increased vulnerability to mood disorders: integrating psychobiology and epidemiology. Depression, 3:3-12.

Brand EF, King CA, Olson E, et al. (1996) Depressed adolescents with a history of sexual abuse: diagnostic comorbidity and suicidality. J Am Acad Child Adolesc Psychiatry, 35:34-41.

Brenner C (1979) Working alliance, therapeutic alliance, and transference. Journal of the American Psychoanalytic Association 27:137-158.

Brent DA, Mann JJ (2005) Family genetic studies, suicide, and suicidal behavior. Am J Med Genet C Semin Med Genet, 133(1):13-24.

Brodsky BS, Kevin KM, Ellis SP, et al. (1997) Characteristics of borderline personality disorder associated with suicidal behavior. Am J Psychiatry, 154(12), 1715-1719.

Bromfield R (1992) Playing for real- The world of a child therapist. Penguin Books, New York, p.77, 99.

References

Burgess JW (1992) Neurocognitive impairment in dramatic personalities: histrionic, narcissistic, borderline, and antisocial disorders. Psychiatry Res, 42:283-290.

Carpy DV (1989) Tolerating the countertransference: a mutative process. International Journal of Psycho-Analysis, 70: 293.

Cashdan S (1988) Object relations therapy, using the relationship. W.W. Norton & Company, New York, pp.6, 41, 52, 55, 71, 121.

Cicchetti D (1987) Developmental psychopathology in infancy: Illustration from the study of maltreated youngsters. Journal of Consulting and Clinical Psychology, 55: 837-845.

Clarkin JF, Levy KN, Lenzenweger MF, Kernberg OF (2007) Evaluating three treatments for borderline personality disorder: A multiwave study. Am J Psychiatry, 164:922-928.

Compass BE, Grant KE, Ey S (1994) Psychosocial stress and child and adolescent depression: Can we be more specific? In W.M. Reynolds & H.F. Johnston (Eds), Handbook of depression in children and adolescents. Plenum Press, New York, pp.509-523.

Conger RD, Neppl T, Kim KJ, et al. (2003) Angry and aggressive behavior across three generations: a prospective, longitudinal study of parents and children. J Abnorm Child Psychology, 31:143-160.

Conrad M, Hammen C (1989) Role of maternal depression in perceptions of child maladjustment. J Consult Clin Psychol, 57:663-667.

Costa PT, McCrae RR (1980) Influence of extraversion and neuroticism on subjective wellbeing: Happy and unhappy people. Journal of Personality and Social Psychology, 38,668-678.

Dinkmeyer D, McKay GD (1989) The parent's handbook-Systematic training for effective parenting (STEP) American guidance services, Inc., p.38.

Dinn WM, Harris CL (2000) Neurocognitive function in antisocial personality disorder. Psychiatry Res, 97:173-190.

Doucet P (1992) The analyst's transference imagery. International Journal of Psycho-Analysis, 73: 657

Downey G, Coyne JC (1990) Children of depressed parents: an integrative review. Psychol Bull, 108(1):50-76.

Dozier M, Bick J (2007) Changing caregivers: coping with early adversity. Psychiatric Annals, 37(6):411-415.

Diagnostic and Statistical Manual of Mental Disorders, 4th edition TR (2000) American Psychiatric Association, Washington, DC.

Drevets WC (1999) Prefrontal cortical amygdalar metabolism in major depression. Ann N Y Acad Sci, 877:614-637.

Ellman SJ (1991) Freud's technique papers-a contemporary perspective. Jason Aronson Inc., New Jersey, p.86, 90.

Elson M (1987) The Kohut seminars: On self psychology and psychotherapy with adolescents and young adults. Norton, New York, p.82.

Erikson EH (1950) Childhood and society. Norton, New York, p.68, 211, 218.

Erikson EH (1968) Identity, youth and crisis. Norton, New York, p. 91, 97, 109.

Favaro A, Ferrara S, Santonastaso P (2007) Self-injurious behavior in a community sample of young women: Relationship with childhood abuse and other types of self-damaging behaviors. J Clin Psychiatry, 68: 122-131.

Fine MA, Sansone RA (1990) Dilemmas in the management of suicidal behavior in individuals with borderline personality disorder. American Journal of Psychotherapy, 44:160-171.

Fischer M, Barkley RA, Smallish L, Fletcher K (2002) Young adult follow-up of hyperactive children: self-reported psychiatric disorders, comorbidity, and the role of childhood conduct problems and teen CD. J Abnorm Child Psychol, 30:463-475.

Freud S (1916 / 1917) Introductory lectures on psycho-analysis. Standard Edition 15 /16.

Freud S (1920) Beyond the pleasure principle. Standard Edition 18: 3-64.

Friedel RO (2004) Dopamine dysfunction in borderline personality disorder: a hypothesis. Neuropsychopharmacology, 29:1029-1039.

Gabbard G (1990) Psychodynamic psychiatry in clinical practice. American Psychiatric Press, Inc. Washington, DC, pp.33-35.

Goldstein RB, Black DW, Nasrallah A, et al. (1991) The prediction of suicide: sensitivity, specificity, and predictive value of a multivariate model applied to suicide among 1906 patients with affective disorders. Archives of General Psychiatry, 48:418-422.

Gordon M (1977) Primary group differentiation in urban Ireland. Social Forces, Vol. 55, March. pp.743-752.

Gordon M (1978) The American Family: past, present and future. Random House, New York, NY, p.41

Gore S, Aseltine RH, Colten ME (1993) Gender, social-relational involvement and depression. Journal of Research on Adolescents, 3: 101-125.

Gould MS, Fisher P, Parides M, et al. (1996) Psychosocial risk factors of child and adolescent complete suicide. Arch Gen Psychiatry, 53:1155-1162.

Grube GMA (1974) Plato's Republic. Hackett Publishing Company, Inc. Indianapolis, Indiana, p.9.

Gunderson JG, Weinberg I, Daversa MT, Kueppenbender KD, Zanarini MC   et al. (2006) Descriptive and longitudinal observations on the relationship of borderline personality disorder and bipolar disorder. Am J Psychiatry, 163:1173-1178.

Guzzetta F, Tondo L, Centorino F, Baldessarini RJ (2007) Lithium treatment   reduces suicide risk in recurrent major depressive disorder. J Clin Psychiatry, 68:380-383.

Hansenne M, Pitchot W, Pinto E, Reggers J, Scantamburlo G, Fuchs S, Pirard S, Ansseau M (2002) 5-HT1A dysfunction in borderline personality disorder. Psychol Med, 32:935-941.

Havens L (1979) Explorations in the uses of language in psychotherapy: complex empathic statements. Psychiatry, 42:40-48.

Hawton K, Harris L (2007) Deliberate self-harm in young people: Characteristics and subsequent mortality in a 20-year cohort of patients presenting to hospital. J Clin Psychiatry, 68:1574-1583.

Hayward M et al. (2006) Personality disorder and unmet needs among psychiatric inpatients. Psychiatric Services, 57:538-543.

Heinrichs M, Wagner D, Schoch W, Soravia L, Hellhammer D, Ehlert U (2005) Predicting posttraumatic stress symptoms from pretraumatic risk factors: A 2-year prospective follow-up study in firefighters. Am J Psychiatry, 162:2276-2286.

Hemfelt R, Minirth F, Meier P (1989) Love Is A Choice- Recovery for codependent relationships. Thomas Nelson Publisher, Nashville, pp. 1.

Hendin H (1981) Psychotherapy and suicide. American Journal of p s y c h o t h e r a p y, 35:469-480.

Henriksson MM, Aro HM, Marttunen MJ, et al. (1993) Mental disorders and   comorbidity in suicide. AM J Psychiatr, 150(6), 935-940.

Hesse H (1968) Narcissus and Goldmund. Bantam Book / published by arrangement with Farrar, Straus and Giroux, Inc. New York, p.44, 171.

His Holiness The Dalai Lama, Cutler HC (1998) The art of happiness. Riverhead Books, New York, NY, pp. 114, 162-171,254.

Hoch J, O'Reilly RL, Carscadden J (2006) Relationship management therapy for patients with borderline personality disorder. Psychiatric Services, 57:179-181.

Hoyert DL, Arias E, and Smith BL (2001) Death: Final data for 1999. National Vital Statistics Report, 49 (8). National Center for Health Statistics, DHHS Publication No. (PHS) 2001-1120, Hyattsville, MD.

Hyde M, McGuiness M (2005) Introducing Jung. Totem Books, UK.

Jacobson E (1964) The self and the object world. International Universities Press, New York.

Jobson KO, Potter WZ (1995) International Psychopharmacology Algorithm Project report. Psychopharmacol Bull, 31:457-507.

References

Johnson JG, Cohen P, Smailes EM, Skodol AE, Brown J, Oldham JM (2001) Childhood verbal abuse and risk for personality disorder during adolescence and early adulthood. Compr Psychiatry, 42:16-23.

Joiner TE, Alfano MS, Metlasky GI (1992) When depression breeds contempt: Reassurance seeking, self-esteem, and rejection of depressed college students by their roommates. Journal of Abnormal Psychology, 101: 165-173.

Kakuzo O (1956) The book of tea. Charles E. Tuttle Co., Inc. Tokyo, Japan.

Kaplan L (1978) Oneness and separateness: From infant to individual. Simon and Schuster (Touchstone Books) New York, p.29.

Kaufman G (1989) The psychology of shame. Theory and treatment of shame-based syndromes. Springer Publishing Company, New York, pp. 61, 27, 34, 183, 210.

Keller MB (2003) Past, present, and future directions for defining optimal treatment outcome in depression: Remission and beyond. Journal of the American Medical Association, 289:3152-3160.

Kenny ME, Moilanen DM, Lomax R, Brabeck MD (1993) Contributions of parental attachment to view of self and depressive symptoms among early adolescents. Journal of Youth and Adolescents, 13, 408-430.

Kerr EM, Bowen M (1988) Family evaluation, W.W. Norton and Company, Inc., New York, NY, pp.44-49, 55-57, 309.

Kernberg OF (1980) Internal world and external reality, object relations theory applied, Jason Aronson Inc. pp. 23, 25, 27, 28.

Kernberg OF (1985) Borderline conditions and pathological narcissism, Jason Aronson Inc. pp. 4-20, 25, 29-30, 56, 80, 213, 229, 237, 331.

Khazaal Y, Zullino D (2006) Topiramate in the treatment of compulsive sexual behavior: case report. BMC Psychiatry, Published online May 23; www.biomecentral.com.

Klatzky SR (1962) Patterns of contact with relatives. American Sociological Association. Washington, DC. pp.241-242.

Klein M (1946) Notes on some schizoid mechanisms. International Journal of Psycho-Analysis, 27:99-110.

Klein M (1952) Some theoretical conclusions regarding the emotional life of the infant. In M. Klein (Ed.), (1975). Envy and gratitude and other works, 1946-1963. Delacorte Press, New York.

Klein M (1955) On identification. In Melanie Klein: Envy and Gratitude and other works. 1946-1963. pp. 141-175. London: Hogarth, 1975.

Knight RP (1953) Borderline States, Bulletin of the Menninger Clinic, 17:1-12.

Kohut H (1976) Creativeness, charisma, group psychology. In: The search for the self. International Universities Press, New York, pp. 804-823.

Kohut H (1977) The restoration of the self. New York: International Press.

Kohut H (1984) How does psychoanalysis cure? Chicago: University of Chicago Press. p.77.

Krampe H et al. (2006) Personality disorder and chronicity of addiction as independent outcome predictors in alcoholism treatment. Psychiatric Services, 57: 708-712.

Larson RJ (1992) Neuroticism and selective encoding and recall of symptoms: Evidence from a combined concurrent retrospective study. Journal of Personality and Social Psychology, 62, 480-488.

Levenson MR, Aldwin CM, Bosse R, Spiro A (1988) Emotionality and mental health: Longitudinal findings from the normative aging study. Journal of Abnormal Psychology, 97, 94-96.

Lewis HB (1971) Shame and guilt in neurosis. New York: International University Press. p.23.

Lieb K, Zanarini MC, Schmahl C, Linehan MM, Bohus M (2004) Borderline personality disorder. Lancet, 364: 453-461.

Lin E, Hwang Y, Tzeng CM (2006) A case study of the utility of the HapMap database for pharmacogenomic haplotype analysis in the Taiwanese population. Mol Diagn Ther, 10(6):367-370.

Linehan MM (1993) Cognitive-behavioral treatment of borderline personality disorder. The Guilford Press. p.42, 55.

Linehan MM et al. (2006) Two-year randomized control trial and follow-up of dialectical behavior therapy vs. therapy by experts for suicidal behaviors and borderline personality disorder. Archives of General Psychiatry, Jul; 63:757-66.

Loew T, Nickel M, Muehlbacher M, Kaplan P, et al. (2006) Topiramate treatment for women with borderline personality disorder: a double-blind, placebo-controlled study. Journal of Clinical Psychopharmacology, 26(February):61-66.

Mahler MS (1974) Symbiosis and individuation: The psychological birth of the human infant. Psychoanalytic Study of the Child, Vol. 29:100.

Mahler MS, Pine F, and Bergman A (1975) The psychological birth of the human infant. New York: Basic Books.

Maltsberger JT (1994) Calculated risk in the treatment of intractably suicidal patients. Psychiatry, 57:199-212.

Mann JJ (2002) A current perspective of suicide and attempted suicide. Ann Int Med, 136(4), 302-311.

Marazziti D, Dell'osso B (2006) Topiramate plus citalopram in the treatment of compulsive-impulsive sexual behaviors. Clinical Practice and Epidemiology in Mental Health, Published online May 22; www.cpementalhealth.com.

Marcus E, Bradley S (1987) Concurrence of Axis I and Axis II illness in treatment-resistant hospitalized patients. Psychiatric Clinic North AM, 10: 177-184

Marmorstein NR, Malone SM, Iacono WG (2004) Psychiatric disorders among offspring of depressed mother: associations with paternal psychopathology. Am J Psychiatry, 161:1588-1594)

Maris RW, Berman AL, Silverman MM (2000) Comprehensive Textbook of Suicidology. New York, Guilford.

Masterson JF, Klein R (1989) Psychotherapy of the disorders of the self, The Masterson Approach. Brunner / Mazel, Inc., New York. p. 36, 70-89, 173, 217.

Mayberg HS, Lozano AM, Voon V, McNeely HE, Seminowicz D, Hamani C, Schwalb JM, Kennedy SH (2005) Deep brain stimulation for treatment-Resistant depression. Neuron, 45:651-660.

McQuillan A, Nicastro R, Guenot F, Girard M, Lissner C, Ferrero F (2005) Intensive dialectical behavior therapy for outpatients with borderline personality disorder who are in crisis. Psychiatric Services, 56:193-197.

Meares R (1993) The metaphor of play-Disruption and restoration in the Borderline experience. Jason Aronson Inc. Northvale, New Jersey. p. 24, 59, 115, 143-144, 156, 170-171, 175-181, 185.

Migone P (1995) Expressed emotion and projective identification: A bridge between psychiatric and psychoanalytic concepts? Contemporary Psychoanalysis, 31: 627.

Miller A (1997) The drama of the gifted child: The search for the true self. Basic Books.

Ney PG (1987) Does verbal abuse leave deeper scars: a study of children and parents. Can J Psychiatry, 32:371-378.

Ney PG, Fung T, Wickett AR (1994) The worst combinations of child abuse and neglect. Child Abuse Negl, 18:705-714.

Nickel M, et al. (2004) Treatment of aggression in female borderline personality patients: a double-blind, placebo-controlled study. Journal of Clinical Psychiatry, 65:1515-1519.

Nickel M, et al. (2005) Treatment of aggression with topiramate in male borderline patients: a double-blind, placebo-controlled study. Biological Psychiatry, 57:495-499.

Nickel M, et al. (2006) Aripiprazole in the treatment of patients with borderline personality disorder: a double-blind, placebo-controlled study. Am J Psychiatry, 163:833-838.

Nickel M, Lowe T (2007) Treatment of aggression with topiramate in male borderline patients, part II: 18-month follow-up. www.sciencedirect.com.

References

Ochsner KN, Ray RD, Cooper JC, Robertson ER, Chopra S, Gabrieli JD, Gross JJ (2004) For better or for worse: Neural systems supporting the cognitive down- and up-regulation of negative emotion. Neuroimage, 23:483-499.

Olino TM, Pettit JW, Klein DN, Allen NB, Seeley JR, Lewinsohn PM (2008) Influence of parental and grandparental major depressive disorder on behavioor problems in early childhood: A three-generation study. J Am Acad. Child Adolesc. Psychiatry, 47(1):53-60.

Oswald M (1962) Aristotle- Nichomachean Ethics. The Bobbs-Merrill Company, Inc. Indianapolis, Indiana, p.282, 286, 288.

Packman WL, Harris EA (1998) Legal issues and risk management in suicidal patients, in Risk Management with Suicidal Patients. Edited by Bougar B, Berman AL, Maris RW, et al. New York, Guilford.

Paris J (2002) Chronic suicidality among patients with borderline personality disorder. Psychiatric Services, 53(6):738-742.

Paris J, Brown R, Nowlis D ((1987) Long-term follow-up of borderline patients in a general hospital. Comprehensive Psychiatry, 28:530-535.

Paris J, Nowlis D, Brown R (1989) Predictors of suicide in borderline personality disorder. Canadian Journal of Psychiatry, 34:8-9.

Paris J, Zweig-Frank H (2001) A 27-year follow-up of patients with borderline personality disorder. Comprehensive Psychiatry, 42:482-487.

Philipsen A, Richter H, Schmahl C, Peters J, et al. (2004) Clonidine in acute aversive inner tension and self-injurious behavior in female patients with borderline personality disorder. Journal of Clinical Psychiatry, 65(October):1414-1419.

Pick IB (1985) Working through in the countertransference. International Journal of Psycho-Analysis, 66: 157-166.

Pokorny AD (1983) Prediction of suicide in psychiatric patients: report of a prospective study. Archives of General Psychiatry, 40:249-257.

Prinstein MJ, Borelli JL, Cheah CSL, Simon VA, Akkins JW (2005) Adolescent girl's interpersonal vulnerability to depressive symptoms: A longitudinal examination of reassurance-seeking and peer relationship. Journal of Abnormal Psychology, 114: 676-688.

Rachlin S (1984) Double jeopardy: suicide and malpractice. General Hospital Psychiatry, 6:302-307.

Rapee RM (1997) Potential role of childrearing practices in the development of anxiety and depression. Clinical Psychology Review, 17:46-47.

Rasmussen P, Gillberg C (2000) Natural outcome of ADHD with developmental coordination disorder at age 22 years: a controlled, longitudinal, community-based study. J Am Acad Child Adolesc Psychiatry, 39:1424-1431.

Rinne T, van den Brink W, Wouters L, van Dyck R (2002) SSRI treatment of borderline personality disorder: a randomized, placebo-controlled trial for female patients with borderline personality disorder. American Journal of Psychiatry, 159(December):2048-2054.

Rose AJ (2002) Co-rumination in the friendships of girls and boys. Child Development, 73:1830-1843.

Rose AJ, Carlso W, Waller EM (2007) Prospective association of co-rumination with friendship and emotional adjustment: considering the socioemotional trade-offs of co-rumination. Developmental Psychology, vol. 43, No.4, 1019-1031.

Ryle A (1994) Projective identification: a particular form of reciprocal role procedure. British Journal of Medical Psychology, 67: 107-114.

Rüsch N, et al. (2007) Shame and implicit self concept in women with borderline personality disorder. Am J Psychiatry, 164:500-508.

Sands S (1997) Self psychology and projective identification-Whither shall they meet? A reply to the editors (1995). Psychoanalytic Dialogue, 7:651-668.

Sameroff AJ, Seifer R, Zax M (1982) Early development of children at risk for emotional disorder. Monogr Soc Res Child Dev, 47(7):1-82.

Serretti A, Artioli P (2004) The pharmacogenomics of selective serotonin reuptake inhibitors. Pharmacogenomics, 4:233-244.

Sharma B, Dunlop BW, Ninan PT, Bradley R (2007) Use of dialectical behavior therapy in borderline personality disorder: A view from residency. Acad Psychiatry, 31:218-224.

Shelton RC, Tollefson GD, Tohen M, Stahl S, Gannon KS, Jacobs TG, et al. (2001) A novel augmentation strategy for treating resistant major depression. American Journal of psychiatry, 158, 131-134.

Shiah I, Chao C, Mao W, Chuang Y (2006) Treatment of paraphilic sexual disorder: the use of topiramate in fetishism. International Clinical Psychopharmacology, 21 (July):241-243.

Siegle GJ (2007) Brain mechanisms of borderline personality disorder at the intersection of cognition, emotion, and the clinic. Am J Psychiatry, 164:1776-1779.

Siegle GJ, Carter CS, Thase ME (2006) Use of fMRI to predict recovery from unipolar depression with cognitive behavior therapy. Am J Psychiatry, 163:735-738.

Soler J, Pascual JC, Campins J, Barrachina J, Puigdemont D, Alvarez E, Pérez V (2005) Double-blind placebo-controlled study of dialectical Behavior therapy plus Olanzapine for borderline personality disorder. Am J Psychiatry, 162:1221-1224.

Soloff PH, Lynch KG, Kelly TM, et al. (2000) Characteristics of suicide attempts of patients with major depressive episode and borderline personality disorder: A comparative study. Am J Psychiatry, 157(4), 601-608.

Southwick S, et al. (1990) Platelet alpha 2-adrenergic receptor binding sites in major depressive disorder and borderline personality disorder. Psychiatry Research, 34:193-203.

Stahl SM (2000) Essential psychopharmacology: Neuroscientific basis and practical applications. Cambridge University Press, New York, p. 271-179, 305-323.

Statham DJ, Heath AC, Madden PAF et al. (1998) Suicidal behavior: an epidemiological and genetic study. Psychol Med, 28:839-855.

Stern A (1938) Psychoanalytical Investigation of and Therapy in the Borderline Group of Neuroses, The psychoanalytical Quarterly, 7: 467-489.

Stern DN (1985) The interpersonal world of the infant, Basic Books, Inc. p. 124-140, 234.

Stone MH (1990) The Fate of Borderline Patients. New York, The Guilford Press.

Stone MH (2006) Relationship of borderline personality disorder and bipolar disorder. Am J Psychiatry, 163:1126-1128.

Strupp HH, Binder Jeffrey L (1984) Psychotherapy in a new key, Basic Books, Inc. p. 32, 141.

Su K, Huang S, Chiu C, Shen W (2003) Omega-3 fatty acids in major depressive disorder: a preliminary double-blind, placebo-controlled trial. European Neuropsychopharmacology, 13(August):267-271.

Sverd J, Dubey DR, Schweitzer R, Ninan R (2003) Pervasive developmental disorders among children and adolescents attending psychiatric day treatment. Psychiatric Services, 54: 1519-1525.

Teicher M, Samson J, Polcari A, McGreenery C (2006) Sticks, and stones, and hurtful words: relative effects of various forms of childhood maltreatment. American Journal of Psychiatry, 163:993-1000.

Thase ME, Greenhouse JB, Frank E, Reynolds CF, Pilkonis PA, Hurley K, et al. (1997) Treatment of major depression with psychotherapy-pharmacotherapy combination, Archives of General Psychiatry, 54, 1009-1015.

Thase ME, Bhargave M, Sachs GS (2003) Treatment of bipolar depression: Current status, continued challenges, and the STEP-BD approach. Psychiatric clinic of North America, 26:495-518.

Thomas AM, Forehand R (1991) The relationship between paternal depressive mood and early adolescent functioning. J Fam Psychol, 4:260-271.

Thornberry TP, Freeman-Gallant A, Lizotte AJ, et al. (2003) Linked lives: The intergenerational transmission of antisocial behavior. J Abnorm Child Psychology, 31:174-184

References

Tice DM, Bratslavsky E, Baumeister RF (2001) Emotional distress regulation takes precedence over impulse control : If you feel bad, do it! J Pers Soc Psychol, 80:53-67.
Tomkin SS (1962) Affect, imagery, consciousness: The positive affects. Vol. 1. Springer, New York.
Tomkin SS (1963) Affect, imagery, consciousness: The negative affects. Vol. 2. Springer, New York, p.118.
Tomkin SS (1987) Shame. In D.L. Nathanson (Ed.), The many faces of shame. Guilford Press, New York.
Tondo L, Ghiani C, Albert M (2001a) Pharmacologic interventions in suicide prevention. J Clin Psychiatry, 62(Suppl 25), 51-55.
Tondo L, Hennen J, Baldessarini RJ (2001b) Lower suicide risk with long-term lithium treatment in major affective illness: A meta-analysis. Acta Psychiatr Scand, 104, 163-172.
Tritt K, Nickel C, Lahmann C, Leiberich P, et al. (2005) Lamotrigine treatment of aggression in female borderline-patients: a randomized, double blind, placebo-controlled study. Journal of Psychopharmacology, 19 (May):287-291.
Vissing YM, Straus MA, Gelles RJ, Harrop JW (1991) Verbal aggression by parents and psychosocial problems of children. Child Abuse Negl, 15:223-238.
Weiner IB (1975) Principles of Psychotherapy, John Wiley and Sons, Inc. p. 74-88.
Weissman MM, Wickramaratne P, Nomura Y, et al. (2005) Families at high and low risk for depression: a three generation study. Arch Gen Psychiatry, 62:29-36.
Winnicott DW (1971) Playing and reality. Tavistock Publications, London, p.5.
Winnicott DW (1965) The maturational process and the facilitating environment: Studies in the theory of emotional development. Hogarth Press, London.
Winnicott DW (1958) The capacity to be alone. The Maturational Process and the Facilitating Environment. New York: International University Press.
Wolf ES (1988) Treating the self, elements of clinical self psychology. The Guilford Press, New York, NY, pp. 11, 13, 25, 28, 29, 38, 91, 100-101.
Yalom ID (1985) The theory and practice of group psychotherapy, Basic Books, Inc. p. 30, 135-198.
Yehuda R, McFarlane AC, Shalev AY (1998) Predicting the development of posttraumatic stress disorder from the acute response to a traumatic event. Biol Psychiatry, 44:1305-1313.
Zanarini M, Frankenburg F (2003) Omega-3 fatty acid treatment of women with women with borderline personality disorder: a double-blind, placebo-controlled pilot study. American Journal of Psychiatry, 160(January):167-169.
Zanarini M, Frankenberg F, Hennen J, Silk K (2003) The longitudinal course of borderline psychopathology: 6-year prospective follow-up of the phenomenology of borderline personality disorder. Am J Psychiatry, 160:274-283.
Zanarini M (2004) Update on pharmacotherapy of borderline personality disorder. Current Psychiatric Reports, 6 (February): 66-70.
Zanarini M, Frankenberg F, Reich D, Silk K, Hudson J, McSweeney L (2007)
The subsyndromal phenomenology of borderline personality disorder: a ten-year follow-up study. Am J Psychiatry, 164:929-935.
Zimmerman M, Mattia JI (1999) Differences between clinical and research practices in diagnosing borderline personality disorder. Am J Psychiatry, 156:1570-1574.
Zimmerman M, Rothschild L, Chelminski I (2005) The prevalence of DSM-IV personality disorders in psychiatric outpatients. Am J Psychiatry, 162:1911-1918.

INDEX

A

accomplishment cycle 188
acting out XI, XIV, 15-26, 34, 44-45, 59-73, 81-110, 116-120, 126, 137, 145-168, 179-220, 231-244, 254-259, 264-280, 288-291, 298-302, 308-310
affect theory of motivation 47
anxiety 20-25, 35, 40-48, 50, 58, 66, 80, 86, 90-104, 110-120, 132, 136, 153, 157, 171-175, 201, 203, 229, 236-237, 244-246, 253, 258, 260, 282-320
archetypal figures 177
aripiprazole 313
attunement 37-42, 85, 126-127, 135, 154, 180, 194, 206, 208, 221, 275, 300
autism spectrum disorders 38, 293, 315
automatic thoughts 47

B

Beck 47, 315
benzodiazepine 212, 309-310
bidirectional projective identification 39
borderline personality organization 44-46, 100, 286
bupropion 312

C

carbamazepine 309, 312
Cashdan 41, 154, 244, 278, 280, 283, 292, 316
celebration 167, 188
chain analysis 223, 286
clonidine 314
coaching 105, 179, 187, 191, 233
co-dependence 89, 189, 292
cognitive behavioral therapy 20-21, 90, 98, 103
cognitive distortion 153, 155
cohesion 15, 43, 72-73, 101, 154, 157, 192, 198-199, 209, 220, 226, 228, 244, 298, 307
common denominator 25, 117, 125, 210

C (continued)

compassion 26, 29, 64-65, 73-77, 103, 105, 108, 123, 136, 169, 183, 194, 205, 214, 219, 226, 231, 241-243, 253, 265-271
control 22, 31-32, 45, 47, 53, 63, 74-93, 126-127, 153, 156-163, 167, 187, 222, 228, 236-237, 253, 256, 263, 269, 284-288, 292, 294, 306, 312, 319, 322
core self 15-16, 83, 86, 119-120, 176, 178, 233
cortisol production 42
co-rumination 171-172, 320
countertransference XIII, 25, 66, 75-76, 85, 134-137, 144, 168, 190, 230, 239, 241, 243, 254, 266, 316, 320

D

death instinct 41, 46, 48, 114, 117, 201, 275, 280
death talk 273
depression 20-24, 31, 42-43, 47, 59, 81, 89-100, 110-121, 144, 161, 171, 183, 187, 236-237, 245-260, 272, 306-322
dialectical behavior therapy XI, 19-22, 198, 268, 305, 314, 319, 321
disintegration 153, 157
disintegration anxiety 157
disruption-restoration cycle 224-225

E

eating disorders 23, 45, 157, 313
ego identity 165
emotional equilibrium 65, 89, 261
emotional field 130, 132
emotional theft 40
empathy 29, 32, 37-40, 66, 73-84, 107-108, 135, 139, 169, 183, 203, 205, 226, 237, 241-243, 253, 260, 265-271, 294
engagement cycle 188
Erikson 38, 42, 46-47, 82, 125-126, 165, 172, 175, 199-200, 316

F

false self 15-16, 21, 71, 73-77, 82-83, 90, 99, 117, 128, 176-180, 198, 236-237, 241, 245
family systems theory 131
family systems therapy 20
fluoxetine 312
fluvoxamine 312
fragmentation 49, 59, 70, 84, 120-121, 127, 139, 151, 157, 178, 191, 193, 220, 228, 233, 244, 253-260, 291, 298, 307-308

323

R

reciprocal interpersonal interaction 31, 41, 127, 227, 229, 298
repetition compulsion 125-126

S

selective serotonin reuptake inhibitor 296, 309, 311
self-injurious behavior 23, 273, 320
selfobject experiences 43, 120, 226, 228, 267, 298
self psychology XIII, 41, 43, 49, 72-75, 83, 89, 139, 157, 192, 198-199, 208, 315-316, 322
sex, drugs and rock and roll 161
shame 36, 47-48, 79, 82-83, 104, 123-124, 136, 153, 156, 163, 166, 179, 190-191, 198-199, 203, 205, 209, 212, 217, 225, 277, 318, 322
Socrates 171
splitting 17, 32-33, 45, 49-52, 64-65, 74, 80, 86-91, 126-127, 133, 165, 170, 175, 178, 191-192, 222-224, 228, 243-244, 266, 275, 278-288, 294, 302
state dependent learning 51-52
Stern 37, 39-40, 44, 321
substance use disorders 45
super-validate 140

T

therapeutic rapport XIII, 29, 33, 69, 78, 101-102, 108-109, 151
therapeutic relationship 20, 28, 32-33, 65, 69-74, 93, 107, 109, 144, 146, 186, 206, 224, 257, 265, 267
time-limited therapy 20
Tomkin 47, 82, 322
topiramate 312, 319, 321
transference XI-XIII, 15, 20-21, 28, 49, 54-56, 58, 66-73, 83, 86, 92, 101, 105, 114, 120, 136, 149-157, 164-168, 173-179, 190, 199-210, 216-217, 219-226, 233-235, 240-241, 246-248, 261-262, 277, 281-284, 287, 289-300, 315-316
transference of creativity 199
transitional object 43, 153-154, 175, 189, 192, 198-201
transitional space 200
transmuting internalization 280
tricyclic antidepressants 311
true self 15-16, 71-74, 80, 90, 126, 176-180, 185, 189, 200-201, 210, 230, 236-237, 287, 296, 301, 319

V

valproic acid 312

W

Winnicott 89, 154, 189, 322

Y

Yalom 63, 92, 322